Emergency Anaesthesia

Edited by

Anthony P Adams MB, BS, PhD, FFARCS

Professor of Anaesthetics, United Medical and Dental Schools of Guy's and St Thomas's Hospitals, University of London; Department of Anaesthetics, Guy's Hospital, London, UK

Penelope B Hewitt MB, BS, FFARCS

Consultant Anaesthetist, Department of Anaesthetics, Guy's Hospital, London, UK

Mark C Rogers MD

Professor of Anesthesiology and Professor of Pediatrics; Chairman Department of Anesthesiology and Critical Care Medicine, The Johns Hopkins Medical Institutions, Baltimore, Maryland, USA

Edward Arnold

© Edward Arnold (Publishers) Ltd 1986

First published in Great Britain 1986 by
Edward Arnold (Publishers) Ltd, 41 Bedford Square, London
WC1B 3DQ

Edward Arnold (Australia) Pty Ltd, 80 Waverley Road,
Caulfield East, Victoria 3145, Australia

British Library Cataloguing in Publication Data
Emergency anaesthesia.
  1. Anaesthesia   2. Emergency medical services
  I. Adams, Anthony P.   II. Hewitt, Penelope B.
  III. Rogers, Mark C.
  617'.96   RD82
  ISBN 0-7131-4505-6

Whilst the advice and information in this book is believed to be
true and accurate at the date of going to press, neither the
authors nor the publisher can accept any legal responsibility or
liability for any errors or omissions that may be made.

Text set in 9/10pt Times Compugraphic
by Colset Private Limited, Singapore.
Printed and bound in Great Britain by
Richard Clay Ltd., Bungay Suffolk.

Contributors

Anthony P. Adams MB, BS, PhD, FFARCS
  Professor of Anaesthetics, United Medical and Dental Schools of Guy's and St Thomas's Hospitals, University of London; Department of Anaesthetics, Guy's Hospital, London, UK
Michael B. Barnett MB, BS, FFARCS
  Consultant Anaesthetist, Department of Anaesthetics, Guy's Hospital, London, UK
Charles Beattie PhD, MD
  Assistant Professor, Director of Critical Care Anesthesia, Department of Anesthesiology and Critical Care Medicine, The Johns Hopkins Medical Institutions, Baltimore, Maryland, USA
Michael P. Broadbent BSc (Hons), FIST, C Biol, M I Biol
  Head Scientific Officer, United Medical and Dental Schools of Guy's and St Thomas's Hospitals; Department of Anaesthetics, Guy's Hospital, London, UK
Elizabeth A. Caffrey MA, MB, BChir, MRCPath
  Department of Haematology, Guy's Hospital, London, UK
Jeremy N. Cashman BSc, MB, BS, FFARCS
  Senior Registrar, Department of Anaesthetics, Guy's Hospital, London, UK
W. Robert Casson MB, ChB, FFARCS
  Senior Registrar, Department of Anaesthetics, Guy's Hospital, London, UK
John H. Cook MB, FRCS, FFARCS, DO
  Consultant Anaesthetist, The District General Hospital, Eastbourne, Sussex, UK
Robert O. Feneck MB, BS, FFARCS
  Consultant Anaesthetist, The London Chest Hospital, London, UK
Shirley Firn MB, BS, FFARCS
  Consultant Anaesthetist, Pinderfields Hospital, Wakefield, Yorkshire, UK
Penelope B. Hewitt MB, BS, FFARCS
  Consultant Anaesthetist, Department of Anaesthetics, Guy's Hospital, London, UK
Ronald M. Jones MB, BS, FFARCS
  Senior Lecturer in Anaesthetics, United Medical and Dental Schools of Guy's and St Thomas's Hospitals; Department of Anaesthetics, Guy's Hospital, London, UK
Robert W. McPherson MD
  Assistant Professor, Anesthesiology and Critical Care Medicine, Department of Anesthesiology and Critical Care Medicine, The Johns Hopkins Medical Institutions, Baltimore, Maryland, USA
Nicholas I. Newton MA, BM, BCh, FFARCS
  Consultant Anaesthetist, Department of Anaesthetics, Guy's Hospital, London, UK
Daniel Nyhan MD
  Department of Anesthesiology and Critical Care Medicine, the Johns Hopkins University School of Medicine and The Johns Hopkins Hospital, Baltimore, Maryland, USA
John S. Paddle MB, BChir, FFARCS
  Consultant Anaesthetist, Department of Anaesthetics, Guy's Hospital London, UK

Gordon M. C. Paterson MB, ChB, FFARCS
Consultant Anaesthetist, Nuffield Department of Anaesthetics, The Radcliffe Infirmary, Oxford, UK

Adrian C. Pearce MB, BChir, FFARCS, MRCP
Senior Registrar, Department of Anaesthetics, Guy's Hospital, London, UK

Frank N. Prior FFARCS
Consultant Anaesthetist, Department of Anaesthetics, Guy's Hospital, London, UK

Elizabeth L. Rogers MD
Associate Professor of Medicine, University of Maryland School of Medicine, The Johns Hopkins University School of Medicine, Baltimore, Maryland, USA

Mark C. Rogers MD
Professor of Anesthesiology and Professor of Pediatrics; Chairman, Department of Anesthesiology and Critical Care Medicine, The Johns Hopkins Medical Institutions, Baltimore, Maryland, USA

James F. Schauble MD
Associate Professor of Anesthesiology, Department of Anesthesiology and Critical Care Medicine, The Johns Hopkins University School of Medicine and The Johns Hopkins Hospital, Baltimore, Maryland, USA

Charles L. Schleien MD
Department of Anesthesiology and Critical Care Medicine, The Johns Hopkins University School of Medicine and the Johns Hopkins Hospital, Baltimore, Maryland, USA

Wendy C. Scott MB ChB, FFARCS
Consultant Anaesthetist, Milton Keynes General Hospital, Milton Keynes, Hertfordshire, UK

Ann M. Skelly BDS (Hons), FDSRCPS
Lecturer in Anaesthetics, United Medical and Dental Schools of Guy's and St Thomas's Hospitals, University of London, Department of Anaesthetics, Guy's Hospital, London, UK

Gerald N. Smith BSc (Hons) MB, BS, PhD, MRCPath
Consultant Haematologist, Department of Haematology, Guy's Hospital, London, UK

Malcolm C. Thompson MB, ChB, FFARCS, DCH, DRCOG, RAMC
Consultant in Anaesthesia and Resuscitation, Duchess of Kent's Military Hospital, Catterick Garrison, North Yorkshire, UK

Raymond M. Towey MB, ChB, FFARCS
Consultant Anaesthetist, Department of Anaesthetics, Guy's Hospital, London, UK

A. Terry Walman MD
Assistant Professor and Co-Director of Critical Care Anesthesia, Department of Anesthesiology and Critical Care Medicine, The Johns Hopkins University School of Medicine and The Johns Hopkins Hospital, Baltimore, Maryland, USA

John R. Wedley MB, ChB, FFARCS
Consultant Anaesthetist, Department of Anaesthetics, Guy's Hospital, London, UK

John P. Williams MD
Assistant Professor of Anesthesiology, University of Texas Health Sciences Center at Houston, Department of Anesthesiology, Hermann Hospital, Houston, Texas, USA

William G. Zitzmann MD
Department of Anesthesiology and Critical Care Medicine, The Johns Hopkins University School of Medicine and the Johns Hopkins Hospital, Baltimore, Maryland, USA

Preface

Messrs Edward Arnold published the first edition of an earlier work entitled *Emergency Anaesthesia* in 1964 under the editorship of Dr HL Thornton and Dr PF Knight. A second edition appeared in 1974 this time with Dr HD Norton-Perkins as co-editor. Dr Thornton's concept over 20 years ago was to emphasize a very important aspect of anaesthetic practice which had not previously received the attention it deserved.

All anaesthetists in every kind of environment are faced with the numerous and varied problems involved when administering anaesthetics for emergency surgery, diagnostic and therapeutic procedures. 'Inexperienced' anaesthetists are liable to have to cope with urgent cases when more experienced colleagues are not available or there is not time to call upon them. Even when 'experienced' anaesthetists are available, emergencies may present strange or unexpected problems which fall outside their current sphere of expertise.

A book designed for anaesthetists who have to deal with emergencies belongs in the pocket rather than in the library so this volume is presented in a completely new and appropriate format. It is not a substitute for asking for help and advice from more senior or experienced colleagues, nor is it intended for planning the management of elective cases or those of a bizarre nature. *Emergency Anaesthesia* is designed to be of particular value to anaesthetists in training, to those who do not have ready access to a wide range of reference books and to those working in difficult situations or in developing countries. References have deliberately been kept to a minimum and are, on the whole, recent important papers with a back-up of reviews and current texts.

The editors have been drastic in their task and are grateful for the cooperation of their team of 32 contributors who have been drawn from the United States of America as well as the British Isles. The result is a text that should have widespread appeal. Every effort has been made to adopt an approach which indicates what the special problems are and how they may be avoided or overcome in the relevant circumstances. The topic of each chapter could, of course, be the subject of a complete book in its own right: the editors' aim has been to emphasize the basic principles of safe and successful patient care whilst avoiding the repetition of descriptions of common anaesthetic practices. The best techniques are usually the ones with which the anaesthetist is most familiar: an emergency situation is not the place to try out a new technique for the first time; experience and practice during elective cases must be obtained first. It is hoped that Senior House Officers, Registrars and Residents will be encouraged to recognize problem situations and to master the variety of techniques mentioned in this book, so that these will stand them in good stead for the future.

A recent study* assessed the job satisfaction of anaesthetists: by far the greatest pleasure was found to be seeing patients wake up safely at the end of an operation. This book is aimed at achieving just that.

London and Baltimore
1986

Anthony P Adams
Penelope B Hewitt, and
Mark C Rogers

Acknowledgements

The editors wish to express their thanks to Mr Jonathan Paddle for his drawings of Figures 1.1, 6.1, 6.2, 6.3 and 6.4.

Figure 1.1 is redrawn with permission of the editor and the publishers (Blackwell Scientific Publications, Oxford) from 'Obstetric Anaesthesia — Safety first' by M Rosen, in *WFSA Lectures* 1984; **2**: 25.

Figure 6.2 is redrawn with permission of the editor of *Anaesthesia* and of the author, Ajeet Singh, of 'Blind nasal intubation. A report of the use of a hook in three cases of ankylosis of the jaw.' in *Anaesthesia* 1966; **21**: 402. Figure 6.4 is redrawn with permission from the International Anaesthesia Research Society from 'New use for Swan–Ganz introducer wire' by KW Roberts, in *Anesthesia and Analgesia* 1981; **60**: 67. Figure 18.1 is reproduced with permission from *Burns – The first 48 hours* by JAD Settle; published by Smith & Nephew Pharmaceuticals Ltd., Romford, Essex, England.

*Klein, L. The role of the anaesthetist: an exploratory study. *The Association of Anaesthetists of Great Britain & Ireland*, 1980.

Contents

Contributors iii

Preface v

Acknowledgements vi

Abbreviations ix

1. General Principles of Emergency Anaesthesia
   Anthony P Adams 1

2. Cardiopulmonary Resuscitation *Daniel Nyhan,
   William G Zitzmann and Mark C Rogers* 14

3. Blood Grouping and Blood Transfusion
   Gerald N Smith 27

4. Blood Disorders *Elizabeth A Caffrey and
   Nicholas I Newton* 44

5. Intravenous Fluids *Anthony P Adams and
   Penelope B Hewitt* 55

6. Practical Procedures *John S Paddle and
   Michael B Barnett* 64

7. Patient Monitoring *Michael P Broadbent and
   Jeremy N Cashman* 81

8. Diagnostic Procedures *Adrian C Pearce* 90

9. General and Abdominal Surgery *Robert O Feneck* 99

10. Orthopaedics *Jeremy N Cashman* 117

11. Neuroanaesthesia and Head Injury
    Robert W McPherson 128

12. Neck Trauma *John P Williams* 140

13. Facio-maxillary, Ear, Nose and Throat Problems
    John R Wedley 155

14. Dental Problems *Ann M Skelly* 164

15. Ophthalmic Emergencies *John H Cook* 173

16. Major Vascular Surgery *Charles Beattie* 180

17. Cardiac and Thoracic Emergencies *James C Schauble* 192

18. Emergency Anaesthesia in Severe Burns
    Shirley Firn 208

19. Military Conflicts and Civil Disasters
    Malcolm C Thompson 222

20. Anaesthesia in Developing Countries
    Raymond M Towey and Frank N Prior   236
21. Regional Anaesthesia   *Gordon MC Patterson*   246
22. Obstetric Emergencies   *W Robert Casson and
    Penelope B Hewitt*   265
23. Paediatric Anaesthesia   *Charles Schleien*   278
24. Emergency Anaesthesia in the Elderly
    Elizabeth L Rogers   289
25. Renal Disease   *W Robert Casson and Ronald M Jones* 300
26. Liver Disease   *Elizabeth L Rogers*   310
27. Respiratory Insufficiency   *A Terry Walman*   326
28. Postoperative Complications   *Wendy Scott*   340
Index   362

Abbreviations

A and E	accident and emergency
α	alpha
~	approximately
AIDS	acquired immune deficiency syndrome
APLS	advanced paediatric life support
ARDS	adult respiratory distress syndrome
ATN	acute tubular necrosis
β	beta
BP	British Pharmacopoeia
BrP	barrier pressure
BSA	body surface area
BSP	bromosulphthalein
c	circa
Ca^{2+}	calcium ion
CAPD	continuous ambulatory peritoneal dialysis
C_4	fourth cervical vertebra
CBF	cerebral blood flow
CDH	congenital diaphragmatic hernia
CFAM	cerebral function analyzing monitor
CFM	cerebral function monitor
CI	cardiac index
$CMRO_2$	cerebral metabolic rate for oxygen
CNS	central nervous system
COHb	carboxyhaemoglobin
CO	cardiac output
CO_2	carbon dioxide
CPAP	continuous positive airway pressure
CPDA	citrate-phosphate-dextrose adenine
CPP	cerebral perfusion pressure
CPPV	continuous positive pressure ventilation
CPR	cardiopulmonary resuscitation

CSF	cerebrospinal fluid
CT	computerized tomography
CVP	central venous pressure
DIC	disseminated intravascular coagulation
2,3–DPG	2,3–diphosphoglycerate
dl	decilitre (= 100 millilitres)
DVT	deep vein thrombosis
ECF	extracellular fluid
ECG	electrocardiogram
EEG	electroencephalogram
EMO	Epstein, Macintosh, Oxford Vaporizer
Eq	equivalent
$\equiv$	equivalent to
F	factor
FEV_1	forced expiratory volume in one second
FDP	fibrin degradation products
FFP	fresh frozen plasma
Fr	French gauge
FRC	functional residual capacity
FIO_2	fraction of inspired oxygen
g	gram
G	gauge
GA	general anaesthesia
GCS	Glasgow Coma Scale
GFR	glomerular filtration rate
G6PD	glucose-6-phosphate dehydrogenase
>	greater than
GI	gastrointestinal
HAS	human albumin solution
Hb	haemoglobin
HES	hydroxyethyl starch
HIV	human immunodeficiency virus
HLA	human lymphocyte antigen
hr	hour
Hct	haematocrit (%)
HPPF	human plasma protein fraction
HTLV III	human T-cell lymphocyte virus III
ICF	intracellular fluid
ICP	intracranial pressure

ICU	intensive care unit
ID	internal diameter
I/E	inspiratory/expiratory ratio
Ig	immunoglobulin
IGP	intragastric pressure
IM	intramuscular
IOP	intraocular pressure
IPNV	intermittent positive–negative ventilation
IPPV	intermittent positive pressure ventilation
i.u.	international unit
IV	intravenous
IVRA	intravenous regional anaesthesia
IVRB	intravenous regional block
K^+	potassium ion
KCl	potassium chloride
KCT	kaolin cephalin time
kg	kilogram
kPa	kilopascal
l	litre
LA	local anaesthesia
LAV	lymphadenopathy associated virus
LISS	low ionic strength saline
LOP	lower oesophageal pressure
LOS	lower oesophageal sphincter
<	less than
LVSWI	left ventricular stroke work index
MAC	minimum alveolar concentration
M	molar
MAPB	mean arterial blood pressure
MCHC	mean corpuscular haemoglobin concentration
MCV	mean corpuscular volume
mg	milligram
min	minute
mmHg	millimetres of mercury
mmol	millimole
mOsm	milliosmole
MTM	Magnesium Trisilicate Mixture
MW	molecular weight
N_2O	nitrous oxide
O_2	oxygen
OD	outside diameter

| OIB | Oxford Inflating Bellows |
| OMV | Oxford Miniature Vaporizer |

P	pressure, tension
Pa_{CO_2}	arterial carbon dioxide tension
PAo	pulmonary artery occluded pressure
Pa_{O_2}	arterial oxygen tension
PCA	patient controlled analgesia
PCV	packed cell volume
PCWP	pulmonary capillary wedge pressure
PEEP	positive end-expiratory pressure
PPF	plasma protein fraction
PT	prothrombin time
PTT	partial thromboplastin time

| R | respiratory quotient |

SAG-M	saline-adenine-glucose-mannitol
SC	subcutaneous
sec	second
SVC	superior vena cava
SVR	systemic vascular resistance

| T_4 | fourth twitch of a train-of-four |
| TOF | train-of-four |

UK	United Kingdom
USAN	United States Adopted Name
USNF	United States National Formulary
USP	United States Pharmacopeia

| $\dot{V}/\dot{Q}$ | ventilation perfusion ratio |

| w/v | weight per volume |

| yr | year(s) |

1

General Principles of Emergency Anaesthesia

Anthony P Adams

Communications
Assistance for the anaesthetist
Equipment
  Suction
Patient assessment
  ASA classification (American Society of Anesthesiologists)
  Cardiovascular disease
  Alcohol
  Trauma
  Critical situations
Rapid-sequence tracheal intubation
  Cricoid pressure (Sellick's manoeuvre[3] Figure 1.1)
  Left lateral head-down position
  Establishment and maintenance of anaesthesia
Inhalation of gastric contents
  Prevention
  Treatment

An emergency anaesthetic is one that is required in the treatment of a patient who has not been scheduled for a booked elective procedure, and this implies that not enough time is available to prepare the patient for operation in the normal way. The patient's condition is often less than optimal and it may not be possible to correct derangements of homeostasis to the desired extent. Also, there may not be enough time to investigate the patient fully by way of laboratory, radiological or other studies.

An urgent anaesthetic is considered by some to be required at once, i.e. an immediately life-threatening situation; however, others consider 'urgent' to be less immediate than 'emergency'. Because of the difficulty in terminology both circumstances are considered to be synonymous in this and the following chapters.

Communications

Immediate and efficient communication systems are absolutely essential, e.g. telephones, radiopagers (list of important numbers). Teamwork on the part of everyone; anaesthetists, surgeons, nurses, radiologists, pathologists etc. is vital so good and happy working relationships need to have been established.

The anaesthetist and his assistant must know where everything is kept so valuable time is not lost in searching for missing items; in particular, knowledge of the storage locations of blood for transfusion. A 'blood bank' refrigerator to store supplies of blood should be close to the operating theatre, and supplies of plasma and plasma substitutes kept immediately available in all areas where resuscitation/anaesthesia for emergency cases is required.

Assistance for the anaesthetist

Trained help for the anaesthetist in an emergency situation is essential. The assistant is needed to assist in setting up systems for patient monitoring and IV fluid therapy, together with connecting or assembling equipment of various kinds and to apply cricoid pressure. The assistant is invaluable in obtaining extra supplies, e.g. more blood.

The anaesthetist, however, is well advised to have with him in the operating theatre immediate supplies of all drugs and equipment that he is likely to require. If he has to fetch something that he ought to have had beforehand, then he has failed. The system used in the USA where a separate cart is used to carry supplies of immediate items (tubes, catheters, airways, connectors, syringes, needles, drugs, anaesthetic sundries, CVP and transfusion sets, filters, IV packs, etc.) has much to commend it. This is because anaesthetic rooms for the induction of anaesthesia are quite uncommon in the USA, so that everything has to be ready and immediately to hand in the operating room.

Equipment

Anaesthetic, resuscitative, suction and monitoring equipment must be checked and kept in readiness for the emergency situation. Some items (e.g. laryngoscopes) should be duplicated or triplicated. In some centres certain drugs are drawn up into syringes in readiness (e.g. obstetric units); clearly agreed policies are essential if this is done in order to prevent accidents.

A serious problem with the British system of using anaesthetic rooms is that anaesthesia is induced in the anaesthetic room and the patient is then transferred to the operating theatre together with all the equipment and monitors necessary. In the emergency situation a number of problems can arise at this juncture and close observation of the patient may be difficult. There is also temptation for the anaesthetist to use less than adequate monitoring in the anaesthetic room because of the nuisance factor of getting the more bulky items of equipment with the patient through the doors into the operating theatre.

- Consider inducing anaesthesia in the operating theatre rather than in the anaesthetic room.
- Be sure that *everything* likely to be needed is immediately available.
- Attach all necessary monitors to the patient and establish baseline measurements before inducing anaesthesia.

Suction

Efficient suction is essential for the anaesthetist in all situations. Careful checking of the adequacy of suction apparatus must be made before anaesthesia is commenced. This includes provision of aspiration jars of adequate capacity, a correctly fitting seal to the cap of these jars, sufficient length of tubing, provision of suction catheters (various lengths and bores) and Yankauer suction ends. The development of sufficient vacuum is tested by occluding the end of the suction tubing and watching the aneroid vacuum gauge. A negative pressure of 100 kPa (760 mmHg) should be adequate for the removal of very viscous material; an adequate suction assembly is one which will aspirate a bowl of porridge in < 5 sec.

The Ambu suction booster is a system where a 250 ml plastic collection bottle – connected to the main suction assembly or to a foot-operated pump – is attached to the endotracheal tube and held in the anaesthetist's hand as intubation is attempted. Should the patient regurgitate or vomit, suction is activated by occlusion of the vent hole on the booster by the anaesthetist's finger so that the vacuum is now directed through the endotracheal tube itself which in effect becomes the sucker tip; aspiration of any vomitus is almost instantaneous (150 ml vomit removed in < 1 sec).[1]

An efficient foot-operated suction assembly should be available in the event of failure of the central vacuum system or electrical supply. Suction systems which work off the anaesthetist's oxygen supply (venturi principle) have the disadvantage that the vacuum produced is usually far from adequate and there is the ever-present risk that the oxygen supply (cylinders) will be depleted just at the time oxygenation of the patient is most needed.

Patient assessment

As much information as possible concerning the patient's medical and surgical condition needs to be gathered in the same way as for any elective procedure. Relevant history about previous anaesthetics, operations, allergies, medication, diseases of the various systems, etc. should be obtained. Clinical examination of the patient should be performed in the usual way. Serious problems can arise in situations when the patient cannot communicate or where there is little or no background information as to his previous medical condition. Patients may carry important medical information (e.g. allergies, special medical conditions) on a neck chain, locket or bracelet such as those provided by the Medic-Alert foundation.

ASA Classification (American Society of Anesthesiologists)

Although this system has drawbacks it is fairly simple to remember and to apply; it has the merit of compelling the anaesthetist to make a decision on the class to which the patient is to be allocated. It should be emphasized that the classification relates to physical status and not to 'risk'.

Class 1   A normal healthy patient
Class 2   A patient with mild systemic disease
Class 3   A patient with severe systemic disease limiting activity but is not incapacitating
Class 4   A patient with incapacitating systemic disease that is a constant threat to life
Class 5   A moribund patient not expected to live 24 hr with or without an operation

The suffix 'E' is used to denote emergency as distinct from elective. The concept of 'risk' is made up of at least three components:

• The risk because of the *clinical status* of the patient
• The risk because of the *operation itself*
• The risk because of the *anaesthetic itself*

Any time available before anaesthesia should be used to the best advantage, i.e. to assess the situation and to complete the most useful investigations first. Indeed, in quite a number of emergency situations especially those of a minor surgical nature all necessary examinations and investigations can be completed before anaesthesia. All patients presenting as emergencies should be regarded as 'unknown quantities' and so kept under surveillance in case their condition deteriorates. This is especially a problem when patients are sent for radiography and it is not uncommon for a crisis to develop during this time (*see* p. 90).

- Appropriate investigations should be made, e.g. radiography, ECG, clinical chemistry, haematology, etc. whenever circumstances permit.

Cardiovascular disease

Cardiovascular diseases present serious problems in emergency situations.[2] In elective cases about 0.15 per cent of adult patients experience myocardial infarction with general anaesthesia and operation; the risk of postoperative myocardial infarction increases to about six per cent in those with arteriosclerotic heart disease (prior myocardial infarction or angina pectoris); there is a 30 per cent risk of recurrent myocardial infarction or cardiac death in patients operated upon within six months of myocardial infarction (32 per cent in the first three months, 15 per cent in the next three months; 2–6 per cent at > 6 months).

- Patients over 70 yr have a 10-times greater risk of myocardial infarction and cardiac death than those < 70 yr.
- The peak time for infarction is between postoperative days three and five, not intra-operatively.
- The risk of cardiac death or postoperative myocardial infarction is four times higher after emergency operations than after elective procedures.
- An 'unplanned' blood pressure reduction of 33 per cent or more for longer than 10 min carries a five-fold increased risk of cardiac-related death.
- Patients with congestive heart failure from other causes also represent increased peri-operative risks.

Prolonged duration of anaesthesia and surgery also influences the incidence of complications.

Other medical problems are considered in general in the following chapters, e.g. diabetes (*see* p. 112), jaundice (*see* p. 114) and pancreatitis (*see* p. 114).

Alcohol

Alcoholic intoxication is a frequent finding in trauma victims, e.g. motor vehicle accidents. Acute intoxication is associated with potent respiratory, cardiovascular and neurological depression; the vasodilatation produced by ethanol often leads to hypothermia by the time the patient reaches the operating theatre.

• Intoxicated patients lack airway protection and are at risk from inhalation of vomitus.

Trauma

All trauma victims and emergency or urgent patients must be assumed to have full stomachs. A meal eaten a short time before the victim has sustained the accident will not be digested and remains in the stomach for many hours. For this reason induction of anaesthesia using rapid-sequence tracheal intubation should be used, together with cricoid pressure unless there is a possibility of cervical vertebral fracture (*see* p. 141); polytrauma concept (*see* p. 123). The passage of a nasogastric tube before anaesthesia and surgery helps to decompress the stomach although absolute reliance cannot be placed on this method; it is of value, however, in all patients with peritonitis or other abdominal emergencies and in any patient in whom there appears to be a prospect of difficult tracheal intubation.

Critical situations

• In an immediately life-threatening situation time should not be wasted performing investigations. The aim is to maintain life and so support of the respiratory and cardiovascular systems and brain function is vital.
• Tracheal intubation should be secured as early as possible in an unconscious patient.
• Blood is taken as soon as possible for grouping and cross-matching (*see* p. 30). Blood, blood substitutes, plasma or crystalloid solutions are given as required. If necessary, uncross-matched blood may need to be given (*see* p. 37).
• Intravenous access with at least one large gauge cannula (14 G) is required; it is often convenient to use a large neck vein for this purpose (external or internal jugular). The Arrow emergency infusion device uses a 'J' tip spring wire guide together with a dilator to facilitate the insertion of a 8.5 Fr (2.85 mm) ID Teflon catheter into the jugular vein. In situations where very major blood loss is being experienced, a cut down to any convenient vein with the insertion of a plastic tube of even larger diameter is valuable; a short length of sterile nasogastric or IV infusion tubing can be used.

A massive blood transfusion may be defined as a rate of 1 ml/kg/min. This represents about 4.2 litre/hr in an adult and 1.1 litre/hr in a 18 kg child. Blood and other infusion fluids should be warmed to 37°C before transfusion to the patient. Care must be taken to prevent air embolism during transfusions; this was a not uncommon problem when a sphygmanometer bulb was used to pressurize blood supplied in glass bottles. Air embolism can still be a problem even with blood and fluids supplied in plastic collapsible packs; three-way stopcocks are the best means of introducing drugs into the infusion line as multiple injections by needles through injection ports can create holes sufficiently large to allow room air to be entrained into the tubing when a fast transfusion is running.

- *In extremis*, do not waste time waiting for the 'correct' IV fluid; give whatever fluid is available within reason.
- In cases with massive blood loss consider collecting shed blood through a filter into a sterile heparinized receptacle (e.g. cardiomyotomy reservoir) and transfusing it to the patient.
- As soon as possible establish a central venous line.

The central venous pressure (CVP) is a good monitor of the transfusion requirement. It is not a guide to the amount of blood lost as is commonly believed, because a hypovolaemic patient may be vasoconstricted to an extent which gives a falsely reassuring CVP measurement. A fast transfusion of 500 ml increases CVP and if the patient is hypovolaemic the CVP falls again. Continue transfusing the patient until the CVP rises and stays at a high value, e.g. about 10 mmHg.

Resuscitation of the patient who has cardiac arrest is discussed in Chapter 2.

Rapid-sequence tracheal intubation

Pre-oxygenation is essential and traditionally is accomplished by the patient breathing 100 per cent oxygen for 5 min. Adequate pre-oxygenation may be achieved faster than this (after only several deep breaths) but only provided that air dilution does not occur during this time; to achieve this a very close fitting face-mask is essential.

- Induction of anaesthesia must only take place when the patient is on an operating table or trolley which can be quickly tipped to the head-down position.

Cricoid pressure (Sellick's manoeuvre[3])

Before induction of anaesthesia, with the patient in the supine and slightly head-down position, the cricoid cartilage is palpated and lightly held by a trained assistant between the thumb and second finger; as the anaesthetic is commenced, pressure is exerted on the cricoid cartilage mainly by the index finger; even a conscious patient can tolerate moderate pressure without discomfort. As soon as consciousness is lost firm pressure can be applied without obstruction of the patient's airway. The oesophagus is compressed between the cricoid ring of cartilage and the vertebral column, thus obstructing the passage of any material regurgitating from the stomach (Fig. 1.1).

Correct application of cricoid pressure pushes the larynx backwards and usually aids visualization of the glottis. Cricoid pressure may also be applied in situations where the patient is in the lateral position; counterpressure is applied by the assistant's other hand to the back of the patient's neck.

Cricoid pressure should not be released until tracheal intubation has been achieved by the cuff of the tube correctly inflated. Cricoid pressure should be released in situations where active vomiting occurs for fear of oesophageal rupture although this complication seems extremely rare.

During cricoid pressure the lungs may be ventilated if the need arises without risk of gastric distension. Indeed, it is of interest that cricoid pressure was originally described to obstruct the entry of air into the stomach where a bellows was used to inflate the lungs of victims of drowning in 18th century Europe.

It was previously thought that the presence of a nasogastric tube renders the manoeuvre ineffective; however, efficient cricoid pressure has now been shown to obliterate the lumen of the oesophagus although the lumen of the nasogastric tube may remain unobstructed.[4] The nasogastric tube must be left unoccluded (i.e. to free drainage) so that it can function as a 'blow-off' valve should a rise in intragastric pressure occur during induction of anaesthesia. The presence of a nasogastric tube in the absence of cricoid pressure makes regurgitation more likely to occur.

Left lateral head-down position

An alternative position of the patient for a rapid-sequence induction of anaesthesia is the left lateral slightly head-down position. This position is favoured for inhalational induction of anaesthesia in the emergency situation; it is also used when difficulty with intubation occurs (*see* p. 73). The position also has considerable merit for the single-handed anaesthetist with no assistant to perform cricoid pressure (although cricoid pressure should be used in this position if possible). The left rather than the right sided posi-

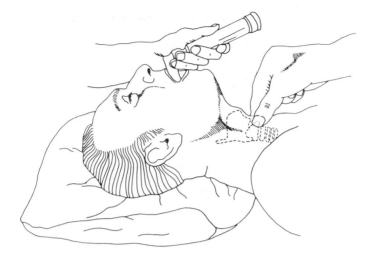

Fig. 1.1 Application of cricoid pressure.

tion is used because the patient's tongue is displaced by gravity to the left of the blade of the laryngoscope (if the patient lies on his right side the tongue lies above the blade and interferes with visualization of the larynx). Practice is required to intubate the trachea of patients in this position but the advantages are that the laryngoscope blade does not have to support the full weight of the jaw so that small left to right, and fore and aft movements of the laryngoscope handle bring the larynx into view.

- The circulation is less compromised with the patient in the head-down position rather than supine. This is important in patients who are hypovolaemic from any cause.
- The left lateral head-down position is very useful in dealing with the child with post-tonsillectomy haemorrhage ('bleeding tonsil'). Blood can run out of the mouth rather than obscure the anaesthetist's view of the larynx (*see* p. 161).

Establishment and maintenance of anaesthesia

- An IV infusion (preferably through a large gauge cannula, e.g. 14 G for an adult) should always be in progress to obtain venous access before commencing anaesthesia whenever possible.
- The nasogastric tube should be aspirated and left unspiggoted.

Anaesthesia is induced with a predetermined dose of IV induction agent (e.g. thiopentone [thiopental], methohexitone [methohexital], etomidate, or propofol) given according to the patient's cardiovascular status, and is immediately followed by suxamethonium (succinylcholine) 1.5–2 mg/kg to facilitate rapid intubation of the trachea. A lower dose of suxamethonium is not recommended because enough of the drug may become hydrolysed in a patient with a slow circulation time to reduce the chances of a swift and sure first attempt at intubation. Ketamine 1–2 mg/kg IV is sometimes favoured for the induction of anaesthesia particularly in the hypotensive patient.

Inhalational methods of induction of anaesthesia have to be used in circumstances where IV induction is not feasible; in this situation there is an increased risk of vomiting or regurgitation and the left-lateral head-down position is recommended (*see* p. 8). Either halothane, enflurane or isoflurane in oxygen are suitable; the addition of N_2O to the mixture accelerates induction. A 50 per cent mixture of cyclopropane in oxygen respired 'to and fro' from a 6 litre bag used to be popular because unconsciousness takes place in three to six breaths; however, the mixture is explosive.

Maintenance of anaesthesia must ensure that severe hyperventilation (with CO_2 washout) does not occur unless there are compelling reasons to the contrary (e.g. head injury, *see* p. 129); cardiac arrest in the hypovolaemic patient is often the result of a further reduction in cardiac output consequent upon a reduced $PaCO_2$ in the presence of high intrathoracic pressures usually associated with IPPV. In such a critical situation the use of IPNV (i.e. a subatmospheric phase during expiration) reduces mean intrathoracic pressure and is of benefit; however, this facility is uncommon in ventilators nowadays and so deliberate or, as is often the case, inadvertent excessive lung ventilation must be avoided. Anaesthetic agents and IV drugs must all be given cautiously in reduced dosage to avoid exacerbation of hypotension. Care also should be taken in the use of drugs known to liberate histamine and thereby produce hypotension (e.g. tubocurarine).

Inhalation of gastric contents

Inhalation of stomach contents is unfortunately still a common problem world-wide, especially associated with emergency anaesthesia. This risk of this occurrence must never be forgotten.

Prevention

Active vomiting and regurgitation of gastric contents with consequent aspiration of foreign material into the lungs may be prevented by:

- Decompressing the stomach as much as possible before anaesthesia and surgery by use of a nasogastric tube or stomach tube; although this is of great help it does not guarantee that the stomach is empty.
- Correct positioning of the patient and the application of cricoid pressure during the induction of anaesthesia.
- Passing a wide-bore stomach tube to empty the stomach as much as possible before extubation is contemplated (this is usually most conveniently performed after induction of anaesthesia when the airway has been secured with a cuffed endotracheal tube).
- Positioning the patient head-down on his side (left side if possible, *see* p. 8) before extubation.

A patient who has anaesthesia for an emergency procedure must not be extubated in the supine position even if consciousness has been regained. The larynx is incompetent after general anaesthesia and gastric contents are likely to be aspirated into the lungs should vomiting or regurgitation occur. If there are circumstances which prevent the patient being turned onto his side (e.g. orthopaedic traction) the stomach must be aspirated with a wide-bore stomach tube of at least 10 mm ID (not a nasogastric tube which is too small in diameter) and then washed out with 30 ml 0.3 M sodium citrate to neutralize any residual acid; remaining solution is then removed by suction, the tube removed and replaced with a conventional nasogastic tube or Salem sump tube.

- If aspiration occurs or is suspected, the pH of tracheal aspirate should be immediately tested using universal indicator or litmus paper.

The acid aspiration syndrome (Mendelson's syndrome) occurs when the pH of the aspirated foreign material is < 2.5. 'Silent' aspiration is common and is unnoticed at the time of occurrence. Symptoms of the acid-aspiration syndrome do not usually present for about six hours when an asthma-like syndrome develops, with wheezing, tachypnoea, tachycardia and the onset of cyanosis. Bronchospasm may be the first sign to indicate that acid-aspiration has occurred.

Treatment

This is directed towards:

- oxygen therapy,
- correction of metabolic acidosis,
- support of the respiratory and cardiovascular systems (IPPV may be necessary, fluid therapy, pharmacological support); treatment of bronchospasm with salbutamol or aminophylline.

Pulmonary lavage is not recommended because of the likelihood of disseminating the acid gastric juice to hitherto uncontaminated regions of the lung. Corticosteroid therapy is sometimes recommended although its benefits are doubtful in the early phases of treatment.

Aspiration of food particles blocks the air passages and causes immediate asphyxia; as much material as possible should be removed by tracheal suction, or bronchoscopy if necessary.

- Antibiotics should be given to combat pulmonary infection and the development of toxic shock once the nature of the organism is known.

References

1. Ruben H, Hansen E, Macnaughton FI. High capacity suction technique. A method of reducing the aspiration hazard during induction. *Anaesthesia* 1979; **34**: 349–51.
2. Foëx P. Anaesthesia and cardiovascular diseases: the importance of preoperative assessment. In: Atkinson RS, Hewer CL (eds). *Recent Advances in Anaesthesia, 14th ed*, London: Churchill Livingstone, 1982: 7–29.
3. Sellick BA. Cricoid pressure to control regurgitation of stomach contents during induction of anaesthesia. *Lancet* 1961; **ii**: 404–6.
4. Salem MR, Joseph NJ, Heyman HJ, Belani B, Paulissian R, Ferrara TP. Cricoid pressure is effective in obliterating the esophageal lumen in the presence of a nasogastric tube. *Anesthesiology* 1985; **63**: 443–6.

Further reading

Dunnill RPH, Colvin MP. *Clinical and Resuscitative Data, 3rd ed.* Oxford: Blackwell, 1985.

Harrison MJ, Jones RM, Pollard BJ. *Anaesthetic Management: A rule based guide.* London: Butterworths, 1986.

Howells TH, Chamney AR, Wraight WJ, Simons RS. The application of cricoid pressure. An assessment and a survey of its practice. *Anaesthesia* 1983; **38**: 457–460.

Katz J. Anesthesia for the trauma patient. *Prog Crit Care Med* 1984; **1**: 218–30.

Katz J, Benumof J, Kadis LB (eds). *Anesthesia and Uncommon Diseases. Pathophysiologic and clinical correlations, 2nd ed.* Philadelphia: Saunders, 1981.

Kaufman L, Sumner E. *Medical Problems and the Anaesthetist.* Current Topics in Anaesthesia – 4. London: Edward Arnold, 1979.

Opie LH. *Drugs and the Heart.* London: The Lancet, 1980.

Prys-Roberts C (ed). *The Circulation in Anaesthesia. Applied physiology and pharmacology.* Oxford: Blackwell, 1980.

Rubinstein D, Wayne D. *Lecture Notes in Clinical Medicine, 3rd ed.* Oxford: Blackwell, 1985.

Vandam LD. *To Make the Patient Ready for Anesthesia: Medical care of the surgical patient.* Menlo Park, California: Addison-Wesley, 1980.

Vickers MD (ed). *Medicine for Anaesthetists, 2nd ed.* Oxford: Blackwell, 1982.

Weatherall DJ, Ledingham JGG, Warrell DA. *Oxford Textbook of Medicine.* Oxford: University Press, 1983.

Wraight WJ, Chamney AR, Howells TH. The determination of an effective cricoid pressure. *Anaesthesia* 1983; **38**: 461–6.

2

Cardiopulmonary Resuscitation

Daniel Nyhan, William G. Zitzmann and Mark C. Rogers

Cardiopulmonary resuscitation in adults
  Basic steps
    airway
    breathing
    circulation
Cardiac arrest in the operating theatre
Paediatric cardiopulmonary resuscitation
  Differences between adult and paediatric patients
  Situations associated with cardiopulmonary arrest in children
  Management of paediatric CPR
  Drugs for resuscitation in children
  Defibrillation
  Complications

The bible records the first reference to mouth-to-mouth resuscitation. Even so, it was only as recently as the 1950s that the studies upon which the modern techniques of successful mouth-to-mouth ventilation are based were performed.[1, 2, 3, 4] In 1960, Kouwenhoven first described closed chest cardiac massage.[5] The potential of combined mouth-to-mouth ventilation and closed chest cardiac massage for improving survival during attempted cardiopulmonary resuscitation (CPR) was increasingly recognized during the 1960s and 1970s. The performance of CPR by lay people was encouraged by the American Heart Association and standards for its practice were published initially in 1974[6] and subsequently updated in 1980.[7] Recent interest in CPR has focused on elucidating the mechanisms determining blood flow in the circulation during conventional CPR, in the hope that the knowledge gained will, in the future, lead to possible alterations in the techniques of CPR, and hence improve survival.

    Cardiopulmonary resuscitation is no more than a temporizing measure. It addresses the most overt manifestation of an underlying disease process but does not address the primary problem. The impact of CPR on overall morbidity and mortality depends not only on the success of CPR *per se* as a temporizing measure, but also on the subsequent successful treatment of the underlying disease. With the increasing understanding of the causes of cardiopulmonary arrest, the importance of successful CPR is readily apparent. In addition to recent advances in understanding the causes of cardiopulmonary arrest, and in the mechanisms underlying CPR, there are an increasing number of pharmacological agents available to the physician. The impact of these latter factors on mortality and morbidity, plus the continued prevalent use of CPR in the community remains to be assessed.

Cardiopulmonary resuscitation in adults

Basic steps

The standardized approach of airway, breathing and circulation (ABC) was developed by the American Heart Association.

Airway

- The first step in CPR is to establish ventilation by means of mouth-to-mouth breathing followed by ventilation with a suitably fitting face-mask as soon as possible.
- Attempts at intubation of the trachea must wait until the patient has undergone a satisfactory period of gas exchange.
- Adequacy of ventilation should be evaluated by noting the rise and fall of the chest and by auscultation of the lungs.[11]
- If adequate gas exchange is not taking place, backward head tilt, jaw lift, and placement of oropharyngeal and nasopharyngeal airways should quickly be employed.
- Victims of cardiac arrest who were hypoxic before the arrest may tolerate only very brief periods of apnoea before irreversible damage ensues.

Breathing

- Once the airway has been established, ventilation should begin with four quick breaths before beginning chest compressions.
- Ventilation should not stop except for attempts at endotracheal intubation, which should not exceed periods of thirty seconds.
- As soon as possible ventilation should be established with 100 per cent oxygen.

- Not all bag and mask systems deliver 100 per cent oxygen and the same meticulous attention to possible disconnections as practised in the operating theatre should be observed in other areas of the hospital.

Circulation

- The carotid pulse should be palpated after a series of four breaths, if the pulse is absent external chest compression should be initiated with a 50 per cent compression and 50 per cent relaxation cycle.
- If a single rescuer is present, a compression to ventilation ratio of 15:2 with a compression rate of 80/min should be employed.
- Two rescuers should use a compression to ventilation ratio of 5:1 with a rate of 60/min.
- Adequacy of chest compressions should be assessed by palpation of femoral and carotid pulses, evaluation of arterial pressure tracing if an arterial line is present and ultimately by improvement in skin colour and constriction of pupils.

Other considerations

Concomitant with the initiation of ventilation, a quick assessment of the patient's airway should be made. Much of the information will need to come from observation of the patient and noting the circumstances of the arrest.

- Cervical spine injury should be suspected in trauma victims and the backward head tilt should not be employed (*see* p. 147).
- Patients being treated on an oncology ward or suffering from hepatic disease have a high risk of bleeding disorders making placement of a nasal airway unwise.
- A basilar skull fracture should raise the possibility of a puncture of the cribriform plate and again contra-indicates placement of any nasal airway.
- Evidence of head and neck surgery should raise the possibility of distorted anatomy with friable tissues secondary to tumour and radiation therapy.

Once the above steps have been taken, a plan for further airway management should be formulated. In the vast majority of cases this will involve standard orotracheal intubation using a laryngoscope and cuffed endotracheal tube.

- Nasal intubation either by the blind route or under direct vision is another option but is contra-indicated in patients with basilar skull fractures and in those with bleeding disorders.
- Multiple attempts at blind nasal intubation should be avoided since brisk bleeding may be initiated even in the patient with normal clotting function making subsequent oral intubation more difficult.
- If intubation of the trachea fails, ventilation may be accomplished by placement of a large bore IV cannula (12–14 G) through the cricothyroid membrane. Anaesthetists must be familiar with one of the several methods of connecting this cannula to a resuscitation bag.

Connexion can be established by use of a Portex paediatric 3.0 mm or 3.5 mm endotracheal tube connector. Alternatively, connexion can be established by use of a syringe barrel and an endotracheal tube connector: 3 ml syringe barrel with 8 mm connector; or 5 to 10 ml syringe with the free end of a British catheter mount (plain or corrugated pattern) pushed down inside the barrel. A 12 G cannula and Portex connector allows a flow of 9 litres/min of oxygen at 30 cmH$_2$O driving pressure.

Cricothyroidotomy involves incision of the cricothyroid membrane with a scalpel and placement of a tracheostomy tube (*see* p. 72). Emergency tracheostomy should be a last resort and performed only rarely. In cardiac arrest associated with massive pulmonary embolus or tracheal trauma, placement of the victim on cardiopulmonary bypass may be the only option.

After basic rescue efforts are underway, placement of a large bore IV or central line should be attempted. The subclavian vein is the preferred choice in this situation since rescue efforts do not have to be interrupted for line placement. Once in place a measurement of central venous pressure can be made and all subsequent administration of drugs should be made through this line.

Cardiac arrest in the operating theatre

In the operating room, cardiac arrest is likely to be encountered associated with an arrhythmia such as asystole, bradycardia and ventricular tachycardia or fibrillation. In the event of *asystole* CPR should be initiated and 1 mg of adrenaline (epinephrine) and 1 mg of atropine should be administered IV. Sodium bicarbonate in a dose of 1 mmol/kg may be given with further amounts governed by results of arterial blood gas measurements. Adrenaline (epinephrine) should be repeated in the same dose at 5 min intervals. If there is no response to the above an isoprenaline (isoproterenol) infusion at 2–20 micrograms/min may be used and consideration given to the placement of a transvenous pacemaker.

Monitored *ventricular fibrillation* should be treated initially with a precordial thump. If there is no change in rhythm the patient should be defibrillated with a direct current countershock delivering 200–300 joules of energy. If there is no change in rhythm after two shocks 1 mg adrenaline (epinephrine) should be given followed by another defibrillation attempt with 360 joules. Results of arterial blood gases and clinical impression may lead to administration of sodium bicarbonate. If there is no response to the third attempt at defibrillation a loading dose of 1 mg/kg lignocaine (lidocaine) or 5 mg/kg bretylium should be given followed by a fourth attempt at defibrillation. Further therapy consists of repeated doses of adrenaline (epinephrine) at five minute intervals and bicarbonate therapy guided by arterial blood gas measurements. Repeated attempts at defibrillation are likely to be useless unless the heart can be oxygenated.

Ventricular tachycardia

The onset of *ventricular tachycardia* in the unconscious patient should be treated with a precordial thump followed by a loading dose of lignocaine (lidocaine) (1 mg/kg). Concurrent with the administration of lignocaine (lidocaine), cardioversion with 200 joules of energy should be attempted. If reversion to normal rhythm occurs a lignocaine (lidocaine) infusion (2–4 mg/min) is begun; if the tachycardia is refractory, bretylium may be infused at a loading dose of 5 mg/kg and cardioversion repeated. Recalcitrant ventricular tachycardia may respond to procainamide or overdrive pacing.

Bradycardia

If *bradycardia* is associated with hypotension atropine (1–2 mg) should be administered. If there is no response an isoprenaline (isoproterenol) infusion (2–20 micrograms/min) should be started. If hypotension persists despite an increase in heart rate, volume infusion or a pressor agent should be added as clinically indicated.

Defibrillators

Defibrillation and cardioversion are mainstays in the treatment of ventricular fibrillation and tachycardia. All operating room areas should have a modern DC monophasic defibrillator easily available and in ready to use condition. Correct use of the defibrillator involves placement of one 13 cm paddle to the right of the sternum below the clavicle and the other to the left of the nipple in the anterior axillary line with delivered energy levels as recommended above.

Open heart defibrillation involves paddle placement over the right atrium and apex of the heart respectively and use of 5–40 joules. The outcome of defibrillation is dependent on the underlying disorder and the presence or absence of hypoxia, electrolyte imbalance and acidosis.

Internal cardiac compression

Open chest cardiac compression is rarely used outside the operating theatre since there is no evidence to indicate it will succeed where closed chest CPR has failed. There are, however, certain indications for open chest CPR:

- Penetrating cardiac injuries (some centres have reported success with emergency room thoracotomy).
- Cardiac arrest with pericardial tamponade.
- Situations where the anatomical characteristics of the chest preclude the application of closed chest CPR.

Drugs used to treat cardiac arrest

The anaesthetist is probably the physician with the most experience in administering the drugs commonly used during CPR. *Atropine* is used to reduce vagal tone and increase heart rate in patients with haemodynamic compromize secondary to bradycardia. Most clinicians feel heart rate is the most important determinant of myocardial oxygen consumption; rate related ischaemia as evidenced by ST segment depression should be noted. *Isoprenaline* (*isoproterenol*) is a β-adrenergic agonist which is used to treat atropine resistant bradycardia and also has a role in regulating heart rate in the transplanted organ. Disadvantages of isoprenaline (isoproterenol) are an increase in myocardial oxygen consumption and often a fall in mean arterial pressure. The dose is 2–20 micrograms/kg/min.

Lignocaine (lidocaine) is the current drug of choice to suppress re-entrant activity that may lead to venticular arrhythmias in the ischaemic myocardium. Adequate blood levels of the drug can be obtained with a bolus dose of 1 mg/kg followed by an infusion of 20–50 micrograms/kg/min. In order to avoid a subtherapeutic drug level a second bolus of 0.5 mg to 1 mg/kg may be given in 8–10 min; only half the loading dose should be given in conditions of congestive cardiac failure, shock and liver dysfunction.

Bretylium tosylate is indicated in the treatment of ventricular tachycardia and ventricular fibrillation refractory to treatment with lignocaine (lidocaine) and DC countershock. Digitalis-induced ventricular tachyarrhythmias are considered a relative contra-indication by some clinicians. The loading dose of bretylium is 5–10 mg/kg, followed by an infusion of 2 mg/min in the adult.

Adrenaline (epinephrine), a mixed α and β agonist is indicated in the treatment of asystole and ventricular fibrillation. The drug produces increases in heart rate and force of myocardial contraction. Adrenaline (epinephrine) is used to convert fine ventricular fibrillation to a coarse pattern considered more likely to respond to electrical countershock. The dose is 0.5–1 mg IV or via the endotracheal tube administered as 5–10 ml of 1:10 000 solution (i.e. 1 mg adrenaline (epinephrine) = 1 ml of 1:1000 strength diluted to 10 ml with isotonic saline). The dose may need to be repeated once or twice at 5 min intervals. Animal studies have shown that *dopamine* is also effective in CPR but that *dobutamine* is not. However, dobutamine is normally used to support the blood pressure once a satisfactory rhythm is established and the circulating volume corrected.

Calcium salts

The efficacy of calcium in resuscitation is doubtful; either calcium gluconate or calcium chloride may be used as both salts are fully ionized in solution, i.e. all the calcium they contain is available immediately. Calcium chloride ($CaCl_2$) is more irritant than calcium gluconate and should be injected very carefully to avoid extravasation. Calcium salts must not be given into an infusion containing bicarbonate as the two compounds react to form an insoluble precipitation of calcium carbonate.

There are various preparations of calcium chloride available in different countries, or even in the same country or hospital. Obviously, great care must be taken to prevent confusion between the solutions available.

Calcium is a divalent ion, thus 2 mEq $Ca^{2+} \equiv 1$ mmol Ca^{2+}. It is much safer to rely on doses in either mEq or mmol, but *not* in terms of mg or volumes (Table 2.1).

Calcium chloride refers to the dihydrate salt (i.e. $CaCl_2 . 2H_2O$), in the British, European and United States Pharmacopoeias. There are other salts of calcium such as the hexahydrate $CaCl_2 . 6H_2O$ and the anhydrous salt $CaCl_2$. Solutions based on anhydrous calcium chloride are not commonly found because calcium chloride is hygroscopic.

Table 2.1 Preparations of calcium chloride

Preparation	Strength	Ca^{2+} Salt	Ca^{2+} Content mmol/ml	mEq/ml
Calcium chloride USP, EP, BP	100 mg/ml (10% w/v)	dihydrate $CaCl_2.2H_2O$	0.68	1.36
Calcium chloride	134 mg/ml (13.4% w/v)	dihydrate $CaCl_2.2H_2O$	0.91	1.80
Calcium chloride	100 mg/ml (10% w/v)	hexahydrate $CaCl_2.6H_2O$	0.46	0.90
Calcium chloride	73.5 mg/ml (7.35% w/v)	dihydrate $CaCl_2.2H_2O$	0.5	1.0
	7.35 mg/ml (0.74% w/v)		0.05	0.1
Calcium chloride	100 mg/ml (10% w/v)	anhydrous $CaCl_2$	0.91	1.8
Calcium gluconate	100 mg/ml (10% w/v)	contains Ca-d-saccharate 0.427% w/v (as stabilizer)	0.25	0.50
		without stabilizer	0.23	0.46

Calcium may be given in the treatment of asystole to improve myocardial tone in an IV dose of 1.5–2.5 mmol/70 kg body weight (3–5 mEq/70 kg) and repeated as necessary at 10 min intervals. It must never be given via the endotracheal tube and great care must be taken with intracardiac injection lest accidental injection into the muscle occurs.

Paediatric cardiopulmonary resuscitation

Cardiopulmonary resuscitation is practised on patients at the extremes of life. Its use is stated to be uncommon after six weeks of life and rare after one year. Even so, with the ever increasing success in treating the chronic diseases of childhood and the concomitant emergence of paediatric intensive care units in many hospitals, the frequency with which cardiopulmonary arrest occurs in the paediatric age group is likely to continue to increase. Furthermore CPR, performed by parents outside hospital, is perhaps one of the few ways of potentially improving the distressingly high mortality associated with sudden infant death syndrome. Advanced paediatric life support (APLS) merely optimizes basic paediatric CPR allowing more time for identification and treatment of the primary cause.

Differences between adult and paediatric patients

The outcome (as defined by successful CPR and eventual percentage of patients leaving hospital) is significantly better for paediatric than adult patients.[8] This is probably due to a number of reasons. Foremost among these include the fact that the single commonest primary cause of arrests in paediatric patients is respiratory in origin, that paediatric patients usually only have one system disease and that unless primarily involved the cardiovascular and nervous sytems in paediatric patients do not usually have underlying disease. Also, of potential importance is the possibility that the developing organs of paediatric patients are more resistant to hypoxia.

Even so, further improvement in paediatric CPR is hampered, at a clinical level by technical obstacles in resuscitating children, and at a research level by the relative lack of understanding of the underlying mechanisms involved.

Situations associated with cardiopulmonary arrest in children

A list of the many causes of cardiopulmonary arrest in children can be found in most paediatric textbooks. It is perhaps more fruitful for the clinician to be acutely aware of the clinical situations where arrests are likely to occur. Since the single commonest primary cause of arrest in children is respiratory in origin, patients at high risk include those undergoing:

- change or withdrawal of ventilatory support
- chest physiotherapy
- airway suctioning
- sedation for minor procedures.

Other paediatric patients at high risk of undergoing a cardiopulmonary arrest include:

- postoperative patients
- patients in coma
- patients with artificial airways (e.g. tracheostomy)
- patients with rapidly progressive respiratory failure
- those subjected to any cause of vagal stimulation
- those with an unstable cardiovascular system.

Signs of impending cardiac arrest in children include changing mental status (e.g. somnolence, irritability, combativeness), heart rate changes (either increases or decreases but especially the latter) and any evidence that the underlying cause is getting acutely worse (e.g. respiratory failure).

Management of paediatric CPR

This follows the lines already described for the adult patient with strict adherence to the principles of airway management, adequate ventilation and circulatory support.

Airway management

In paediatric basic CPR this consists of excluding airway obstruction (e.g. due to a foreign body in the pharynx) and ensuring airway patency by appropriate head tilt/lift and chin tilt/lift. Ventilation is carried out using mouth-to-mouth ventilation at a rate of 16/min in children and 20/min in infants. Mouth-to-mouth ventilation delivers no more than 16–18 per cent oxygen to the patient. The circulation is supported by chest compression at a rate of 100/min in infants and 80/min in children with downward compression lasting 50 per cent of each cycle.

Attention to additional details must be paid if it is hoped to effect forward circulation during paediatric CPR.

- The patient should be on a firm surface.
- The point of compression should be mid-sternum. At this point the heart lies between the sternum and the spine.
- Chest compression should consist of ¾ inch (in infants) and 1½ inches (in children) perpendicular depressions of the sternum.

Advanced paediatric life support

Appropriate equipment necessary for the proper conduct of advanced paediatric life support is usually readily available in settings where its use is likely (e.g. operating theatre, paediatric intensive care unit, emergency room). Such equipment should include an Ambu or similar bag (with a nonrebreathing valve, e.g. Ruben valve) delivering 100 per cent oxygen, appropriately sized face-masks, suction, oro- and nasopharyngeal airways, laryngo-scope with appropriately sized blades and endotracheal tubes (recommended size = $\dfrac{16 + \text{age of patient}}{4}$).

Muscle relaxants should be available to facilitate intubation when appropriate. Recommended dose of suxamethonium (succinylcholine) is 1 mg/kg and of pancuronium 0.1 mg/kg.

Drugs for resuscitation in children

The indications for the use of specific resuscitative drugs are outlined in the section dealing with adult CPR.

The recommended dosage of *atropine* is 0.01 mg/kg with a minimum total dose of 0.15 mg. It should be given IV but otherwise may be administered intralingually or via the endotracheal tube. *Calcium chloride* should be given in a dose of 0.14 mEq/kg (0.07 mmol/kg) and only IV since IM administration or administration via the endotracheal tube leads to tissue necrosis. Its use is contra-indicated in ventricular fibrillation.

Adrenaline (*epinephrine*) should be given at a dose of 10 micrograms/kg (i.e. 0.1 ml/kg of a 1/10 000 solution). It can be given IV or if necessary IM or intracardiac and every 3–5 min in an arrest situation. It is incompatible with $NaHCO_3$ and its efficacy depends on the patient not being acidotic.

Sodium bicarbonate ($NaHCO_3$) should be given at a dose of 1 mmol/kg, IV only. It is incompatible with most drugs, so IV lines should be flushed after its administration. If given intratracheally, it deactivates surfactant leading to atelectasis. Sodium bicarbonate can cause intracranial haemorrhage in infants because of its hypertonicity. It should therefore be diluted 1:1 in 5 per cent dextrose solution or sterile water.

Lignocaine (*lidocaine*) should be given by infusion at a rate of 20–50 micrograms/kg/min after an initial loading dose of 1 mg/kg. A bolus may be given IV or if necessary via the endotracheal tube. Lignocaine (lidocaine) is incompatible with $NaHCO_3$ and its use should be discontinued if the PR interval or QRS complex widen.

Defibrillation

Electrical defibrillation is used to treat ventricular fibrillation after failure of a precordial thump. The success and safe use of electrical defibrillation depends on attention to certain details not always adhered to. The recommended energy is 1–2 joules/kg and defibrillation is recommended during expiration when transthoracic impedance is at its lowest. One paddle should be placed to the right of the upper sternum and the other at the apex such that current 'flows across the heart.' Large paddles with paste or saline should be used to decrease skin resistance and the paddles should be held with firm pressure during defibrillation. It should also be noted that defibrillation even with the same energy, may be successful on repeated attempts because previous defibrillation decreases transthoracic impedance. The success of cardioversion is inversely related to the duration of the arrhythmia. Excess electrode paste may cause short-circuiting. The use of excess electricity during defibrillation may cause skin burns or myocardial damage.

Complications

The complications of CPR can be classified into those secondary to hypoxia (e.g. brain damage, renal failure, etc.) and those secondary to the actual performance of the procedure itself (e.g. fractured rib, ruptured liver, pneumothorax, cardiac tamponade). These latter complications should always be kept in mind when CPR is seemingly unsuccessful and appropriate therapeutic meassures embarked upon where possible (e.g. placement of chest tube for a pneumothorax).

Future of paediatric CPR: the mechanisms determining blood flow in paediatric CPR are not as well understood as in adults. The effectiveness of spontaneous ventilation circulation CPR [SVC–CPR] in paediatrics, and its precise parameters remain to be established.

References

1. Elam JO, Brown ES, Elder JD Jr. Artificial respiration by mouth to mask method. A study of the respiratory gas exchange of paralyzed patients ventilated by operator's expired air. *N. Eng. J. Med.* 1954; **250**: 749.
2. Safar P, Escarraga LA, Elam JO. A comparison of the mouth to mouth and mouth to airway methods of artificial respiration with the chest-pressure arm-lift methods. *N. Eng. J. Med.* 1958; **258**: 671.
3. Gordon AS, Frye CW, Gittelson L, Sadova MS, Beattie ES Jr. Mouth to mouth versus manual artificial respiration for children and adults. *JAMA* 1958; **167**: 320.
4. Safar P, Redding J. The 'tight jaw' in resuscitation. *Anesthesiology* 1959: **20**: 701.
5. Kouwenhoven WB, Jude JR, Knickerbocker GG. Closed-chest cardiac massage. *JAMA* 1960; **173**: 1064.
6. Standards for cardiopulmonary resuscitation (CPR) and emergency cardiac care (ECC). *JAMA (suppl.)* 1974; **227**: 833.
7. Standards and guidelines for cardiopulmonary resuscitation (CPR) and emergency cardiac care (ECC). *JAMA* 1980; **244**: 453–509.

8. DeGard ML. Cardiopulmonary resuscitation: analysis of six years experience and review of literature. *Ann. Emerg. Med.* 1981; **10**: 408–16.

Further reading

Safar P. *Cardiopulmonary Cerebral Resuscitation. A manual for physicians and paramedical instructors*, prepared for the World Federation of Societies of Anaesthesiologists. Stavanger, Norway: AS Laerdal, 1981; and Philadelphia: WB Saunders.
Wilson F, Park WG. *Basic Resuscitation and Primary Care.* Lancaster, England: MTP Press, 1980.

3

Blood Grouping and Blood Transfusion

Gerald N Smith

Blood transfusion serology
  The ABO blood group system
  The Rhesus (Rh) blood group system
  Other blood group systems
Laboratory aspects
  Blood grouping
  Direct compatibility (cross-match) tests
  Antibody screening tests
  Antibody identification
Blood donors
Blood and blood products
  Anticoagulants
  Red cells suspended in saline-adenine-glucose-mannitol
    (SAG-M)
  Storage of blood and blood products
Clinical aspects of transfusion
  Patient identification
  Blood samples
  The request form
  Degree of urgency
  Infusion flow rates
  Preparation for surgery
  Acute blood loss
Massive blood transfusion
  Hypothermia
  Citrate toxicity
  Hyperkalaemia
  Bleeding
  Microaggregate infusion
  High affinity haemoglobin
Adverse reactions to blood and blood products
  Severe immediate reactions
  Moderate or minor reactions
  Delayed reactions

Paediatric practice
Sickle cell disease
Autotransfusion

Blood transfusion serology

The ABO blood group system

ABO blood groups are of major importance because of the invariable presence of naturally-occurring anti-A and anti-B in the serum of individuals lacking the corresponding red cell antigens (Table 3.1) and the potentially lethal effects of ABO-incompatible blood transfusions.

An individual may inherit an *A*, *B* or *O* gene from each parent, giving rise to six possible genotypes (*AA*, *AO*, *OO*, *BO*, *BB*, *AB*) and four phenotypes or 'groups' (A, O, B, AB). The *A* and *B* genes code for enzymes which convert a precursor substance, H, into A or B substances. The O gene is an amorph which leaves H unchanged. Red cells and some other tissues carry these antigens, and A, B and H substances are found in plasma and in some secretions. A and B subgroups (e.g. A_1, A_2) are recognized but are of little clinical significance.

Anti-A and anti-B are complement-binding antibodies. *In vivo*, they cause intravascular lysis of red cells bearing the A and B antigens. The life-threatening consequences of ABO-incompatible transfusions, however, result from the effects of complement activation and the release of vasoactive and thromboplastic substances rather than haemoglobinaemia or haemoglobinuria.

Table 3.1   ABO blood groups

Blood group	Plasma antibody	Blood group frequency*	Compatible donor red cells
A	anti-B(β)	47%	A (O)†
O	{ anti-A(α) anti-B(β)	42%	O
B	anti-A(α)	8%	B (O)†
AB	none	3%	AB (A, B, O)†

* English population
† Give correct ABO group whenever possible to conserve group O blood for group O recipients and to avoid problems with transfused anti-A and anti-B.

The Rhesus (Rh) blood group system

The importance of this system stems from the frequency with which Rh-negative individuals make antibody in response to Rh-positive red cells – either as a consequence of transfusion or of fetomaternal bleeding. Rh antibodies are predominantly IgG, they can cross the placenta, and are the commonest cause of haemolytic disease of the newborn. When bound to Rh-positive red cells, they interact with receptors on mononuclear phagocytes in the spleen, liver and elsewhere, causing red cell sequestration and destruction (extravascular haemolysis). Rhesus antibodies do not activate complement but they may cause severe transfusion reactions.

Rhesus is a complex antigen of which D is a part. For historical reasons and because of the importance of D, the terms Rh-positive and D-positive are used interchangeably. Rhesus(D)-negative individuals lack the D antigen. Family studies have shown that D-positive individuals may be either homozygous (*DD*) or heterozygous (*Dd*), but the product implied by *d* has never been demonstrated serologically, i.e. anti-d has not been found. Some 83 per cent of the English population are Rh(D)-positive.

The other parts of the Rh complex are governed by two genetic loci closely linked to D. The common alleles are designated *C*, *c* and *E*, *e* respectively. Because of the close linkage, the Rh alleles on a given chromosome are passed from parent to offspring as a triplet, e.g. *CDe*, *cde*, etc.

A common variant of the Rh antigen, D^u, may be considered as a weak form of D, with fewer antigenic determinants on each red cell. Rare types of D^u individual may form anti-D if given Rh-positive blood. It is customary, therefore, to treat D^u recipients of blood as if they were Rh-negative, and D^u donors as Rh-positive.

Rhesus antigens are found only on red cells.

Other blood group systems

These are quantitatively less important in blood transfusion practice for several reasons. If naturally-occurring antibodies are found (e.g. anti-Lewis), they are usually IgM, they do not cross the placenta, and they are mostly inactive at physiological temperatures. Alloantibodies are relatively uncommon because most of the antigens are poor immunogens. Nevertheless, antibodies of clinical significance do occur in these systems, and examples of the more commonly encountered specificities are shown in Table 3.2. Most are IgG and may therefore cause haemolytic disease of the newborn. A few bind complement and may cause severe transfusion reactions with intravascular haemolysis. One purpose of the

Table 3.2 Some important alloantibodies

Alloantibody		Percentage of blood donors lacking the relevant antigen
Rhesus:	anti-D	15
	anti-C	30
	anti-e	2
Anti-Kell (K)		91
Anti-Duffy (Fy^a)		35
Anti-Kidd (Jk^a)		23

routine cross–match and antibody screening tests is to avoid these incompatibilities.

Laboratory aspects

Blood grouping

ABO grouping tests are usually done at room temperature with an hour's incubation. The patient's red cells are tested with anti-A and anti-B reagents, and the presence of the corresponding antibodies (*see* Table 3.1) in the patient's serum provides an invaluable check on the results of the cell grouping. In emergency, the results of a cell group can be known in a few minutes.

Rhesus(D) grouping is more problematic in that anti-D is usually an incomplete antibody and routine tests require incubation at 37°C for satisfactory cell coating, followed by another procedure, such as the addition of albumin, to produce agglutination. Two different anti-D reagents are normally used in separate tests on a given blood sample. There is no serum group check. For emergency work, special reagents have to be used which cause rapid direct agglutination of Rh-positive cells.

Direct compatibility (cross-match) tests

These tests with the recipient's serum and the donor red cells serve as an additional check on ABO compatibility (against errors of donor or recipient group), and aim to detect antibodies which may react with other antigens on the donor cells. Several different methods of antibody detection have to be used when testing each donor unit because an unknown antibody may react only by one or other of these, e.g. papain or indirect antiglobulin tests. If incubation times of less than 20 min are used, the sensitivity of the haemagglutination tests is greatly diminished and antibodies may escape detection. In some laboratories methods using a low ionic strength saline (LISS) are employed to reduce incubation time in these tests.

In the UK, there is no statutory requirement for tests to be done at the bedside to detect ABO incompatibility. In France and Spain, where this practice has been followed, opinions differ concerning its value in preventing serious transfusion reactions. If well-defined clinical and laboratory procedures are followed, bedside testing would seem to be an unnecessary complication, especially in emergency practice.

Antibody screening tests

Tests between recipient's serum and reagent red cells known to express most of the clinically important antigens are particularly useful when done well in advance of the cross-match tests so that, in the event of a positive result, futher investigations may be undertaken to identify the antibody and select appropriate blood.

Antibody identification

This is required only if unexpected antibodies have been found in the cross-matching or antibody screening tests. A panel of typed cells is used to define the antibody specificity.

Blood donors

Details about the recruitment and selection of blood donors are given by Barbara.[1] In emergency, the collection of blood from donors for immediate use is impractical for most hospitals, and is rarely justifiable. The urgent grouping of donors presents another potential source of error, and the results of the recommended tests for hepatitis B, syphilis and anti-HIV(LAV/HTLVIII) cannot be obtained rapidly. Supplies are best provided from central stocks; in the UK these are held by the National Blood Transfusion Service, who will make provision for their urgent replacement.

Blood and blood products

Over the last decade, the availability of closed-system blood collection packs and the development of automated plasmapheresis have made possible the production of a variety of blood components, each intended to meet particular therapeutic needs. During emergency treatment, it is often important to know the detailed specification of the products available for transfusion. General information about anticoagulants is given here, followed by a summary list of blood products likely to be used in emergency (Table 3.3). In special cases, leukocyte-poor blood, coagulation factor concentrates or other preparations not shown in the table may be needed. These cases should be discussed with the haematologist.

Anticoagulants

Citrate solutions have been used almost exclusively for the collection of blood for transfusion. Several formulations incorporating dextrose and phosphate, and more recently, adenine, have been developed with the aim of preserving red cell viability during storage and prolonging shelf-life. The majority of whole blood donations are now collected into 63 ml of citrate-phosphate dextrose-adenine, formula 1 (CPDA-1), which contains:

trisodium citrate, $2H_2O$	1660 mg (5.65 mmol)
citric acid, H_2O	206 mg (1.03 mmol)
sodium dihydrogen phosphate, H_2O	140 mg (1.01 mmol)
dextrose, anhydrous	1830 mg (10.17 mmol)
adenine	17.3 mg (0.13 mmol)

The conversion of citrated to heparinized blood immediately before transfusion is now rarely requested. If required, 500 i.u. heparin is added to the unit (500 ml) of *whole blood*, followed by 5 mmol Ca^{2+} (Calcium Chloride Injection) (*see* p. 20).

Red cells suspended in saline-adenine-glucose-mannitol (SAG-M)

Many blood donations now have most of the citrated plasma removed for component production. To maintain the viability of the remaining red cells, and to improve the flow characteristics, 100 ml SAG-M solution containing the following, is added to the packed cells:

sodium chloride	877 mg (15 mmol)
adenine	16.9 mg (0.125 mmol)
glucose, anhydrous	818 mg (4.54 mmol)
mannitol	525 mg (2.88 mmol)

Because of the low protein content of SAG-M blood, no more than 4 units should normally be used for replacement in acute blood loss in adults. It should not be used in hypoalbuminaemia.

Storage of blood and blood products

Products containing red cells must be stored at 4–6°C in a

Table 3.3 Blood and blood products — some important characteristics

Item	Volume	Storage	Description	Compatibility	Uses
(1) Citrated whole blood CPDA-1	500 ml	4–6°C	Unprocessed blood donation, PCV 0.4	Group and cross-match	Acute, large volume blood loss.
(2) SAG-M blood	400 ml	4–6°C	See text. PCV 0.5	Group and cross-match	Acute blood loss, especially cover for surgery: maximum 4 unit transfusion.
(3) Plasma-reduced blood	300 ml	4–6°C	Product (1) from which 180–220 ml plasma has been removed. PCV 0.6	Group and cross-match	Correction of anaemia; acute blood loss and cover for surgery, but watch PCV.
(4) Concentrated (packed) red cells	250 ml	4–6°C	Products (1)–(3) from which most of the plasma has been removed immediately before use. PCV 0.7–0.8.	Group and cross-match	Correction of anaemia in normovolaemic recipient.
(5) Platelet concentrates	50 ml	22°C, gentle mixing	Platelets from product (1) in citrated plasma. Pool of several units may be supplied. Contain small numbers of red cells.	ABO essential, Rh desirable; no cross-match.	Bleeding due to thrombocytopenia and to qualitative platelet defects. Use special giving set, no additional filters. No aspirin, etc.

Table 3.3 – *continued*

Item	Volume	Storage	Description	Compatibility	Uses
(6) Fresh-frozen plasma (FFP)	200 ml	−30°C	Plasma from product (1) separated and frozen shortly after donation. All coagulation factor activity retained.	ABO essential*, Rh desirable.	Minor bleeds in some congenital coagulation deficiencies. Acquired multiple factor deficiencies e.g. DIC, warfarin treatment.
(7) Cryoprecipitate	20 ml	−30°C	Proteins precipitated at low temperature from citrated plasma. Contains VIII, von Willebrand factor, fibrinogen and fibronectin.	ABO* and Rh desirable.	Classical haemophilia, von Willebrand's disease, hypofibrino-genaemia. Consult haematologist.
(8) Cryoprecipitate-poor plasma (expander/ exhausted plasma)	200 ml	−30°C	Supernatant plasma from cryoprecipitate, lacking VIII etc,	ABO* and Rh desirable.	Plasma volume replacement. Burns and other acute protein-losing conditions.
(9) Anti-Rh(D) immunoglobulin	1 ml or 2 ml	4–6°C	IgG preparation containing 250 or 500 i.u. anti-D. Not for intravenous use.	Rh(D)-negative recipients only.	Prophylaxis against primary Rh alloimmunization due to pregnancy or transfusion. Consult haematologist.

(10) Human Albumin Solution (HAS)**†(4.5%)	100 ml, 400 ml 500 ml	2–25°C in the dark	Solution containing 4.3–4.5 g protein/dl (not less than 90% albumin); 130–160 mmol Na$^+$/litre; not more than 2 mmol potassium/litre; 7.2 mmol n-octanoate/litre. Heated to destroy Hepatitis-B virus.	All groups	Acute hypovolaemia, burns, crush injuries etc. NB: Has lower colloid osmotic potential than plasma; diuretics may be used to reduce fluid and electrolyte load in appropriate cases.
(11) Human Albumin BP (salt-poor albumin)†	100 ml	2–25°C in the dark	Each 100 ml contains 20 g protein (not less than 95% albumin); 130 mmol Na$^+$/litre; 10 mmol potassium/litre. Otherwise as HPPF	All groups.	Acute/subacute hypoalbuminaemia (<20 g/litre). For average adult, one bottle will raise serum albumin by 3 g/litre; aim to raise level above 30 g/litre. NB: Because of high osmotic potential, give total dose over not <12 hr.

* For these *plasma* products, ABO compatibility refers to *donor plasma* and *recipient red cells*, e.g. *AB plasma* may be given to all groups, group *O plasma* must only be given to group O recipients.

† UK National Blood Transfusion Service. Similar products are available commercially.

** Human Albumin Solution (HAS), previously known as Human Plasma Protein Fraction.

refrigerator fitted with a temperature recorder and an alarm system. Above the recommended temperature, red cell ATP and 2,3-diphosphoglycerate (2,3-DPG) are less well maintained, potassium is lost at a greater rate, and there is impaired red cell survival following transfusion. There is also an increased risk of bacterial growth. Citrated blood freezes at $-0.5°C$ and is lysed. Where relevant, expiry dates are shown on product labels. The red cell preparations in Table 3.3 have a shelf-life of 35 days. If the closed pack has to be opened for washing or other procedures, then transfusion of the unit must be completed within 12 hr.

Platelet function deteriorates in a few days even under optimum storage conditions (22°C with continous gentle mixing) and platelet concentrates should be used as soon as possible after preparation. Similarly, the frozen coagulation factor preparations should be transfused without delay once they have been thawed.

Clinical aspects of transfusion

Patient identification

The full name, date of birth and unique hospital case number of the patient must all appear on the blood specimen and on the request form. Particular care is needed with unidentified, unconscious patients.

Blood samples

Whenever possible, a blood sample should be taken for grouping and cross-matching before any intravenous infusions are given, as these may compromise the interpretation of tests taken subsequently. Ten ml clotted blood is sufficient for grouping and for cross-matching 5 units of blood. Allow an extra 1 ml for each additional unit requested.

The request form

The laboratory will often be able to respond more quickly to requests if information is given about the current clinical problem, previous blood transfusions or pregnancies, and details of any medications which may give abnormal serological results (e.g. α-methyl dopa or high dose penicillin causing positive direct antiglobulin tests).

Degree of urgency

The following options are associated with a progressive increase in the risk of serological incompatibility:

- Full group and 1 hr cross-match: time taken *from receipt of specimen* – 2 hr.
- Rapid group and 20 min cross-match: time taken – 45 min.
- Rapid group for the selection of uncross-matched blood of the same ABO and Rh groups: time taken 5–10 min.
- Uncross-matched group O Rh-negative blood.

The last two options are rarely warranted provided that plasma substitutes or albumin are to hand. Shorter cross-match times will be needed if LISS methods are used (*see* p. 31).

Infusion flow rates

Maximum infusion rates are largely determined by the size of cannula or catheter used. As a general guide, flow rates of about 250 ml/min are possible using a 14 G cannula (1.5 mm ID), and about 70 ml/min through an 18 G (0.8 mm ID). Flow rates may be increased by compression of plastic blood bags by use of a simple inflatable pressure cuff or a spring driven plate in a metal chamber or box, or a roller pump may be used on the infusion line tubing. Whenever positive pressure is used, extra care must be taken to prevent air embolism (*see* p. 7).

Standard infusion sets have an integral clot filter with a mesh size of 170 μm. Sets may need to be changed frequently when large volume transfusions are being given so that the flow rate can be maintained. In any event, sets should be changed every 12–24 hr to avoid complications from bacterial contamination. Micro-aggregate in–line filters which remove particles above 20–40 μm size are used by many anaesthetists in an effort to avoid 'shock lung' especially when many units of blood are given (see below).

Preparation for surgery

While the need for action in emergency will often override the following considerations, it is nevertheless true that some patients will present with chronic anaemias and should be treated accordingly if at all possible.

In chronic anaemia, when the haemoglobin falls below 10 g/dl, cardiac output at rest increases and there is an exaggerated cardiac response to stress. Although there is some evidence to suggest that in the absence of cardiac, respiratory and renal abnormality, a haemoglobin level of 7 g/dl is well tolerated during surgery,[2] it is common anaesthetic practice to require a pre-operative level of 10 g/dl or more.

When time permits, it is preferable to treat deficiency anaemias with the relevant haematinic. If transfusion is essential, an interval of 48 hr between transfusion and surgery is desirable to allow equilibration. Plasma-reduced or packed red cells may be given to a normovolaemic recipient over two to four hours, but if there is any degree of cardiovascular compromise, a more cautious approach may be needed. Diuretics (e.g. frusemide, 40 mg IV) may be given before transfusion and repeated as necessary. No more than one-third of the recipient's blood volume should be given at one transfusion.

Acute blood loss

The rapid removal of 15 per cent of the blood volume is generally well tolerated in healthy adults, but additional factors such as trauma, may contribute to the hypotensive effects of acute blood loss. Hypotension in the face of bleeding demands urgent measures to raise and maintain the systolic blood pressure above 100 mmHg.

Massive blood transfusion (*see* p. 6)

The provision of blood under these circumstances is sometimes dictated by whatever comes to hand, but if possible, blood less than two weeks old is to be preferred. There is no evidence, however, that 'fresh' blood offers any advantage over the proper use of blood components.

Hypothermia

Body core temperature may fall below 30°C following the massive transfusion of cold blood. As the temperature falls, sino-atrial bradycardia develops and ventricular fibrillation may occur. Cooling is readily prevented by passing the blood through a thermostatically controlled heat exchanger in the transfusion line. Several devices are available. Units of blood should not be pre-heated by immersion in a bath of warm water: not only may access ports be contaminated and labels rendered illegible, but if the blood is inadvertently heated above 40°C, red cell survival may be impaired.

Citrate toxicity

Following massive transfusion with citrated whole blood

(13 mmol citrate/litre), plasma citrate may rise to 5 mmol/litre or more (normal, 0.05 mmol/litre). With CPDA-1 anticoagulant, acidosis is not a significant problem, nor is the potential alkalosis following the conversion of citrate to bicarbonate. The main toxic effect is due to a reduction in ionized plasma calcium causing impaired myocardial function. Hypocalcaemia augments the adverse effects of hyperkalaemia (*see* below) so that the control of citrate toxicity assumes an added importance. If citrated whole blood is transfused at a rate of 100 ml/min or more, 10 ml of 10 per cent Calcium Gluconate Injection (2.23 mmol Ca^{2+}) should be given – slowly, and through a different vein (not a central catheter) – after every unit transfused.

Hyperkalaemia

The amount of potassium in the plasma from a unit of CPDA-1 blood shortly after collection is about 1.5 mmol. By 14 days this has risen to 4.5 mmol, and by 21 days to 6 mmol. Provided that hypocalcaemia is prevented, massive transfusion with blood less than two weeks old is unlikely to cause serious hyperkalaemia, unless the picture is complicated by renal failure or diabetes, for example, when emergency treatment with insulin and glucose may be required. As plasma potassium levels *in vivo* rise above 6 mmol/litre, there is progressive T wave peaking, P wave depression and QRS-T fusion on ECG.

At 9–10 mmol potassium/litre, asystole or ventricular fibrillation may occur (*see* p. 58).

Bleeding

Citrated blood rapidly loses coagulation factors V and VIII activity, and platelet function deteriorates. Patients requiring massive transfusion may develop bleeding problems due to these deficiencies. Following extensive wounds or surgery, and associated with some pathological conditions, there may also be a degree of disseminated intravascular coagulation (DIC).

Two units of fresh frozen plasma (FFP) should be given after every 8 units of stored blood. Thrombocytopenic bleeding should be treated with platelet concentrates. Platelet function may be impaired following extracorporeal circulation or as a consequence of aspirin or other medications, and again, platelet transfusions may be needed.

Microaggregate infusion

There is no evidence that microaggregate infusion causes any ill effect at normal rates of transfusion. The suggestion that it may be important in the pathogenesis of respiratory problems seen after massive transfusion is controversial.[3] It is doubtful whether the use of in-line filters in these circumstances serves any purpose. Inevitably, transfusion flow rates will be impaired by their use.

High affinity haemoglobin

The new blood storage media, CPDA-1 and SAG-M, maintain ATP and 2,3-DPG levels in red cells at or above normal for 7–10 days. By the end of their shelf-life, however, most red cell preparations are low in the organic phosphates and the affinity of haemoglobin for oxygen is increased. Theoretically, this could impair tissue oxygenation following massive blood transfusion, but conclusive evidence for a clinically significant effect is lacking.[4]

Adverse reactions to blood and blood products

Severe immediate reactions

Severe reactions occurring immediately, or within a short time of transfusion, are usually due to antibody-mediated complement-dependent interactions between recipient antibodies and donor antigens. ABO incompatibility is usually implicated, but other red cell antibodies and other causes of complement activation may produce a similar picture. Rare individuals with total IgA deficiency and complement-binding anti-IgA antibodies may suffer severe anaphylaxis if transfused with blood containing even minute amounts of IgA. The donor blood may be heavily contaminated with bacteria and cause severe endotoxic shock.

Symptoms are variable, but may include pain at the site of infusion, loin pain, dyspnoea and chest pain, rigors, nausea and vomiting, and collapse. In the unconscious or anaesthetized patient, hypotension or abnormal bleeding may be the only signs of this type of reaction.

- The transfusion must be stopped immediately and the unit of blood and attached giving set removed.
- Other units already cross-matched must not be used until it has been shown that it is safe to do so.
- The haematologist must be informed.
- Blood samples must be taken for testing as soon as possible from a vein other than that used for transfusion.

- Serological tests will include a direct antiglobulin test, repeat grouping of the patient and the donor unit, and repeat cross-match of all suspect units.
- Plasma and any urine passed subsequently should be examined for haemoglobin.
- In the absence of positive serological findings, bacteriological examination of the unit and giving set must be pursued.

The main complications of this type of reaction are renal failure and DIC. The latter is usually short-lived once the transfusion has been stopped. Treatment, if needed, is with FFP and platelet concentrates. Incipient renal failure should be anticipated, an IV injection of frusemide (furosemide), 80–120 mg, should be given in an attempt to provoke a diuresis, and fluid balance maintained with IV infusions if necessary. In the face of anuria or oliguria, the advice of a renal physician should be sought. Careful attention to fluid and electrolyte balance and treatment by diet, cation exchange resin or dialysis will be needed.

Moderate or minor reactions

Less severe reactions manifested as fever, chills, urticaria and other rashes occur quite often during transfusion. Red cell incompatibility is rarely implicated. Although leukocyte and platelet alloantibodies (usually HLA) are commonly found, their relevance to this type of reaction is not always clear and the immediate cause is often elusive.[5]

Treatment with antipyretics and antihistamines is usually effective and should be given prophylactically if further transfusions are needed. If symptoms persist, and particularly if leukocyte or platelet antibodies have been found, then leukocyte-poor blood should be tried.

Delayed reactions

Delayed transfusion reactions due to the production of red cell alloantibodies days or even weeks after transfusion may be recognized by an unaccountable fall in haemoglobin, the appearance of spherocytes in the blood film or mild, transient jaundice. In most cases, the event passes unnoticed. It is important to investigate suspected cases in anticipation of further transfusions and to assess the relevance of any antibodies to future pregnancies.

Infections transmitted by transfusion have been reviewed by Soulier.[6]

Paediatric practice

Major surgery or exchange transfusions in neonates and infants pose special problems because of the small blood volume and the nature of the procedure being undertaken. In general, the freshest blood available is used (< five days old) to avoid significant storage effects. The use of components such as FFP and platelet concentrates may also be required.

Sickle cell disease

Elective major surgery in homozygous (HbSS) patients with sickle cell disease is best done following a transfusion programme aimed at raising the proportion of HbA to about 60 per cent. In emergency, exchange transfusion may be indicated. With or without transfusion, extra care is needed in these cases to avoid hypoxia and acidosis (*see* p. 51).

In sickle trait (HbAS), attention to good oxygenation and hydration is usually all that is required unless procedures involving occlusion with tourniquets are involved when transfusion may be indicated. These and other sickle syndrome cases (e.g. HbSC, HbS-β-thalassaemia) should be discussed with the haematologist.

Autotransfusion

Some cardiothoracic units collect 500 ml citrated blood from patients shortly before going on bypass, for use in the immediate postoperative period as a source of fresh blood. Elective autologous transfusion may be essential in patients with rare alloantibodies to high frequency blood group antigens. In these cases, red cells may be accumulated over several weeks or months and stored frozen.

The salvaging of blood shed into the operation site for immediate return requires special equipment and is still largely experimental.[7]

References

1. Barbara, JAJ. *Microbiology in Blood Transfusion*. Bristol: Wright-PSG, 1983.
2. Moore, FD. Transcapillary refill, the unrepaired anaemia and clinical haemodilution. *Surg. Gynec. Obstet.* 1974; **56**: 521.
3. International forum: When is the microfiltration of whole blood and red cell concentrates essential? When is it superfluous? *Vox Sang.* 1986; **50**: 54.
4. International Forum. What is the clinical important of altera-

tions of the haemoglobin oxygen affinity in preserved blood? *Vox Sang*. 1978; **34**: 11.

5. Minchinton, RM, Waters, AH. The occurrence and significance of neutrophil antibodies. Annotation. *Brit. J. Haemat*. 1984; **56**: 521.

6. Soulier, JP. Diseases transmissible by blood transfusion. *Vox Sang*. 1984; **47**: 1.

7. Hauer, JM, Thurer, RL. Controversies in autotransfusion. *Vox Sang*. 1984; **46**: 8.

Further reading

Mollison, PL. *Blood Transfusion in Clinical Medicine, 7th ed*. Oxford: Blackwell Scientific Publications, 1983.

4

Blood Disorders

Elizabeth A. Caffrey and Nicholas I. Newton

Bleeding disorders
   Emergency tests for haemostatic disorders
   Replacement therapy for haemostatic disorders
   Anaesthetic considerations
   Selected disorders
Anaemias
   Anaesthetic considerations
   Selected anaemias
Polycythaemia

Bleeding disorders

Clinically significant bleeding disorders may be inherited or acquired. Successful management relies on correct interpretation of laboratory tests and the appropriate use of blood products.

Emergency tests for haemostatic disorders

- *Platelet count*: most modern methods use particle counters; results may be falsely low if the platelets are clumped or increased if red cell fragments are present.
- *The bleeding time* is a convenient test of platelet function, but is also likely to be abnormal if there is significant thrombocytopenia.
- *The partial thromboplastin time (PTT)/ Kaolin cephalin time (KCT)* measures the intrinsic and common pathways of coagulation. It is sensitive to reduced levels of all plasma factors except VII.
- *The prothrombin time (PT)* measures the extrinsic and common pathways of coagulation. It is sensitive to reduced levels of factors, V, VII, X, prothrombin and fibrinogen.
- *The thrombin time* measures the conversion of fibrinogen to

fibrin. It is prolonged by heparin, fibrin degradation products (FDP) and hypofibrinogenaemia.
- *Reptilase time.* Reptilase is a snake venom with thrombin-like activity. The reptilase time is prolonged by FDP but not by heparin.
- *Fibrinogen estimation.* The amount of fibrinogen in blood may be directly measured, or inferred from indirect observations (e.g. fibrinogen titre). The concentration may be reduced as a result of defective production (e.g. liver disease), increased consumption (e.g. intravascular coagulation), or increased destruction (lysis).

Replacement therapy for haemostatic disorders

- *Fresh frozen plasma* (FFP) contains all plasma clotting factors. It should be ABO compatible with the patient's red cells and is thawed immediately before use to retain maximum activity. Allergic reactions to plasma may occur, and are sometimes serious.
- *Cryoprecipitate*, the cryoprotein fraction of plasma, contains F VIII, fibrinogen and F XIII. It is thawed immediately before use.
- *Factor concentrates* are freeze-dried products prepared from fresh, pooled human plasma. They are stored at 4°C and reconstituted with water for injection. There is a high risk of transmission of hepatitis from their use, and a few cases of acquired immune deficiency syndrome (AIDS) have been associated with their administration to haemophiliacs: heat treatment is now being used to avert this hazard.

   Factor VIII concentrate is used for the treatment of haemophilia A, and F IX concentrate for the treatment of haemophilia B. Most preparations of F IX also contain F II, F X and some F VII.
- *Platelet concentrate* is prepared from small donor pools or single donors and has a relatively short shelf-life, at best several days. It should be kept at room temperature and be ABO compatible with the recipient's plasma.

Anaesthetic considerations

- Intramuscular injections may lead to extensive, potentially serious haematomata and should never be used.
- Regional nerve blocks should be avoided. Spinal and epidural blocks are absolutely contra-indicated.

- Intubation is only employed when essential; the nasal route is contra-indicated.
- Internal jugular vein cannulation carries the risk that inadvertent haematoma formation may cause tracheal compression.
- Care in handling the unconscious patient is important to prevent bruising and haemarthroses in haemophiliacs.

Selected disorders

Platelet abnormalities

Thrombocytopenia
Thrombocytopenia is the commonest cause of a haemorrhagic state. It may be due to deficient production (aplasia, cytotoxics), increased consumption (intravascular coagulation), immune destruction (drugs, idiopathic), massive transfusion or extracorporeal circulation.

Where possible correct the underlying cause before surgery. Replacement with platelet concentrate may be effective but the response is sometimes disappointing, especially when platelet antibodies are present. Platelets should be given during, rather than before surgery as their survival in the circulation may be short.

Qualitative platelet defects
Impaired platelet function may result from uraemia, extracorporeal circulation, paraproteinaemia and the effects of drugs (e.g. aspirin). Platelets with abnormal function are commonly found in myeloproliferative syndromes. Inherited abnormalities (e.g. Glanzmann's thrombasthenia) are rare.

Platelet transfusion may be necessary despite normal numbers, but isologous platelets may also become defective e.g. in uraemia, myeloma.

Inherited plasma abnormalities

Haemophilia A (Classical haemophilia)
This is the commonest inherited bleeding disorder. Most patients are male but F VIII levels in female carriers are sometimes low enough to cause a bleeding tendency. Thirty per cent have no family history, and mildly affected cases may be undiagnosed until major trauma or surgery.

The PTT is prolonged; PT and bleeding time are both normal. Severe cases with F VIII clotting activity $< 1\%$ (0.01 i.u./ml) usually have a characteristic history of spontaneous haemarthroses, deep haemorrhages and/or prolonged bleeding from even trivial wounds. Though functionally abnormal in clotting assays, the amount of factor VIII protein in plasma is usually normal when measured by immunological methods.

The clotting defect may be corrected by factor VIII concentrate or cryoprecipitate by IV injection. For major surgery the required dose depends on body weight and baseline F VIII level. Adequacy of dose is assessed by pre and post dose assays. The plasma half-life of F VIII is short (8 hr), so repeated injections are necessary to maintain haemostatic levels until healing occurs.

Antifibrinolytic therapy with tranexamic acid is contra-indicated if there is a possibility of internal bleeding or haematuria, but may be helpful in the management of dental haemorrhage or epistaxis.

Factor VIII inhibitors. Six per cent of haemophiliacs have circulating antibodies to F VIII. Test for inhibitors must be performed before operation, and if present, only life-saving surgery should be contemplated. Treatment is difficult; possibilities include massive doses of F VIII, porcine F VIII, prothrombin complex concentrates and plasma exchange.

Haemophilia B (Christmas disease)

This affects 15 per cent of all haemophiliacs. The haemostatic defect is due to deficiency of F IX, but the condition is clinically identical to haemophilia A.

Treatment is similar to haemophilia A, but using reconstituted F IX concentrate. Antibodies to F IX are rare.

Other factor deficiencies

Inherited deficiencies of each of the clotting factors have been reported. They are extremely rare, and are treated with specific concentrates or fresh plasma as necessary.

Von Willebrand's disease

This includes a number of syndromes with overlapping haematological features. Their inheritance is not sex linked. Clinical manifestations include a tendency to bruising, epistaxis, menorrhagia, GI bleeding and excessive blood loss after surgery or childbirth. Most patients are mildly affected and spontaneous haemarthroses and muscle haematomata are rare.

The bleeding time and PTT are prolonged due to a defect of platelet function and reduced F VIII clotting activity. F VIII protein is also reduced, in contrast to haemophilia A in which it is qualitatively rather than quantitatively abnormal.

In an emergency the haemostatic defects may be corrected by plasma or cryoprecipitate. Their administration causes an initial rise in plasma F VIII and stimulates a temporary increase in the production of this protein over the following 24 hr. If only super-ficial bleeding is anticipated antifibrinolytic drugs may be helpful.

Acquired plasma abnormalities

Liver disease

All coagulation factors with the possible exception of F VIII are synthesized in the liver. Prolongation of clotting tests may be an early indication of hepatocellular damage. In obstructive jaundice failure to absorb vitamin K results in reduced levels of factors II, VII, IX and X.

In severe liver disease, quantitative and qualitative abnormali-ties of clotting factor synthesis, intravascular coagulation, the anticoagulant effects of FDP and thrombocytopenia may all con-tribute to the haemostatic disorder.

Treatment depends upon the correction of the underlying patho-logy. The administration of vitamin K, FFP and/or platelets may be necessary if bleeding occurs or is anticipated.

Oral anticoagulants

The vitamin K antagonists interfere with the hepatic synthesis of factors II, VII, IX and X. The plasma levels of these proteins fall, and abnormal molecules which lack coagulant activity are produced.

Warfarin causes few adverse reactions and is the drug of choice. Because of the long half-life of some of the vitamin K dependent factors adequate anticoagulation takes two to three days to achieve. Plasma clotting factors return to normal within a few days of stopping treatment.

Treatment is monitored by the PT; the therapeutic range is 2–4½ times the normal control using reagents which conform to British or International standards. For minor surgery/dental extractions ensure PT is less than 2½ times the normal control.

For major surgery reverse the warfarin effect and consider pro-phylactic heparin for the peri-operative period.

Warfarin may be reversed by fresh plasma which has an imme-diate but short lived effect. Vitamin K reverses the clotting defect but its maximum effect is delayed (c12 hr). Use small doses (up to 2 mg) if the anticoagulant is to be continued. Gross overdosage (attempted suicide) may require large doses of vitamin K.

Heparin

This rapidly activates antithrombin III, a natural anticoagulant. It has an anti F Xa effect which is the basis of its use in low dose pro-phylaxis. Larger doses cause neutralization of thrombin, thereby preventing the conversion of fibrinogen to fibrin and inhibiting thrombus formation.

For prophylaxis give 5000 i.u. SC every 8–12 hr. This dose does not usually prolong routine clotting tests.

Full anticoagulation may need doses of the order of 40 000 i.u./24 hr. Continuous IV infusion is the recommended method of administration. Treatment is monitored by the PTT which should be kept within 1½–2½ times the normal control.

Since the half-life of heparin is short (1½ hr), stopping treatment may be adequate for overdose. For immediate reversal protamine sulphate is effective, but in excess has anticoagulant properties.

Disseminated intravascular coagulation (DIC)

Increased consumption of platelets and plasma clotting factors with intravascular deposition of thrombi may occur from many causes; e.g. amniotic fluid embolism, Gram-negative septicaemia, major trauma and disseminated malignancy. There may be an enhanced fibrinolytic response leading to formation of FDPs, some of which have anticoagulant properties.

In acute disseminated intravascular coagulation there may be overt bleeding even from venepuncture sites. Screening tests of haemostasis are all abnormal and the platelet count is low. The blood may be incoagulable due to complete defibrination.

In chronic forms the levels of plasma clotting factors may be normal or raised due to a compensatory increase in production.

Treatment is the correction of the underlying cause. Blood, fresh plasma and platelets may be needed to correct life threatening haemostatic defects.

The place of heparin in the treatment of DIC remains controversial.

Anaemias

Anaesthetic considerations

Oxygen delivery to the tissues depends upon the haemoglobin level, its percentage saturation and the cardiac output.

The lowest acceptable haemoglobin level for anaesthesia is determined by the patient's age, co-existing heart or respiratory disease and by the urgency of the surgery.

Haemoglobin levels above 9–10 g/dl normally carry minimal risk (with the exception of B_{12} or folate deficiency, *see* p. 53).

In patients with haemoglobin levels below 8–9 g/dl the cardiac output rises and the oxygen dissociation curve is shifted to the right. Many patients with chronic anaemias, e.g. renal failure, are safely anaesthetized with values of 6–8 g/dl when the following measures are adopted.

- Pre-oxygenation prior to induction of anaesthesia.
- High inspired oxygen concentration throughout.
- Respiratory and cardiovascular depression are avoided.
- Complete reversal of neuromuscular blockade at the end of surgery.
- Minimal use of intravenous opiates and inhalational anaesthetic agents to avoid prolonged recovery.
- Administration of oxygen postoperatively.

Selected anaemias

Abnormal haemoglobins

There are many inherited qualitative defects of globin structure. The majority are benign. Common haemoglobins likely to cause clinical problems are haemoglobins S and C. Both are predominantly seen in subjects of African extraction. The gene for HbS is also present in high frequency in some Arab populations.

Simple haemoglobin traits (HbAS or HbAC)
Subjects are heterozygous for HbA and either HbS or HbC. There is no anaemia and no clinical consequence. Individuals with HbS trait (HbAS) do not sickle under normal physiological conditions. Well conducted anaesthesia carries no greater risk for these patients than normal; adequate hydration must be ensured.

Homozygous states
- *Sickle cell anaemia (HbSS).* There is a severe lifelong haemolytic anaemia (6–9 g/dl). Patients suffer from recurrent, painful crises due to infarction of bones and viscera. Symptoms may mimic the 'acute abdomen'. Crises are often precipitated by infection, exercise or pregnancy. Skeletal and sexual development are delayed. The enlarged spleen atrophies during childhood due to repeated infarction. There is an increased susceptibility to infection.
- *HbC disease (HbCC).* There is a mild haemolytic anaemia with no distinctive symptoms. (Sickling does not occur.)

Compound haemoglobinopathy
1. *HbSC disease (HbS plus HbC).* This condition is of variable severity. The diagnosis is easily overlooked because patients

are often not anaemic; growth and development are normal. However, painful sickling crises do occur, especially during surgery and pregnancy.

2. *HbS/thalassaemia (HbS plus thalassaemia)*. Severe forms are similar to sickle cell anaemia and are difficult to distinguish from it both clinically and haematologically. In other cases the condition is milder and may be almost symptom free.

Diagnosis
In all states where HbS is present the solubility (screening) test is positive. It is quick and reliable in an emergency. Precise diagnosis requires detailed haemoglobin typing and, in some cases, family studies.

If there is significant anaemia and/or marked red cell morphological abnormalities, assume the patient has a major sickling disorder until proved otherwise.

If the blood count and film appearances are normal it is likely that the patient has the simple trait. (At least eight per cent of the patients of African origin in UK and USA carry the gene for HbS).

Treatment
Painful vaso-occlusive crises need prompt rehydration, adequate analgesia and antibiotics, if appropriate. Transfusion may be necessary in severe cases if symptoms persist and major organ damage is suspected.

Blood transfusion reduces the percentage of HbS-containing cells by dilution and temporarily suppresses their production. Oxygen delivery to the tissues is improved and the deoxygenated blood is less viscous. Planned transfusion before surgery and during pregnancy significantly reduces the risk of sickling. Patients with SC disease or S/thalassaemia, who are not anaemic, need partial exchange transfusion.

Anaesthetic considerations
Patients with sickle cell diseases are at particular risk both during anaesthesia and in the postoperative period.

The following measures reduce the incidence of severe sickling crises:

- Pre-operative transfusion is of prime importance.
- Maintenance of a high inspired oxygen concentration, with intubation to avoid respiratory obstruction.
- Prevention of hypotension, vasoconstriction and dehydration.
- A warming coil for IV fluids, and warming mattress should be employed.
- Tourniquets must not be used.

- Postoperative ventilation is beneficial following prolonged surgery.
- Prophylactic antibiotic therapy and chest physiotherapy are important postoperatively.

Thalassaemias

A group of disorders in which there is deficient production of either α- or β-globin chains. It is widespread throughout the Mediterranean, Middle East and Asia.

Beta thalassaemia major
A profound anaemia develops in the first year of life (3–6 g/dl). There is gross hepatosplenomegaly. Characteristic bony deformities develop due to massive marrow expansion e.g. frontal bossing, prognathous jaw. Fractures may follow minor trauma. Organ and endocrine failure occurs with advancing age due to haemosiderosis. Death occurs in the second decade, usually from cardiac complications.

HbH disease
There is a significant deficiency of alpha chains. The excess beta chains form tetramers (HbH). Clinical features vary from little disability to those of beta thalassaemia major. Anaemia is moderately severe (7–10 g/dl). Approximately 20 per cent of the haemoglobin is HbH. Its oxygen affinity is 10-times that of HbA, as a result oxygen delivery in the tissues is impaired.

Thalassaemia minor (α- or β-thalassaemia trait)
These are benign conditions. Anaemia, if present, is mild. They are sometimes mistaken for iron deficiency. Iron supplements cannot improve the haemoglobin level and are contra-indicated.

Diagnosis
The red cells are hypochromic (low MCH) and microcytic (low MCV). Precise diagnosis is by haemoglobin studies. In contrast to iron deficiency, the serum iron levels are normal or raised.

Glucose-6-phosphate dehydrogenase deficiency

More than 70 variants of this enzyme are described; many are entirely benign. Clinical manifestations are variable and depend on enzyme type:

Neonatal jaundice (G6PD Canton)
Favism (G6PD Mediterranean)
Drug sensitivity (G6PD A⁻). This variant is commonly found
in subjects of African extraction.

Haemolysis is provoked both by infection and by many substances including sulphonamides, nitrofurantoin and some anti-
malarials. Common anaesthetic drugs are not known to precipitate
an attack. There is a theoretical risk with the use of prilocaine.

Because the gene for this enzyme is sex linked, most patients
with clinical deficiency are male. In spite of the high frequency of
enzyme defect, remarkably few problems occur in practice if
known precipitants of haemolysis are avoided.

Iron deficiency

Anaemia caused by iron lack is usually due to chronic blood loss
e.g. peptic ulcer, menorrhagia. The red cells are hypochromic and
microcytic. If there is substantial recent bleeding, platelet and
white cell counts may also be elevated. In an emergency, blood
transfusion may be necessary. When bleeding has ceased oral iron
corrects the anaemia by 1 g/week.

Hereditary haemorrhagic telangiectasia is a rare cause of
chronic bleeding. Characteristic lesions in the mouth may complicate intubation.

Similar red cell indices in thalassaemia minor may be misinter-
preted as iron deficiency.

Vitamin B₁₂ or folate deficiency

Deficiency of either vitamin causes a macrocytic anaemia (high
MCV). The marrow is megaloblastic. In severe cases platelet and
white cell counts are low.

Patients are often in incipient cardiac failure; transfusion
should be avoided whenever possible.

Lack of these co-enzymes affects metabolism in all tissues; drugs
which modify cardiac function may precipitate severe cardiac
arrhythmias.

Surgery should be postponed, at least until appropriate replacement therapy has begun, even if the anaemia is slight.

Pancytopenia

Anaemia is complicated by thrombocytopenia and leucopenia.
Excessive bleeding and/or infection may complicate surgery.

Causes include:

- lymphoma or leukaemia
- aplasia, idiopathic or drug induced
- severe B_{12} or folate deficiency
- secondary tumour. Red and white cell precursors in the peripheral blood are often indicative of metastatic marrow deposits (leucoerythroblastic change).

Polycythaemia

Spuriously high haemoglobin levels occur in dehydration e.g. excessive use of diuretics.

In *true* polycythaemia the total red cell mass is increased. It is usually secondary to chronic hypoxia associated with cardiopulmonary disease. Treatment is that of the underlying cause.

Polycythaemia rubra vera is a primary myeloproliferative disorder in which there is inappropriate excessive production of *all* marrow elements. Platelet and white cell counts are elevated. Haemorrhagic as well as thrombotic complications are common; surgery should be avoided in untreated individuals. If time allows, normal haematological values are restored using alkylating agents or radioactive phosphorus. In an emergency, venesection will reduce the red cell mass but does not correct the thrombocytosis.

Further reading

Aldrete JA, Guerra F. Hematologic diseases. In: Katz J, Benumof J, Kadis LB (eds) *Anesthesia and Uncommon Diseases: Pathophysiologic and clinical correlations, 2nd ed*. Philadelphia; W B Saunders, 1981: 313–83.

Chanarin I, Brozović M, Tidmarsh E, Waters DAW. *Blood and its Diseases, 2nd ed*. Edinburgh; Churchill Livingstone, 1980.

5

Intravenous Fluids

Anthony P Adams and Penelope B Hewitt

Crystalloids
    Water depletion
    Salt depletion
    Potassium
    Water excess
Special solutions
    Mannitol
Colloids
    Plasma expanders and substitutes
    Human plasma derivatives
Artificial blood substitutes

Patients presenting for emergency anaesthesia and surgery will usually require intravenous fluid therapy. The choice of an appropriate fluid regimen will depend on the clinical status of the patient. This may range from a minimal disturbance to a severe water, electrolyte and acid–base abnormality related to the surgical pathology. In turn this may be complicated by an underlying therapy (e.g. diuretics) or disease (e.g. chronic obstructive airway disease). A thorough history and careful clinical examination will give the basic (and best) assessment of the fluid and electrolyte status, and this should be confirmed by plasma and urine biochemical measurements. The assessment and correction of these disturbances before surgery is essential to ensure maximum benefit to the patient.

In this chapter we are not concerned with blood, blood products (*see* Chapter 3) or intravenous nutrition but with 'clear fluids': crystalloids and colloids.

Crystalloids

Crystalloids are solutions of electrolytes and/or dextrose in water which in general are rapidly redistributed throughout the extra-cellular fluid (ECF) and intracellular fluid (ICF) and are then rapidly excreted. The colloids, on the other hand, because of their structure, tend to stay longer in the intravascular compartment before being excreted, and so support the circulation for longer.

Patients with minimal fluid disturbance will require only maintenance volumes of fluids and electrolytes, these may be calculated as follows:

Water: 24-hr requirement:
100 ml/kg for 1st 10 kg
50 ml/kg for 2nd 10 kg
25 ml/kg for all subsequent kg
e.g. 80 kg man requires:

1000 ml	(100×10)
500 ml	(50×10)
1500 ml	(25×60)
3000 ml	

Sodium: 24-hr requirement:
2–3 mmol/kg
Potassium: 24-hr requirement:
0.5–1.0 mmol/kg

Patients with more severe disturbances will require more drastic treatment.

Water depletion

This is almost always caused by a failure of water intake. Water is lost from the ECF causing an increase in osmolality, which in turn draws water from the cells producing an intracellular dehydration with a relatively small reduction in the extracellular volume. Thirst is intense but blood pressure is well maintained until relatively late; urine output falls, the serum urea rises early as do most of the serum electrolyte values. This is a prerenal renal failure. The treatment is water replacement by mouth, or intravenously with a dextrose solution.

Salt depletion

This condition is usually due to excessive losses from the intestine (vomiting, diarrhoea, obstruction), from the kidneys (diabetic ketosis) or from the circulation (haemorrhage, burns). It is clearly associated with water deficiency. There is an increasing reduction in plasma volume and the symptoms and signs depend entirely on the severity, ranging from mild thirst to complete circulatory collapse. The treatment is to replace both salt and water at the appropriate rate: the faster the loss the faster the replacement. Care must be taken to avoid overload of the circulation. Auscultation of the chest, measurement of the central venous pressure, or in severe cardiovascular disease, measurement of the pulmonary wedge pressure is necessary.

Potassium

Depletion

This usually occurs as a result of excessive loss through the kidneys or the intestinal tract aggravated by inadequate replacement. Hypokalaemia has a profound effect on smooth muscle in general and on the myocardium in particular, producing arrhythmias, hypotension, and the possibility of cardiac arrest in diastole. The ECG shows lowering of the T waves; tall U waves may be seen. At very low serum potassium levels (<3 mmol/litre) ST segments are depressed. Supraventricular ectopic rhythms are common. It is essential that hypokalaemia is treated prior to surgery. The simplest and fastest method is via the IV route at a rate that should not exceed 20 mmol/hr unless the ECG is monitored (*see* p. 84). Serum potassium measurements should also be made.

Excess

This is almost always due to a failure to excrete potassium ions. If unrelieved, hyperkalaemia usually causes death in cardiac asystole but ventricular fibrillation occurs occasionally. Hyperkalaemia is usually associated with metabolic acidosis. The ECG changes seen are narrow, peaked T waves and a reduction in the QT interval. Intraventricular conduction disturbances occur followed by prolongation of the PR interval and eventually by loss of the P waves and development of a slow idioventricular rhythm.

- Treatment is urgent. If the cause is prerenal failure then a diuresis should be induced by IV fluids (5 per cent dextrose). If the cause is renal or postrenal then the following regimen should be instituted: 20 ml of 10 per cent calcium gluconate (5 mmol Ca^{2+}; *see* p. 20) (to protect the heart from arrhythmias). Sodium bicarbonate 8.4 per cent IV using ECG monitoring until T waves return to normal.

Alternatively, 50 g glucose and 20 i.u. insulin can be given by a single IV bolus, followed by 20 g glucose (50 per cent solution) and

5–20 i.u. insulin hourly by infusion according to blood glucose levels. This produces a shift of glucose from extracellular to intracellular compartments taking potassium ions with it. Thus, the extracellular concentration of potassium ions is lowered and the dangerous effects on the myocardium reduced. More long-term management includes ion exchange resins, dialysis or the surgical relief of urinary tract obstruction.

Table 5.1   Electrolyte content of crystalloid solutions

| | Millimoles/litre | | | | |
	Na^+	K^+	HCO_3^-	Cl^-	Ca^{2+}
Mean normal plasma values (approx)	142	4.5	26	103	2.5
Sodium chloride 0.9% (isotonic saline)	150	—	—	150	—
Compound sodium lactate (Hartmann's)	131	5	29	111	2
Sodium chloride 0.18% and glucose 4.3%	30	—	—	30	—
Potassium chloride and glucose	—	40	—	40	—
Potassium chloride and sodium chloride	150	40	—	190	—
Sodium bicarbonate 1.4% (0.17 mmol/ml)	167	—	167	—	—
Sodium bicarbonate 8.4% (1 mmol/ml)	1000	—	1000	—	—
Sodium lactate M/6	167	—	167	—	—
Ammonium chloride M/6	—	—	—	167	—
Sodium chloride 1.8% (hypertonic)	300	—	—	300	—
Dextrose 5% or 10%; Mannitol 10%, 15%, 20%, 25%.	—	—	—	—	—

Water excess

This is nearly always iatrogenic usually following large intakes of non-electrolyte fluid or excessive water absorption during bladder irrigation. There is a profound decrease in osmolality in the ECF, which leads to intracellular oedema accounting for the symptoms of:

- confusion
- headaches
- cerebral oedema
- convulsions
- coma

Treatment is to give hypertonic saline (1.8 per cent NaCl) and if necessary a diuretic. 'At risk' patients should be carefully monitored to avoid circulatory overload (*see* p. 82).

Special solutions

Mannitol

Mannitol is a sugar (and a crystalloid) usually available as a 10 or 20 per cent solution. It is used principally in the treatment of cerebral oedema (*see* p. 136). Mannitol is hypertonic and therefore acts transiently as a plasma expander. The solution is irritant should extravasation occur. Mannitol must always be used with extreme care: the main disadvantages are the risk of producing a subdural haemorrhage (as the brain shrinks) and the occurrence of a 'rebound' rise in intracranial pressure because some of the drug penetrates the brain eventually.

Mannitol is also a powerful osmotic diuretic because of decreased salt absorption from the loop of Henle. However, there are other safer agents which can be used to promote diuresis.

Colloids

Plasma expanders and substitutes

The dextrans

These are polysaccharides of average MW of either 40 000, 70 000 or 110 000 and are commonly referred to as dextran 40, 70 or 110 (Table 5.2). The greater the average MW the longer the dextran remains in the circulation (Figure 5.1).

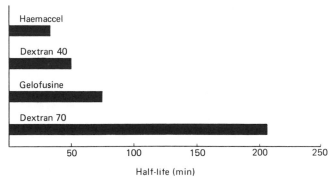

Fig. 5.1 Relative duration of action of colloids.

These dextrans are prepared in either 5 per cent dextrose or saline and are hypertonic with respect to plasma; solutions in dextrose may be preferred because of their low sodium content. Not only do dextran solutions increase the circulating volume by virtue of the volume infused, but their hypertonicity draws fluid into the vascular compartment from the cells, almost doubling the expansion effect of the infusion. The dextrans also reduce red blood cell adhesiveness and so prevent agglutination.

Indications

- Treatment of hypovolaemia
- Normovolaemic haemodilution for certain major surgical emergencies
- Prevention of thrombo-embolic complications

Table 5.2   The dextran preparations
Care must be taken in patients vulnerable to vascular overloading, e.g. congestive heart failure, renal failure. Contra-indications: patients with severe bleeding tendency.

Preparation		Dextran concentration (g/litre)	NaCl (g/litre)	Dextrose (g/litre)
Dextran 40	10% in dextrose 5%	100	—	50
(Rheomacrodex; Lomodex)	10% in saline	100	9	—

Correct dehydration before giving dextran 40. Adults: reduced capillary circulation in shock, 500–1000 ml IV over 30–60 min, plus a further 500 ml the same day; thereafter 500 ml/day for up to five days. Do not use in patients with renal failure with blood urea levels > 10 mmol/litre (60 mg/100 ml), or whose urine output cannot be maintained > 1500 ml/day.

Dextran 70	6% in dextrose 5%	60	—	50
(Macrodex)	6% in saline	60	9	—

In hypovolaemic shock 500–1000 ml may be given initially at a rate depending on the patient's needs. Thereafter given equal volumes of dextran 70 and blood. Total dose not to exceed 2500 ml in adults.

Dextran 110	6% in saline	60	9	—
(Dextraven 110)				

In moderate blood loss 500 ml may be infused in 15 min; a further 500 ml more slowly (30–45 min). In severe haemorrhage, 1 litre infused rapidly and a further 500 ml more slowly may be given.

Complications

Allergic reactions may rarely occur (e.g. spontaneous hypersensitivity reactions: rigors, flushing – occasionally with asthma and hypotension, urticaria, erythema). The patient should be closely observed for signs of untoward effects especially within a few minutes of starting the infusion.

Difficulties with cross-matching blood for transfusion

- Always take blood for this purpose before infusing dextran.

Gelatin derivatives

Gelofusine, and polygeline (Haemaccel) are commonly used and contain no preservatives (Table 5.3). They have an average MW of 30 000–35 000 and thus their duration of action is shorter than the dextrans. As with the dextrans the plasma expansion exceeds the infused volume. Both these gelatins have a shelf-life of eight years at room temperature (five years in the tropics) which makes them useful in difficult situations (*see* p. 236).

Complications

These are extremely rare; very rapid infusion of gelatins (especially to normovolaemic patients) may be associated with release of vasoactive substances. The gelatins should not be used to prevent falls in arterial pressure consequent upon spinal or epidural anaesthesia. The exact mechanism of such histamine release has not been determined. Histamine release may be especially hazardous in patients with known allergic conditions e.g. asthma.

Not more than 1.5 litres of gelatin should be given to an adult (30 ml/kg in children) unless blood is unavailable.

Hydroxyethyl starch (HES)

This is a starch based compound with a haemodynamic action similar to dextran 70. The interesting difference is that while small molecules are excreted through the kidneys, the larger ones are gradually degraded and taken up by the reticulo-endothelial system. Hydroxyethyl starch provides rapid volume expansion lasting 24 hr or longer and maintains a plasma oncotic pressure similar to human albumin solution (*see* p. 35) remaining in the vasculature and minimizing the risk of pulmonary oedema.

Complications

There is a low incidence of allergic reactions and minimal effects on coagulation and on cross-matching of blood.

Table 5.3 The modified gelatin derivatives

	Modified gelatin concentration (g/litre)	Average MW	Colloid osmotic pressure (@ 37°C) mm H_2O	Na$^+$ mmol/l	K$^+$ mmol/l	Ca^{2+} mmol/l	Cl$^-$ mmol/l
Gelofusine 4% colloidal solution	40	30 000	465	154	0.4	0.4	125
Polygeline (Haemaccel) 3.5% colloidal solution	35	35 000	350–390	145	5.1	6.25	145

Human plasma derivatives (*see* p. 34)

Artificial blood substitutes

The fluorocarbons

Fluorocarbons, usually as an emulsion with surfactant and electrolytes, have the ability to bind oxygen and carbon dioxide reversibly. These products are still experimental.

Further reading

Doenicke A, Grote B, Lorenz W. Blood and blood substitutes. *Br. J. Anaesth.* 1977; **49**: 681–8.

Marshall M, Bird T. *Blood Loss and Replacement.* London: Edward Arnold, 1983.

Twigley AJ, Hillman KM. The end of the crystalloid era? A new approach to peri-operative fluid administration. *Anaesthesia* 1985; **40**: 860–71.

Willatts SM. *Lecture Notes on Fluid and Electrolyte Balance, 2nd ed.* Oxford: Blackwell, 1986.

6

Practical Procedures

John S Paddle and Michael B Barnett

Central venous cannulation
  Purpose
  Choice of technique
  Choice of cannula
  Positioning
  Preparation
  Techniques
  Difficulties
  Multiple cannulation
Percutaneous arterial cannulation
  Purpose
  Sites
  Collateral circulation in the hand and foot
  Choice of cannula
  Preparation
  Technique
  Difficulties
Insertion of a pleural drain
  Purpose
  Site of drain
  Choice of drain
  Technique
Cricothyroidotomy
  Purpose
  Equipment
  Technique
Difficult intubation
  Intubation under direct vision
  Blind nasal intubation under general anaesthesia
  Blind nasal intubation under local anaesthesia
  Retrograde intubation

Central venous cannulation

Purpose

Emergency cannulation of a central vein is needed for measurement of right atrial pressure, for the administration of certain drugs and to provide intravenous access when peripheral venous cannulation is not possible. Less common emergency uses include the insertion of a pulmonary artery catheter, the insertion of a temporary transvenous cardiac pacemaker and the aspiration of an air embolus.

Choice of technique

Several different techniques for cannulation have been described,[1] although many are very similar. Consistent successful cannulation and a low incidence of complications is best achieved by becoming familiar with one or two techniques. Although cannulation of a central vein may be achieved from the femoral vein or the basilic vein, it is generally easier and more reliable using the internal jugular or subclavian vein. The safest technique is probably via the right internal jugular vein.

Choice of cannula

There are many suitable varieties of cannula available. The final choice of length and diameter will depend on the size of the patient, the purpose for which the cannula is required and the technique chosen. Some commonly used sizes are listed below according to the age of the patient. It is of course better to use too long a cannula and not insert it completely than be left with only the tip of a short cannula in a vein.

Cannula for direct insertion

	Gauge	Length
Adults	14–16 G	12–14 cm
Children	16–18 G	5–14 cm
Neonates	20–22 G	5 cm

Catheter over guidewire devices (Seldinger method)

Although very large diameter catheters can be inserted either surgically or by techniques that progressively dilate the site of venous access to the size required, for general use the size of catheter that can be introduced by this method is limited to the size of needle that can easily be inserted first.

	Needle gauge and catheter gauge	Catheter length
Adults	14–16 G	15–20 cm
Children	16–18 G	10–15 cm
Neonates	20–22 G	5–10 cm

Positioning

Care and time must be spent in appropriate positioning of the patient. Lack of success in cannulation is often related to hasty attempts made with a badly positioned patient.

The position for *internal jugular vein cannulation* (upper and posterior approaches) is the same.

- The patient lies supine.
- Any head pillow is removed and for children and neonates a support is placed under the shoulders so as to extend the neck.
- The head is rotated to the contralateral side.
- In adults the use of some head-down tilt and in children and neonates the application of firm pressure on the liver by an assistant will help to raise the pressure in, and therefore the diameter of, the veins in the neck.

The position for *subclavian vein cannulation* is slightly different.

- The patient lies supine.
- Place a support between the shoulders so as to drop the right shoulder.
- A pillow may be placed under the patient's head.

Preparation

Appropriate skin preparation and towelling should be undertaken. Gloves should be worn. Intradermal and subcutaneous local anaesthetics should be used for conscious patients. Some children may also require heavy sedation in order to ensure they lie still enough. Attempts at cannulation in a restless child are dangerous.

Techniques

The internal jugular vein (upper approach)

Palpate, if possible, but do not retract, the carotid artery. Insert the cannula and needle at a point midway between the tip of the mastoid process and the sternoclavicular joint. Advance caudally keeping lateral to the carotid artery and posteriorly at about 30° to the coronal plane. When the internal jugular vein has been punctured, further advance the cannula over the needle (Fig. 6.1).

The junction of the internal jugular vein with the subclavian vein (posterior approach)

This approach is useful where the carotid artery is difficult to palpate, or in short or bull-necked individuals. The point of entry is 2–3 cm above the midpoint of the clavicle. Avoiding the external jugular vein, the cannula and needle are advanced *anteriorly* towards the ipsilateral sternoclavicular joint until the vein is punctured. Advance the cannula over the needle, do not advance the needle beyond this point. Remember that it is better to aim too anteriorly and to hit bone than to aim too posteriorly and risk arterial puncture; pneumothorax is also a risk.

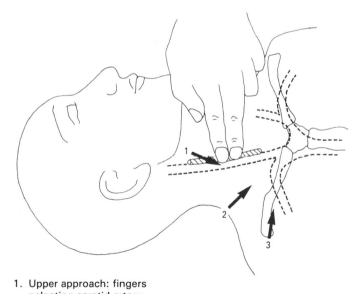

1. Upper approach: fingers
   palpating carotid artery
2. Posterior approach
3. Infraclavicular approach

Fig. 6.1 Cannulation of the internal jugular and subclavian veins.

The right subclavian vein

Insert the needle and cannula at a point immediately below the junction of the lateral and middle-thirds of the clavicle. Direct the needle and cannula *under* the clavicle towards the suprasternal notch but not beyond it. When the vein is identified by aspiration of blood advance the cannula over the needle into the vein.

Difficulties

Two main difficulties may be encountered. Firstly a vein may not be punctured and secondly, following successful puncture of a vein, there may be difficulty in advancing the cannula into the vein. Some hints are offered for overcoming these problems.

Failure to puncture a vein

- Review the positioning of the patient and the identification of the landmarks.
- Withdraw the cannula and needle *to the skin* in the *same line as the first attempt* and then make a small change in the angle of approach for the next attempt.
- Check that the cannula and needle are still patent.
- Finally try a different technique.

Failure to cannulate after successful puncture

- With the needle tip still in the vein, alter the angle of the needle and cannula.
- Rotate the needle in the vein.
- Repuncture the vein at a slightly different point.
- Try to thread a wire down the needle, then remove the needle and pass a cannula over the wire into the vein (Seldinger method).

Difficulties in cannulating the right subclavian vein

- If the needle and cannula strike the first rib and will not pass between it and the clavicle then try a more lateral point of entry under the clavicle.
- If the vein cannot be identified then try a more medial point of entry under the clavicle. Remember that as the needle and cannula pass under the clavicle, their direction towards the suprasternal notch must be constantly maintained.

Multiple cannulation

If multiple central venous cannulae are required then consider the use of a double or triple lumen catheter. Alternatively the same vein may be cannulated more than once.

Double cannulation of the same vein

Keep the first cannula and needle in the vein. Advance the second cannula and needle underneath the first, in the *same line* and with the bevel of the second needle facing the first cannula. Failure to advance in the same line or to hold the bevel facing the first cannula may easily lead to damage of the first cannula. It is a useful technique but must be undertaken with great care.

Percutaneous arterial cannulation

Purpose

Arterial cannulation provides a direct and continuous means of recording arterial pressure for use during surgery when heavy blood loss may occur or when hypotensive anaesthetic techniques are to be used. It also provides access for arterial sampling.

Sites

- Radial artery
- Ulnar artery
- Brachial artery
- Dorsalis pedis artery
- Femoral artery

Collateral circulation in the hand and foot

The collateral circulation in a well perfused hand or foot virtually ensures that the presence of a cannula in the radial, ulnar or dorsalis pedis is unlikely to jeopardize the distal circulation. Where perfusion is poor, the collateral circulation of the hand may be tested by a modified Allen's test. Ask the patient to clench his fist and hold his hand up. Occlude the radial and ulnar arteries and ask the patient to extend his fingers. Release the pressure over the *ulnar* artery. Immediate flushing of the hand confirms the patency of the ulnar–radial collateral circulation. In an unconscious patient, elevate the hand and exsanguinate the forearm and hand using an Esmark bandage before proceeding to occlude the radial and ulnar arteries.

Choice of cannula

Adult – 20 G Teflon e.g. 32 mm or 2 inch Abbocath.
Child – 22 G Teflon e.g. 32 mm Abbocath.
Neonate – 22 G Teflon e.g. 32 mm Abbocath.
Neonate – 22 G polypropylene e.g. 1 inch Medicut.
Neonate – 24 G Teflon e.g. 19 mm Jelco.
Guide wire e.g. Vygon Leadercath 0.5 mm external diameter for use with 20 G and 22 G cannulae.

Preparation

For the radial or ulnar artery, place the supinated arm on a board with a gauze roll under the wrist. Tape the extended fingers and abducted thumb to the board. Clean the skin with chlorhexidine in spirit.

Technique

- Palpate the radial or ulnar artery.
- If the patient is conscious, infiltrate the skin with local anaesthetic just distal to the intended point of entry of the artery.
- Make a small transverse skin incision with the point of a scalpel blade.
- Insert the cannula at an angle of 30° or less to the forearm and enter the artery by either:
    Direct cannulation, as the arterial blood fills the hub, gently advance the cannula over the needle, or
    Transfixion through the posterior wall of the artery. Withdraw the cannula and arterial blood will fill the hub when the tip lies within the lumen. Now slide the cannula over the needle.
- Connect the cannula to a previously prepared system for providing an intermittent or continuous flush of heparinized saline. All connections in the system should incorporate a Luer lock. Disconnection of an arterial line may rapidly lead to disastrous effects.

Difficulties

- Although blood may appear in the hub, the cannula may impinge on the vessel wall and refuse to slide over the needle into the vessel lumen. Reinsert the needle, transfix the posterior wall, remove the needle and slowly withdraw the cannula until arterial blood pulses back and then gently attempt to slide the cannula up.

- If this fails, try threading a Seldinger wire through the needle, then remove the needle and feed a cannula over the wire into the artery.
- If a haematoma appears, withdraw the cannula, compress the site for at least 5 min and use an alternative artery.
- A low blood pressure may make both palpation and cannulation of arteries difficult. Therefore consider appropriate measures for raising the blood pressure.
- If percutaneous cannulation is not possible consider a formal surgical approach to the artery.

Insertion of a pleural drain

Purpose

Emergency drainage of the pleural space is usually required to remove blood or air. It may also be necessary for the removal of effusions, pus, chyle or oesophageal contents.

Site of drain

Although the emergency drainage of a pneumothorax may be achieved through the second intercostal space in the midclavicular line, the best place to insert a pleural drain is through the fourth intercostal space in the midaxillary line.[2] This is generally the safest, most comfortable and most effective site.

If there are adhesions between the pleural layers, or the chest has recently been surgically explored or normal anatomy has been distorted by trauma then the choice of site for a pleural drain should be made on the basis of a careful clinical examination, good quality radiographs and needle aspiration.

Choice of drain

The drain should be as wide as can easily be inserted particularly for the removal of fluid or blood. A trocar is required for the insertion of the drain and the most commonly used drain is supplied with its own indwelling trocar e.g. Argyle pattern. A 12 or 14 G intravenous cannula may be used to achieve temporary drainage of a pneumothorax.

Technique

- Prepare the skin with an antiseptic and drape with sterile towels.
- Infiltrate the layers of the chest wall through to the pleura with 15–20 ml of 1 per cent lignocaine (lidocaine).
- Incise the skin widely enough to accommodate the drain.
- Place one securing suture for the drain and a second suture to close the drainage site when the drain is eventually removed.
- Deepen the incision towards but not as far as the pleura.
- Insert the blunt point of a pair of forceps (e.g. Spencer Wells) and spread the tissues and create a passage through into the pleural space large enough to accommodate the drain.
- To prevent a sudden overshoot of the trocar, clamp the tube and trocar with a pair of forceps at a distance from the tip equal to a little more than the estimated distance from skin to pleura.
- Insert the tube and trocar, remove the pair of forceps and advance the tube over the trocar towards the apex for removal of air and towards the most dependent part of the pleural space for removal of blood or fluid.
- Remove the trocar, temporarily clamp the tube and tie the tube to the chest wall using the suture placed there earlier.
- Connect the tube to an underwater seal and tape the tube securely to the chest wall.
- Check that air, blood or fluid drains freely and that the water column in the underwater seal system oscillates with respiration.
- Finally check the position of the drain with a radiograph.

Cricothyroidotomy

Purpose

Cricothyroidotomy is undertaken for the relief of upper airway obstruction at or above the level of the larynx when attempts at removal of the cause of the obstruction and/or endotracheal intubation have failed. The procedure is quicker and safer to perform than a tracheostomy especially in the hands of those with little surgical experience.

Equipment

- A scalpel blade and handle.
- A pair of artery forceps e.g. Spencer Wells.

- A *small* cuffed tracheostomy or endotracheal tube e.g. size 5.0 mm for an adult. (Note that it is essential to use a small endotracheal tube as the hole created by this technique is likely to be small and will not accommodate the normal size of tracheostomy or endotracheal tube easily.)
- An oxygen supply and the appropriate bag and connections for manual lung inflation.
- Suction facilities.

Technique

- Place the patient supine with a sandbag under the shoulders so as to achieve maximum head and neck extension.
- Holding the larynx with the thumb and middle finger, identify the cricothyroid membrane with the index finger.
- Make a 3 cm horizontal incision through the skin and stab the cricothyroid membrane with the scalpel blade.
- Dilate the opening with a pair of artery forceps.
- Insert the tracheostomy or endotracheal tube.
- Connect the tracheostomy tube to the means of manual lung inflation.

Difficult intubation

A variety of conditions may make intubation difficult. If upper airway obstruction is present, tracheostomy or 'awake' intubation under local anaesthesia should be considered before induction of general anaesthesia. As a *guiding rule*, before attempts are made at intubation, muscle relaxants should *not* be used until it has been clearly demonstrated that the patient can be ventilated using a facemask *without* the use of a muscle relaxant.

The following techniques for intubation are described:

- Intubation under direct vision.
- Blind nasal intubation under general anaesthesia.
- Blind nasal intubation under local anaesthesia.
- Retrograde intubation under local anaesthesia.

Intubation under direct vision

Good analgesia and full relaxation under general anaesthesia often permit intubation when vision of the larynx is difficult. The use of a lubricated gum elastic catheter or a suitable introducer e.g. Mallinckrodt 'satin-slip' intubating stylet inside a smaller bore endotracheal tube than would usually be chosen may also facilitate intubation. A large adult Macintosh larynogoscope blade may help in bull necked and massive patients.

Where no more than the upper surface of the epiglottis is viewed, a nasotracheal tube may enter the larynx more readily than an oral tracheal tube.

Where there is a limitation of opening the mouth, the use of a *fibreoptic bronchoscope* as an introducer through a nasotracheal tube offers a good solution to the problem of difficult intubation. The fibreoptic bronchoscope is preferred to the fibreoptic laryngoscope because of its suction facilities. Much practice and expertise are required in its use but the authors wish to recommend that such practice should be part of anaesthetic training.

Where *trismus* is present, provided upper airway obstruction does not preclude the induction of general anaesthesia, a Ferguson mouth gag may permit the mouth to open sufficiently to insert a laryngoscope and intubate the patient.

Blind nasal intubation under general anaesthesia

This may be performed using relaxant drugs or under deep inhalational anaesthesia with spontaneous breathing. The former method is quicker but less certain of success.

Position

Place the patient supine with one pillow under the head and with the head fully extended.

Techniques

Before induction, each nasal airway should be sprayed with 0.5 ml cocaine, 5 per cent, or phenylephrine hydrochloride 0.25 per cent solution to decongest the mucosa. The patient should be warned of the bitter taste.

When performed with spontaneous breathing, the level of anaesthesia must be deepened to obtund the laryngeal reflexes. Five per cent CO_2 may be added for up to two minutes to encourage hyperventilation on a mixture of 30 per cent O_2 and 70 per cent N_2O with 1.5–2 per cent halothane. It may take from 5–10 min to achieve the correct depth; ECG monitoring is important. Choose an uncuffed tube which will easily pass the nares e.g. 7.0 mm in an adult man or a 6.0 mm in an adult woman; the curvature of the tube should be apropriate to the patient's shape, *viz* a greater curve is necessary for a patient with a short neck. Pass the tube into the nasopharynx, shut the mouth and occlude the opposite nostril so that *breath sounds* can be clearly heard through the tube. With the other hand or with help of an assistant push the larynx to the left, right or backwards to find the position in which as the tube is advanced, the breath sounds are loudest. It is worth remembering that a nasal tube often passes lateral to the larynx unless intentionally manoeuvred towards the opposite side. On an inspiration, try intubation.

Blind intubation may also be successful using a relaxant technique such as intravenous thiopentone and suxamethonium with face-mask oxygenation. The same points concerning the direction of the tip of the tube, the curvature of the tube and the mobilization of the larynx apply as for spontaneous breathing.

Difficulties

The tube may impinge on the anterior surface of the larynx: the use of a soft tube makes this less likely. Conversely, intubation of the oesophagus will indicate the need for a tube with a greater curvature.

Use of a wire hook[3] (Fig. 6.2) will assist both in lifting the tube

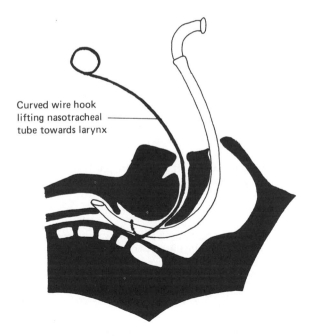

Curved wire hook lifting nasotracheal tube towards larynx

Fig. 6.2 Blind nasal intubation facilitated by use of a wire hook.

anteriorly and in keeping it in the midline. Pass the hook over the dorsum of the tongue as far as the posterior pharyngeal wall before introducing the nasotracheal tube. The tip of the hook should have a shallow curve to permit its withdrawal after successful intubation.

Blind nasal intubation under local anaesthesia

Such intubation will require anaesthesia of the larynx above and below the vocal cords, the pharynx and posterior part of the tongue and of the nasal airways.

Block of the internal branch of the superior laryngeal nerve from inside the mouth may be difficult if there is restricted opening of the mouth and therefore an external approach is also described.

When local anaesthesia is established, blind nasal intubation is performed applying the same principles as when performed under general anaesthesia with spontaneous breathing.

Sedation
Most patients will require sedation to allay anxiety e.g. 5–10 mg Diazemuls (diazepam) or 2–5 mg midazolam IV.

Secretions
Reduction of secretions is advisable with atropine 0.6 mg IM or hyoscine 0.2 mg IM, but this should be given *after* the sucking of an anaesthetic lozenge otherwise the mouth will be too dry to dissolve the lozenge.

Technique of local anaesthesia

Nasal airways
Spray 0.5 ml 5 per cent cocaine or 0.25 per cent phenylephrine into each nostril on an inspiration. The patient should be warned of the bitter taste.

Oropharynx
Fifteen to twenty minutes before the vocal cords and supraglottic region are anaesthetized, give the patient an anaesthetic lozenge to suck, e.g. amethocaine lozenge (60 mg) or benzocaine lozenge (100 mg). Alternatively, 10 ml of 2 per cent viscous lignocaine (lidocaine) may be gargled and spat out.

Vocal cords and supraglottic region
Oral approach. Sit the patient up and instruct him to mouth breathe. Take a swab, roll it and clamp it in Krause's forceps or

Moynihan's cholecystectomy forceps. Dip the swab in 4 per cent lignocaine (lidocaine) and gently squeeze it out. With the left hand pull the tongue forward gripping it in a damp swab. With the right hand, pass the Krause forceps diagonally over the back of the tongue so that the lignocaine (lidocaine) swab rests in the pyriform fossa, pressing the forceps gently downwards on the tongue. Hold the swab in the pyriform fossa for 2–3 minutes. Repeat the procedure on the other side.

If the patient gags, spray the palate and the fauces with 1–2 ml of 4 per cent lignocaine. If there is restricted opening of the mouth, use the external approach.

External approach. Place the patient supine with a sandbag under the shoulders to extend the neck as much as possible.

Clean the skin of the neck with chlorhexidine in spirit. With the finger and thumb of the left hand, identify the hyoid cartilage and trace it backwards to the most posterior part which is its greater cornu. With a 21 G needle attached to a 10 ml syringe containing 10 ml 1 per cent lignocaine (lidocaine) approach from laterally to enter the skin just inferior to the greater cornu whilst retracting the carotid sheath posteriorly with the index finger (Fig. 6.3). Pierce the thyrohyoid membrane which lies at a depth of 1–1.5 cm. Aspirate for blood to ensure no vessel is punctured and for air to ensure the needle has not entered the pharynx.

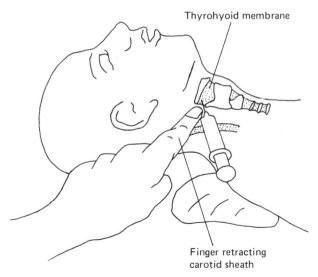

Thyrohyoid membrane

Finger retracting
carotid sheath

Fig. 6.3 Local anaesthesia of the larynx by the external approach.

Inject 5 ml lignocaine (lidocaine) and repeat the procedure on the other side.

If the hyoid is difficult to palpate, identify the greater cornu of the thyroid cartilage. The thyrohyoid membrane may then be approached by sliding the needle off the greater cornu of the thyroid cartilage in a cephalad direction.

Transtracheal injection. Sit the patient up. Clean the skin over the cricothyroid membrane with chlorhexidine in spirit.

Raise a bleb of local anaesthetic in the skin over the cricothyroid membrane. Attach a 21 G needle *firmly* to a 2 ml syringe containing 2 ml 4 per cent lignocaine (lidocaine). Warn the patient that the procedure will make him cough. Advance the 21 G needle directly backwards (about 1 cm) to puncture the cricothyroid membrane and *aspirate for air*. Instruct the patient to breathe out and at the end of expiration, inject the 2 ml of lignocaine (lidocaine) quickly. With the left hand holding the hub of the needle and the right hand holding the barrel of the syringe, withdraw both rapidly – before the patient takes a deep breath and starts expulsive coughing.

Retrograde intubation

This should be performed under local anaesthesia of the pharynx, larynx and nasal airways and should be considered for patients with marked restriction in opening the mouth and as an alternative to blind nasal intubation.

Equipment

- 16 G cannula (e.g. 16 G Abbocath).
- Introducer wire of pulmonary balloon-flotation catheter (USCI Bard, Teflon coated spring guide 007045 120 cm)[4].
- Oral or nasal endotracheal tube preferably with Murphy's eye (side hole).

Technique

- Local anaesthesia of the nasal airways, pharynx and larynx is required as described above.
- Clean the skin over the cricothyroid membrane with chlorhexidine in spirit and infiltrate the skin with 1 ml 2 per cent lignocaine (lidocaine).
- Introduce the 16 G cannula into the subglottic airway through the cricothyroid membrane directing the cannula upwards towards the pharynx. Withdraw the stylet and pass the soft flexible end of a pulmonary balloon-flotation catheter

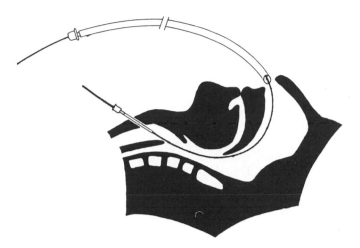

Fig. 6.4   Tracheal intubation using retrograde insertion of guide wire.

introducer wire through the cannula. Continue passing the wire either out through the mouth or into the nasopharynx and out through the nose. Thread the wire through the lumen of the endotracheal tube via its bevelled end and pass the tube over the guide wire into the larynx (Fig. 6.4).

Difficulty
If the endotracheal tube sticks on the epiglottis or the arytenoids or slips out when the introducer wire is removed, thread the introducer wire through the Murphy's eye of the endotracheal tube instead of through its bevelled end.[5] This gives an extra 1 cm in length to the tip of the advancing endotracheal tube.

References

1. Rosen M, Latto IP, Ng WS. *Handbook of Percutaneous Central Venous Catheterisation.* London:W. B. Saunders, 1981.
2. Firmin RK, Welch JD. Insertion of a chest drain. *Hospital Update* 1980; **6**(5): 481–6.
3. Singh A. Blind nasal intubation. *Anaesthesia* 1966; **21**: 400–402.
4. Robets KW. New use for Swan-Ganz introducer wire. *Anesthesia & Analgesia* 1981; **60**: 67.

5. Bourke D, Levesque PR. Modification of retrograde guide for endotracheal intubation. *Anesthesia & Analgesia* 1974; **53**: 1013–14.

Further reading

Latto IP, Rosen M. *Difficulties in Tracheal Intubation*. London: Baillière Tindall, 1985.

7

Patient Monitoring

Michael P Broadbent and Jeremy N Cashman

Cardiovascular monitoring
  Arterial pressure
  Central venous pressure
  Electrocardiography
Respiratory monitoring
  Auscultation
  Capnography
  Transcutaneous CO_2 and O_2 monitoring
  Pulse oximetry
  Ventilator alarms
  Blood gases
Neurophysiological monitoring
  Intracranial pressure
  Electroencephalography
  Sensory evoked potentials (SEPs)
  Neuromuscular function
Temperature monitoring
Electrolytes and glucose
  Electrolytes
  Glucose
Oncotic pressure
Newer techniques
  The niroscope
  Ion-selective electrodes
  Computerization of monitoring

The use of monitoring during emergency anaesthesia is often dictated by the relative urgency of the surgical situation and should provide information that aids clinical decision making and prompts therapeutic intervention. This chapter outlines both the minimal monitoring requirements needed to provide the anaesthetist with sufficient information to ensure support of vital physiological functions and details more specialized facilities for use if circumstances permit.

Monitoring blood pressure and ECG have been suggested as the basic requirement for the practice of safe anaesthesia. We suggest that monitoring temperature and at least one respiratory parameter should complete the series of absolute mandatory measurements for all emergency anaesthesia.

Cardiovascular monitoring

Arterial pressure

Arterial pressure may be measured either directly or indirectly. Direct measurement, which requires specialized equipment, should give a beat-to-beat record of arterial pressure and waveform and provides the most comprehensive amount of information regarding the patient's circulatory status but the overall technique may be subject to technical difficulties. The ability to monitor blood gas levels easily (*see* below) from the inserted cannula is advantageous. Indirect methods, which may be manual or automated, are generally only of use over a limited range of pressures.

When sophisticated monitoring equipment or technical expertise is not readily available it is still possible to measure arterial pressure directly by use of a pressure line-air bubble technique.[1, 2] An arterial cannula is connected to a short length of manometer tube containing heparinized saline, in which there is a single small air bubble. The bubble will oscillate with arterial pulsation; inflation of a blood pressure cuff placed over the upper arm will cause the oscillations to cease when systolic pressure is exceeded. The Pressurveil system is a similar mechanical arrangement whereby mean arterial pressure is read on an aneroid gauge (Fig. 7.1).

Central venous pressure

Central venous pressure provides an indication of right heart filling pressure. In the majority of patients this will be an adequate reflection of left sided filling pressure and will provide sufficient information for the management of most patients. Placement of pulmonary artery pressure lines should be reserved for patients subsequently suspected of having mismatch between right and left heart filling pressures.

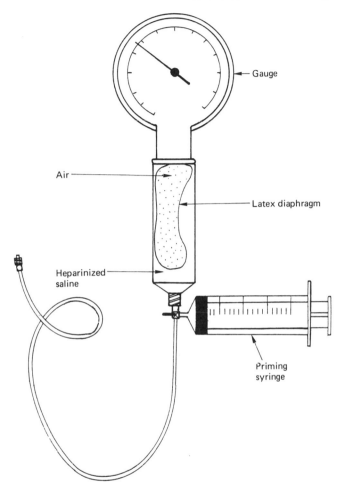

Fig. 7.1 Closed pressure monitoring system (Pressurveil): latex diaphragm separates heparinized saline in intravascular catheter from air in contact with pressure gauge.

Electrocardiography

The ECG allows continuous monitoring of the electrical activity of the heart giving an assessment of heart rate and rhythm and additionally providing evidence of ischaemia. It also provides valuable continuous monitoring of IV potassium therapy (*see* p. 57); the development of hyperkalaemia being associated with peaked T waves in the ECG. The CM_5 lead is ideally suited for monitoring all of these parameters in the operating room. (*C*entral *M*anubrium; 5th intercostal space in the anterior axillary line.)

Respiratory monitoring

Auscultation

This is performed as part of the physical examination in all patients. Intra-operative precordial and oesophageal stethoscopes may be employed, especially in circumstances where there is high risk of air embolism. The latter is minimally invasive and the potential for multiparameter monitoring, incorporating the display of heart and breath sounds, temperature and ECG has added attractions. However, auscultation can provide only limited information of the patient's respiratory status since it does not quantify the adequacy of alveolar ventilation. This parameter may be derived from measurement of respiratory rate and tidal volume (*spirometry*). Despite apparently adequate alveolar ventilation, gas exchange may be impaired.

Specialized equipment is available for the noninvasive measurement of carbon dioxide production and oxygen utilization as indicators of alveolar gas exchange. The integrity of the anaesthetic equipment also needs to be monitored.

Capnography

Monitoring of variations in the exhaled CO_2 waveform can indicate changes in not only CO_2 production but also CO_2 transport, regional changes in lung function and impairment of CO_2 elimination. Capnography is invaluable in the management of the head-injured patient (*see* p. 129), and may provide much useful information in many other anaesthetic situations.

Transcutaneous CO_2 and O_2 monitoring

These have limitations (notably a slow response time), but may be useful in specific cases such as monitoring the neonate. Transcutaneous oxygen analysers detect capillary oxygen but have limited usefulness in certain disease states and in obese patients. They are also subject to intra-operative interference by anaesthetic vapours. Avoiding delivery of hypoxic gas mixtures can be assisted by the use of an oxygen analyser in the inspiratory limb of the breathing circuit.

Pulse oximetry

These instruments (e.g. Nellcor oximeter) measure oxyhaemoglobin saturation, but may be subject to interference by carboxyhaemoglobin. They are especially useful in patients with pigmented skin. In those centres where mass spectrometry is available, it is possible to separate the individual components of complex gas mixtures according to their mass and charge.

Ventilator alarms

Anaesthetic ventilators should always be used in combination with disconnect alarms, although such threshold alarms are not failsafe. Most ventilators will incorporate an airway pressure manometer, although a high-pressure monitor, warning of airway obstruction, may be more useful.

Blood gases

The sampling of arterial blood for measurement of acid–base status and gas analysis allows for more direct monitoring of the adequacy of ventilation and to optimize pH. Glass syringes are to be preferred to plastic, the amount of heparin should only be sufficient to occupy the syringe dead space and meticulous care should be taken to exclude all air bubbles. Samples may be stored at 4°C for up to 3 hr.[3] Modern blood gas analysers measure pH, P_{CO_2} and P_{O_2} directly and calculate other parameters algorithmically.

Neurophysiological monitoring

Intracranial pressure

Intracranial pressure (ICP) may be monitored by means of a ventricular catheter, subarachnoid screw or extradural transducer. The normal mean value is 10 mmHg (1.3 kPa), but this fluctuates with ventilation, coughing, straining etc. It is recommended that a target level for treatment should be set at 25 mmHg (>3.3 kPa). This value is below the level of decompensation on the pressure/volume curve.

Electroencephalography

The conventional electroencephalogram (EEG) has only limited use in routine anaesthesia. The Compressed Spectral Array (CSA),

Cerebral Function Monitor (CFM) and the newer Cerebral Function Analysing Monitor (CFAM) process data in a more interpretable form. The CSA converts EEG data from a time to a frequency domain and displays this in the form of a three-dimensional graph. The CFM gives a crude measure of electrical activity without discriminating between the contribution of the different frequencies, and produces a display of variations in EEG amplitude. Intraoperative events such as epileptiform seizures are easily recognizable whereas an assessment of depth of anaesthesia is more difficult.

Sensory evoked potentials (SEPs)

Auditory, visual and somatosensory SEPs each monitor a different aspect of electrical activity in the central nervous system.[4] The somatosensory evoked potential is likely to be encountered by the anaesthetist during surgery for spinal cord injury, the visual evoked response is used to assess the integrity of the optic pathway during surgery in the proximity of the optic chiasma, whilst auditory evoked responses can be used to monitor brain stem function. A stimulus applied to a sensory nerve will induce an evoked potential in the relevant part of the sensory cortex which can be picked up by a modified EEG. This provides information not only about the integrity of the sensory pathway but also of cortical function. Many of the commonly used anaesthetic drugs, especially the inhalational agents, cause a dose related suppression of the cortical response. Interpretation of SEPs may be difficult.

Neuromuscular function

The train-of-four (TOF) pattern of stimulation is the most sensitive technique for monitoring of neuromuscular function in clinical practice.[5] Measuring the response to stimulation may not be straightforward. Mechanomyography (the measuring of the evoked force of muscle contraction using a force displacement transducer), is too cumbersome a technique to apply in the emergency situation. Electromyography (the recording of the electrical activity of an appropriate muscle), is an easier technique to apply and is becoming increasingly available. However, for most clinical purposes merely counting the number of twitches in the TOF response may allow the anaesthetist to quantify the extent of block. During onset of neuromuscular blockade the fourth twitch in the TOF is lost at approximately 75 per cent depression of the first twitch, the third at 80 per cent and the second at 90 per cent depression of the first (these values may vary slightly depending on the individual relaxant used); during recovery good correlation with clinical signs of adequate return of muscle power has been found if the amplitude of the fourth to the first twitch of the TOF exceeds 60 per cent.

Temperature monitoring

The standard mercury-in-glass thermometer and skin temperature sensitive pad are not suitable due to lack of sensitivity. Core temperature may be measured by thermistor or thermocouple probes placed in the nasopharynx, external auditory meatus, oesophagus (at the level of the heart) or rectum. In addition, a skin probe (usually positioned on the great toe) allows a core–skin gradient to be obtained. This simply derived information can be extremely sensitive in mirroring deterioration in cardiac output. A fall in toe temperature (reflecting a reduction in femoral blood flow), to less than 27°C indicates a cardiac output of roughly half normal. Instability of body temperature will occur in malignant hyperpyrexia.

Electrolytes and glucose

These are normally analysed in the laboratory, but may easily be measured by the clinician.

Electrolytes

Most laboratories tend to employ ion-specific electrodes for electrolyte measurement. An alternative technique is flame photometry; either serum or plasma is suitable for this analysis.

Glucose

The commercially available 'glucose sticks' consist of a cellulose strip impregnated with glucose oxidase, a chromogen indicator system, and coated with a semi-permeable membrane. A fixed contact time is allowed for blood (arterial or venous) to permeate the strip.

Glucose oxidase is specific for glucose, releasing hydrogen peroxide which yields a colour change on reaction with the chromogen. The development of colour is compared with a chart. Accuracy can be improved by employing a photometric 'glucose meter'.

Oncotic pressure

The measurement of colloidal osmotic (oncotic) pressure and the estimation of urinary osmolality are effective indicators of a patient's state of hydration. Measured by the method of freezing point depression, they provide invaluable clinical information in the treatment of diabetes insipidus, acute renal failure and hyperosmolar coma.

Newer techniques

The Niroscope

This instrument (*N*ear *I*nfra*R*ed *O*xygen *S*ufficiency *scope*) is a new development in neurophysiological monitoring,[6] which will allow direct assessment, on a continual basis, of oxygenation of the cerebral cortex to a depth of 3–4 cm. It employs the principle of reflectance spectrophotometry of near infra-red light, of a wavelength which can pass through a 'window' in the skull. Mitochondrial cytochrome c' oxidase weakly absorbs this light. The amount of reflected photons gives an indication of the oxygen status of the cell.

Ion-selective electrodes

The ability to monitor continuously, specific ions intravascularly will have applications not only in the intensive care unit, but also in the operating theatre. Devices based upon silicon gate technology usually comprise a silicon chip embedded in an unreactive resin. An ion-specific membrane encloses the chip and its surrounding pocket of sensing fluid. These membranes may only admit molecules up to a certain size or may be impregnated with enzymes reacting with a specific substrate. Miniaturization of these and their attachment inside catheters may offer a cheap and effective means of measuring circulating ions of importance to the anaesthetist in the emergency situation.

Computerization of monitoring

Many of the existing monitors of anaesthetic parameters have the ability to digitalize their output and to route data via appropriate interfaces for computerization. The increasing amount of data that will inevitably follow from more extensive monitoring will need to be sympathetically handled by computers so that its full significance may be appreciated.

References

1. Gilston A. A simple method of monitoring the arterial blood pressure. *Br. J. Anaesth.* 1972; **44**: 1334.
2. Zorab JSM. Continuous display of the arterial pressure. A simple manometric technique. *Anaesthesia.* 1969; **24**: 431–7.
3. Adams AP, Hahn CEW. *Principles and Practice of Blood-gas Analysis, 2nd ed* London: Churchill-Livingstone, 1982.
4. Grundy BL. Intraoperative monitoring of sensory-evoked potentials. *Anesthesiology* 1983; **58**: 72–87.
5. Ali HH. Mechanomyography and electromyography. In: *Muscle Relaxation.* New York: Georg Thieme, 1981: 82–8.
6. Fox EJ. The monitor of the future. (Editorial) *Anaesthesia* 1983; **38**: 433.

Further reading

Blitt CD (ed). *Monitoring in Anesthesia and Critical Care Medicine.* London: Churchill-Livingstone, 1985.

Spence AA (ed). *Respiratory Monitoring in Intensive Care.* Clinics in Critical Care Medicine – 4. London: Churchill-Livingstone, 1982.

Steward DJ. Patient monitoring during pediatric anaesthesia. In: Katz RL (ed). *Seminars in Anesthesia* 1984; **3**(1): 43–9.

Monitoring and anaesthesia. Conference summary. *Can. Anaesth. Soc. J.* 1984: **31**: 395–406.

The anaesthetic monitors. A panel discussion. *Can. Anaesth. Soc. J.* 1984: **31**: 294–8.

8

Diagnostic Procedures

Adrian C Pearce

General considerations
Anaesthetic considerations
 Nervous system
 Cardiovascular system
 Computerized tomography
 Angiography
 Cardiac catheterization and dye studies
 Magnetic resonance
Effects of contrast medium

Emergency diagnostic procedures which require anaesthesia are concerned mainly with invasive or noninvasive imaging of the cardiovascular and nervous systems. Procedures involved include computerized tomography, cerebral and major vessel angiography, cardiac catheterization and magnetic resonance studies. These investigations are undertaken in or near the radiology department.

General considerations

The familiar surroundings of the anaesthetic or operating room are usually replaced by a poorly lit, cold room not designed for the administration of general anaesthetics. Following induction of anaesthesia in these difficult circumstances the patient may be placed, occasionally without warning, into a variety of positions for a procedure of indeterminate duration. Therefore, check the anaesthetic machine, breathing systems and gas supplies with special care, make immediately available all equipment and drugs that are likely to be required and check the location and function of resuscitation apparatus (including the defibrillator) and suction apparatus.

Induction of anaesthesia is best carried out on the *tilting* bed or stretcher used for transporting the patient to the radiology department. This allows better patient access during induction (for turning or tilting head down) than the encumbered, nontilting radiology table. Endotracheal intubation will guarantee and protect the airway and is usually advisable in these emergency patients. One of the members of the radiology department should be instructed in cricoid pressure, if trained anaesthetic assistance is not available.

The anaesthetic breathing system must accommodate patient positioning and repositioning. A long, lightweight, flexible Bain type co-axial system is ideal. Explosive anaesthetic agents must not be used. If extensive movement of the table is anticipated, use a trial run to check the length and freedom of movement of the breathing system and monitoring cables.

Patient monitors should have displays which are visible in the dark or at great distance and incorporate alarms. Space and equipment are often at a premium in the radiology department, but an ECG and intermittent measurement of blood pressure provide a minimum degree of patient supervision. A reliable peripheral pulse monitor or oximeter gives additional, helpful information. Rectal or oesophageal temperature must be monitored in all babies and ideally in all patients, since hypothermia is prone to occur. Patient colour may be difficult to determine in the gloom; use a torch or other light source.

The procedures are often concerned purely with diagnosis. The underlying pathology will not be ameliorated by the investigation and may be substantially worsened. Emergency patients exhibit greater derangement of function of the system under investigation than those undergoing routine screening and may also have significant disease in other systems – for example head, chest, abdominal and limb injuries in the trauma patient. Management and monitoring of these patients must be appropriately intense (e.g. direct arterial, pulmonary artery pressure, end-tidal CO_2 or blood gas tension measurements), otherwise serious deterioration of the patient will occur. If the patient has come from the ICU, it is useful for the ICU nurse to accompany the patient and help with this intensive management.

- Never underestimate the difficulties that may occur in the simplest radiological procedure.

Anaesthetic considerations

Nervous system

- *Thiopentone* (thiopental) decreases intracranial pressure

(ICP) and may cause a small increase in cerebral perfusion pressure (CPP).

- *Volatile agents* increase ICP (least marked with isoflurane).
- *Muscle relaxation and hyperventilation* decrease ICP and increase CPP.
- N_2O causes a small increase in ICP, and a large increase if there is an air-containing cavity within the CNS.

Cardiovascular system

- A decrease in systemic vascular resistance (SVR) (volatile agents especially isoflurane, droperidol, pethidine, chlorpromazine) and an increase in pulmonary vascular resistance (PVR) (crying, IPPV, hypoxia, hypercarbia) promote right-to-left shunting with increasing cyanosis.
- *Volatile agents* decrease myocardial contractility: enflurane and halothane more than isoflurane.
- *Heart rate* tends to increase with isoflurane and enflurane but decreases with halothane.
- *Fentanyl/alfentanil and sufentanil* have little effect on the cardiovascular system, although an initial reduction in blood pressure is not uncommonly seen.
- *Lignocaine (lidocaine)* 1.0–1.5 mg/kg IV to decrease the response to intubation has gained wide acceptance in the USA but not in the UK.

Computerized tomography (CT)

Emergency CT scans are usually of the head, chest or abdomen. The procedure is noninvasive and therefore painless but requires absolute stillness during each 'slice' (15–60 sec) and relative stillness during the whole procedure (10–30 min). Anaesthetic assistance will be sought in those patients who are unable to lie supine in safety and keep still for this length of time. The following approaches are useful.

Firm strapping of the head/body
Strapping without sedation or anaesthesia is suitable for neonates (with a pacifier if crying) and drowsy children or adults. Intermittently restless patients may be managed by timing the slices with periods of quiescence. Check between slices that airway obstruction has not occurred in the supine position; a lignocaine (lidocaine) coated oral airway may help in these circumstances.

Sedation
Sedation with a benzodiazepine, e.g. diazepam 0.05–0.2 mg/kg or

midazolam 0.02–0.1 mg/kg IV may help anxious patients. Restlessness may be due to hypoxia, pain or hypotension and in these circumstances should not be treated with pure sedation. In patients with a head injury it carries a high risk of decreasing the level of consciousness so that respiration or airway maintenance is impaired with disastrous consequences. Make certain that chest movement is visible at all times and check the patient closely between each slice.

General anaesthesia

This, along with endotracheal intubation, is the only safe course in those patients who cannot safely be sedated. An anaesthetic technique appropriate to the likely pathology and length of scan should be adopted. If raised ICP is suspected, induction with thiopentone (thiopental), suxamethonium (succinylcholine) and endotracheal intubation should be followed by maintenance with O_2/N_2O and increments of thiopentone and controlled ventilation to a Pa_{CO_2} of approximately 30 mmHg (4.0 kPa). Muscle relaxation can either be provided by further doses of suxamethonium, atracurium or vecuronium. The most modern scanners can complete a study in under 10 min. Nitrous oxide should be avoided if an air space within the cranium is present or suspected. Respiratory movements will not usually interfere with a CT scan of the head, but may lower resolution during a scan of the chest or upper abdomen; muscle relaxation and controlled ventilation will allow suitably timed periods of apnoea.

Sedation using infusions of anaesthetic agents is not recommended unless great experience has been gained in elective procedures.

Angiography

Cerebral

Well-motivated conscious adults will tolerate unilateral carotid angiography under sedation only; the majority of other patients require general anaesthesia. The investigation is usually performed in adults to delineate abnormal vessels following subarachnoid haemorrhage. Access to the carotid artery is usually by direct puncture in the neck, and to the vertebral artery by retrograde cannulation from the femoral artery. Bilateral carotid and vertebral angiography performed by this retrograde technique may not require general anaesthesia.

Intra-cranial vessel spasm is commonly found in association

with the bleeding vessel and may be increased by the contrast medium.

- Hypertension at any stage of the procedure carries the risk of further bleeding and hypotension the danger of cerebral infarction.

Moderate hyperventilation produces good quality pictures without reducing cerebral blood flow to an unacceptable degree. A capnograph is a very useful monitor (*see* p. 84). A suggested technique is:

- Preoxygenate, record baseline pulse rate and blood pressure.
- Intravenous induction of anaesthesia with fentanyl 1–1.5 micrograms/kg, thiopentone (thiopental) 3–6 mg/kg followed by suxamethonium (succinylcholine) 1–1.5 mg/kg and oral intubation with a cuffed tube. (Topical 4 per cent lignocaine spray to the larynx and trachea, if advisable.) Further muscle paralysis with a nondepolarizing relaxant, bearing in mind the known cardiovascular effects of each and the likely length of the procedure (1–3 hr). Vecuronium shows the greatest degree of cardiovascular stability but is short acting. Alcuronium represents a reasonable compromise, but all muscle relaxants have been used in this situation.
- Maintenance of anaesthesia with O_2/N_2O and *low* levels of volatile agent titrated to keep the blood pressure within acceptable limits, without greatly affecting cerebrovascular haemodynamics. Enflurane or isoflurane ensures a more rapid recovery than halothane. If seizure activity has been prominent prior to the investigation, it seems prudent to avoid enflurane. Moderate hyperventilation to a Pa_{CO_2} 30–34 mmHg (4.0–4.5 kPa). At the end of the study, the muscle relaxant should be reversed and the patient extubated. Prolonged coughing on the tube should be avoided. The investigation sometimes causes a major deterioration in the patient's condition.

Major and limb vessel

The pain on injection of large volumes of older types of contrast media meant that general anaesthesia was routinely required. With the newer agents (*see* below) IV sedation/analgesia is often sufficient if vessel access is covered by local anaesthetic infiltration.

General anaesthesia is usually provided for translumbar aortography because involuntary patient movement may cause the needle to tear through the aorta. Endotracheal intubation is required, as the prone position is adopted. Bearing in mind the high incidence of coronary artery disease in these patients, a suitable technique is induction with fentanyl and thiopentone or etomidate, suxamethonium and endotracheal intubation followed by maintenance with O_2/N_2O and volatile agent or narcotic. If the chest and pelvis are supported, leaving the abdomen free, spontaneous respiration can be maintained although muscle relaxation and IPPV may be preferable. In the latter situation vecuronium and atracurium have the most appropriate duration as the procedure commonly takes 15–45 min.

Regional blocks may be useful e.g. brachial plexus for upper limb and epidural anaesthesia for lower limb angiography.

Cardiac catheterization and dye studies

Cardiac catheterization is painless apart from arterial and venous access, which may be covered by infiltration of local anaesthetic. Injection of contrast medium into the major vessels, chambers of the heart or coronary arteries is associated with flushing, burning and nausea and may require sedation or anaesthesia, otherwise patient movement will occur.

The measurements of pressure or oxygen saturations within the chambers are made sequentially and so the cardiovascular system should remain stable and near normal for the duration of the procedure. Sedation with the patient breathing air, or oxygen enriched air, is as near ideal as possible. Sick patients do not tolerate heavy sedation and it is more important to keep the patient alive than to obtain these ideal conditions. Intubation, muscle relaxation and IPPV is the safest technique and does not generally result in misdiagnosis of congenital abnormalities provided that it is instituted prior to, rather than during, the measurements.

- Monitor rectal temperature, ECG and blood pressure – by cuff or directly from intravascular catheter.
- Give maintenance IV fluids, assess blood loss (via sampling and leakage around catheters) as a proportion of total blood volume, measure and correct blood glucose and acid–base balance.
- Full facilities for resuscitation must be immediately available.

Neonates

Feed 2 hr prior to procedure with a clear dextrose containing fluid to avert hypoglycaemia and crying due to hunger. Keep warm with gamgee/foil around the legs and head. Strap to a crucifix splint and supply a pacifier. No anaesthesia or sedation given.

Infants and young children (< 15 kg)

Possibilities include:

- *Pethidine Co.* (pethidine (demerol) 25 mg, promethazine 6.25 mg and chlorpromazine 6.25 mg/ml). The full sedative dose (0.1 ml/kg) must be reduced in the more sick emergency patient. Give 0.05 ml/kg IM 30 min prior to procedure with incremental intra-operative sedation with diazepam 0.05 mg/kg or ketamine 0.5 mg/kg. Watch for respiratory depression and be ready to intubate and ventilate.
- *Ketamine* 1–2 mg/kg IV or 5 mg/kg IM with 1 mg/kg increments. The airway and respiration are usually, but not always maintained, therefore an anaesthetist should be available. The hypertension and tachycardia that occur on injection have largely settled after 10 min and do not seem to recur after reinjection. Salivation may be profuse and detrimental to airway maintenance. An antisialogogue orally or IM is valuable – atropine 0.015 mg/kg or glycopyrronium (glycopyrrolate) 0.007 mg/kg. Eye opening, vocalizing and limb movements are common. Additional diazepam 0.1–0.2 mg/kg IV provides smoother conditions and reduces the cumulative dose of ketamine. Recovery may be quite prolonged once the dose of ketamine exceeds 10 mg/kg.
- *General anaesthesia.* Oxygen/nitrous oxide, low levels of volatile agent and spontaneous respiration is only suitable for fitter, older children. Generally, intubation, muscle relaxation and IPPV is the safest course. A smooth induction without crying or struggling helps maintain pulmonary blood flow, often reduced in congenital heart disease. Intravenous, inhalation agents or intramuscular ketamine have all been used successfully, the latter being particularly useful in chubby babies without prior IV access. The mean intrathoracic pressure must be kept as low as possible (adequate expiratory time, no PEEP, muscle relaxation) and the FIO_2 adjusted to maintain a normal, not elevated, PaO_2. Usually an FIO_2 0.35–0.50 will assure oxygenation of all blood passing through the lung. In moribund, cyanosed children, 100 per cent oxygen is usually given.

Anaesthesia is maintained with nitrous oxide, low levels of volatile agent or IV narcotic. The PaO_2 and $PaCO_2$ must be checked and adjustments made. Vecuronium or pancuronium are the most useful relaxants, depending on the likely length of the procedure and possibility of continuing IPPV.

Older children and adults

Sedation is usually best achieved with oral/IV diazepam or papavaretum 0.3 mg/kg with hyoscine 0.006 mg/kg IM. Most procedures (coronary angiography, pressure studies) can be undertaken with this basal sedation, supplemented with an intravenous benzodiazepine. A brief period of anaesthesia, e.g. to cover left ventricular angiography, may be obtained with a small dose of thiopentone (thiopental). Increasing restlessness during a procedure may be due to pulmonary oedema/hypotension/hypoxia and pure sedation is inappropriate.

Magnetic resonance

This facility is presently only available at a few centres. A strong magnetic field and radiofrequency pulses are used to generate images. Ferrous metal contained in monitoring leads or anaesthetic equipment may distort the magnetic field. Wires attached to the patient and leaving the scanner may pick up stray radiofrequency signals. Both these effects lower resolution. A blood pressure cuff with plastic connectors and ECG telemetry overcome some of the monitoring problems although the magnetic field and radiofrequency pulses interfere with the ECG display. Plastic connectors and valves should be used in the anaesthetic breathing systems.

Effects of contrast medium

These agents are hyperosmolar and contain iodine. The former property is responsible for most of the adverse effects. Older type contrast media solutions (Hypaque, Conray) have osmolarities of 1000–1500 mOsmol/l, i.e. four to five times that of plasma. One ml/kg of these solutions will raise plasma osmolarity by 30 mOsmol/litre 5 min after injection. In large vessel studies, 3–4 ml/kg may be injected. This large osmolar load causes initially an increase in intravascular volume, followed by a brisk osmotic diuresis with resulting dehydration. Direct myocardial depression and a decrease in SVR can also be demonstrated. These effects are poorly tolerated, especially in sick neonates with cardiovascular disease. Most recent media (metrizamide, Hexabrix) have lower osmolarities (470–490 mOsmol/l) and are much safer in this respect. Patients receiving neuroleptics and antidepressants are at risk if thoracic or cervical (but not lumbar) myelography or ventriculography is performed using metrizamide; lowered seizure thresholds have been demonstrated in animal experiments and in some patients there have been indications of a similar mechanism. Diazepam may be used if the patient needs a sedative.

All media are associated with other reactions. These may be minor – flushing, nausea, vomiting, urticaria, or life-threatening – hypotension, bronchospasm, upper airway oedema, cardiac arrhythmias. Approximately 500 fatalities associated with intravascular contrast media occur in the USA per year. Severe reactions should be treated with oxygen, IV fluids, adrenaline (epinephrine) 1–5 micrograms/kg and hydrocortisone 200–500 mg. Predominant wheezing without hypotension will respond to aminophylline 3–5 mg/kg.

Patients who have reacted previously to contrast medium and require a radiological procedure should be pretreated to reduce the incidence and severity of a reaction. If time permits, a combination of prednisone 50 mg orally six-hourly for two to three doses and diphenhydramine 50 mg IM given before the procedure is effective. In the emergency situation this will not be appropriate. It seems prudent to give hydrocortisone 200–500 mg IV before giving one of the newer contrast media. Pretreatment with H_1 and H_2 receptor antagonists (diphenhydramine 25–50 mg and cimetidine 200–400 mg) is supported by animal work but unproven in man. It is worth considering if a previous life–threatening reaction has occurred. An indwelling cannula and full facilities for resuscitation are, of course, mandatory for any radiological investigation requiring contrast medium.

Further reading

Branthwaite MA. Anaesthesia for diagnostic procedures. *Anaesthesia for Cardiac Surgery and Allied Procedures*. Oxford: Blackwell Scientific Publications, 1984; 39–58.

Campkin TV, Turner JM. Anaesthesia for neuroradiology. *Neurosurgical Anaesthesia and Intensive Care*. London: Butterworths, 1980; 71–84.

Goldberg M. Systemic reactions to intravascular contrast media. *Anesthesiology* 1984; **60**: 46–56.

9

General and Abdominal Surgery

Robert O Feneck

Pre-operative assessment and preparation
    Fluid and electrolyte balance
    Respiratory disease
    Cardiovascular disease
    Renal disease
    Other problems
Pre-operative laboratory investigations
Premedication
    Analgesics
    Anticholinergic drugs
    Benzodiazepines
    Phenothiazines
    Metoclopramide
    H_2-receptor antagonists
Anaesthetic considerations
    Regional or general anaesthesia
    Induction of anaesthesia
    Maintenance of anaesthesia
    Fluid balance during anaesthesia
    Termination of anaesthesia
Postoperative considerations
    Fluid balance
    Analgesia
    Physiotherapy
Implications of special conditions
    Diabetes
    Burst abdomen
    Acute pancreatitis
    The jaundiced patient

Pre-operative assessment and preparation

Fluid and electrolyte balance

Any ill patient will have a reduced or absent oral fluid intake; in combination with insensible losses this will lead eventually to abnormalities of fluid and electrolyte balance.

The gastrointestinal tract secretes eight litres of fluid every day, most of which is reabsorbed. Gastric juice is made up of two components. The secretion of the parietal or oxyntic cells consists of an isotonic solution of HCl, with a small and variable amount of NaCl and KCl, depending on the overall rate of secretion. The mucus secretion of the epithelial cells is rich in Na^+, K^+, and Cl^-, but this secretion is quantitatively much less than that of the oxyntic cells.

Mechanical obstruction at or near the pylorus produces repetitive vomiting and a loss predominantly of H^+ ions, Cl^- and water. Alkaline pancreatic and duodenal secretions are retained, and therefore the loss of H^+ ions produces a metabolic alkalosis. The loss of large amounts of Cl^- in the vomitus affects the renal handling of Na^+. Reabsorption of Na^+ takes place in the proximal tubules, for which Cl^- needs to be available since the only other anion present in significant amounts is HCO_3^- which cannot as easily pass the proximal tubular cell wall.

Therefore reabsorption of Na^+ now takes place lower in the tubule by exchange for K^+, and eventually for H^+ ions, resulting in the inappropriate secretion of an acid urine in a patient with a metabolic alkalosis.

The hypokalaemia is largely due to renal mechanisms, i.e. following low Cl^- concentration, with consequent exchange of Na^+ for K^+, and in response to secondary hyperaldosteronism following the loss of water. Also, any inherent acid–base converting ability within the kidney will be reduced by the lowered glomerular filtration rate following the loss of water.

High small intestinal obstruction presents a different picture. Absorption of saliva, bile, gastric, pancreatic and duodenal secretions is deranged causing a large loss of fluid. The loss of alkaline intestinal secretions as well as acid gastric secretions prevents the development of a metabolic alkalosis.

Indeed, the loss of such a large volume of fluid may produce peripheral circulatory failure and a metabolic acidosis. Loss of K^+ is marked; plasma K^+ levels are often very low. The loss of large volumes of fluid into the gut produces severe pain, abdominal distension and vomiting. The distension further stimulates intestinal secretion, and the gut wall becomes inflamed and swollen with protein-rich fluid, loses its muscle tone, and areas of patchy necrosis may develop which eventually will perforate.

The pre-operative management of these conditions is fortunately relatively straightforward. A nasogastric or wider bore oesophageal tube (e.g. size 12 – diameter 7 mm) is passed in order to empty the stomach. This helps to prevent repetitive vomiting, and decompresses the bowel rendering ischaemic necrosis less likely. The lost fluid should be replaced with isotonic (0.9 per cent) NaCl. This will replace losses of Na^+, Cl^-, and H_2O, and the improvement in the circulation will enable the kidney to convert the electrolyte and acid–base imbalance. Large volumes of NaCl are occasionally needed, but usually 1 litre should suffice. It is advisable to pass a urinary catheter to monitor urine output.

If hypokalaemia is present KCl should be added to the infusion to be given slowly, i.e. not more than 40 mmol K^+ / litre concentration, at a rate not exceeding 40 mmol K^+ /hr; use lower concentrations and rates of infusion whenever possible. Monitoring of serum K^+ concentration is by observation of the ECG (oscilloscope) and serial serum K^+ measurements. The serum K^+ should *always* be corrected before anaesthesia since hypokalaemia may cause cardiac dysrhythmias, hypotension and cardiac arrest. *Never* replace gastrointestinal losses with IV fluids containing no or low Na^+; this causes relative hyponatraemia.

Low small bowel obstruction presents a milder problem biochemically, as solutes and water are frequently reabsorbed above the obstruction.

Large bowel obstruction classically presents with pain, distension and relative or absolute constipation. Electrolyte imbalance and dehydration do not normally occur as a result of fluid losses; they may occur following reduced intake or for other reasons.

In addition to loss of extracellular fluid (ECF), blood may be lost into the gut lumen (haematemesis/melaena) or into the peritoneal cavity (trauma/bowel perforation, etc.). Circulatory volume deficit may be estimated from haemodynamic parameters; when severe, CVP monitoring is necessary. Adequate resuscitation of circulatory volume prior to anaesthesia is essential.

Respiratory disease

Abdominal distension causes elevation of the diaphragm, basal collapse with ventilation/perfusion mismatch and arterial hypoxaemia. This in combination with pain and anxiety produces a shallow rapid breathing and hypocapnia.

Many patients exhibit these features, but only occasionally is controlled oxygen therapy required. When oxygen is necessary, it should be humidified to minimize losses of heat and water vapour.

The respiratory consequences of the acute abdomen may be enough to precipitate acute respiratory failure in patients with chronic lung disease and poor respiratory reserve. Similarly, respiratory failure may develop postoperatively as a result of the residual effects of the anaesthetic, poor sputum clearance and inhibition of respiratory movement due to the abdominal incision (*see* Chapter 27).

Formal and comprehensive respiratory function tests are rarely possible or of great value in the emergency situation. A good assessment can be made by a history of the degree and duration of symptoms (cough, sputum production, dyspnoea) and of effort tolerance, and by clinical examination. Arterial blood gas analysis is often helpful; peak expiratory flow rate analysis, forced vital capacity and FEV_1 may be useful, but need patient co-operation. A pre-operative chest radiograph is mandatory.

At this stage, decisions on aspects of postoperative management should be taken; consider:

- a period of supportive intermittent positive pressure ventilation (IPPV)
- regional postoperative analgesia, e.g. continuous epidural block thus minimizing opiate-induced respiratory depression and maximizing pain relief and chest movement for physiotherapy
- intercostal blockade as an alternative.

Cardiovascular disease

Minor disturbances of cardiovascular function are not uncommon, usually as a result of fluid and electrolyte imbalance, and respond to simple treatment. Occasionally, large losses of ECF and K^+ cause severe hypotension and arrhythmias which may then become the presenting feature of the illness. Only when the haemodynamic disturbance is corrected is the acute abdomen unmasked.

More severe disturbances may be due to a number of factors, e.g. septicaemia, pulmonary embolus, myocardial infarction, etc. These patients may need pre-operative inotropic support, and extensive monitoring facilities should be available in the operating theatre. Anaesthesia for acute abdominal emergency surgery in the presence of recent myocardial infarction represents a considerable risk – much greater than that of myocardial revascularization procedures (*see* p. 5).

Patients with pre-existing valvular heart disease should be considered at risk from subacute bacterial endocarditis whatever operative procedure is undertaken. Appropriate antibiotics should be prescribed pre-operatively.

Patients with mesenteric embolus present a difficult problem. The fluid and electrolyte losses are often severe, and toxaemia develops due to bowel necrosis. In addition, the source of the embolus is often a complicating factor, i.e. from left atrium (due to atrial fibrillation from whatever cause), left ventricle (mural thrombus following recent infarction, LV aneurysm, etc) or rarely, disease of the mitral or aortic valves. Thus the clinical picture is of a severely ill patient, complicated by pre-existing cardiovascular disease. Full monitoring and supportive facilities should be available – the prognosis is often very poor.

Renal disease

In previously healthy individuals, losses of ECF and electrolytes will cause a degree of renal dysfunction which usually responds to simple treatment.

Patients with pre-existing renal disease may have an increased risk of developing an acute abdomen, for example due to adhesion formation from previous surgery, or following drug treatment (steroids, etc; *see* Chapter 25).

Other problems

The special problems of the diabetic and jaundiced patient are discussed on pp. 112 and 114.

Age-related neurological disease may co-exist in elderly patients with an acute abdomen. Problems of movement and physio-therapy in the postoperative period should be anticipated and minimized whenever possible.

Patients with Munchausen and other deceiver-syndromes present typically with an 'acute abdomen' since it is one of the easiest conditions to fake. These patients have no special anaesthetic implications.

Pre-operative laboratory investigations

* Haemoglobin concentration (Hb), packed cell volume (PCV) or haematocrit should be measured. In all but the simplest cases, blood should be taken for grouping; where necessary blood should be cross-matched.

- Blood urea and electrolyte measurements should be performed. This is especially *important* in patients with obstructed bowel or paralytic ileus.
- Liver function tests and blood sugar measurements should be carried out where appropriate (*see* p. 313).
- Serum amylase measurements should be made on any patients presenting as an atypical abdominal emergency in order to exclude acute haemorrhagic pancreatitis (*see* p. 114).
- Pre-operative chest radiography should be performed at the same time.
- Twelve-lead ECG and rhythm strip if appropriate.
- Simple respiratory function tests (FVC, FEV_1, peak expiratory flow rate) and arterial blood gas analysis as appropriate.
- Plain abdominal radiography used to be virtually the only surgical pre-operative investigation of an acute abdomen. Many procedures such as endoscopy, diagnostic real-time ultrasound, mesenteric angiography, CT scanning etc. are increasingly used as diagnostic aids.

Premedication

Analgesics

Severe visceral pain responds poorly to simple anti-inflammatory analgesics; morphine, pethidine (demerol) or their derivatives are more effective and in addition have a useful sedative and euphoric effect.

Morphine causes a greater increase in biliary pressure than pethidine, and causes an increase in poorly co-ordinated bowel contractility. Pethidine (demerol) may be preferred therefore for patients undergoing biliary surgery, or (more controversially), colonic anastomoses.

- All opiate drugs delay gastric emptying.
- All opiates have an emetic effect; there is little evidence to suggest that any one drug is better or worse in this respect.

Anticholinergic drugs

Anticholinergic drugs are frequently used to reduce salivary secretions, and to block the cardiac effects of vagal stimulation. This latter effect may be especially useful in patients undergoing laparotomy with peritoneal traction and consequent vagal stimulation.

Atropine and more particularly hyoscine (scopolamine) both cross the blood–brain barrier; hyoscine has the stronger sedative and anti-emetic effect, but may be poorly tolerated in the elderly. Glycopyrronium (glycopyrrolate) has a more prolonged action, but does not cross the blood–brain barrier and therefore exhibits no central effects.

All anticholinergic drugs decrease the tone of the lower oesophageal sphincter (LOS) thereby theoretically enhancing the danger of regurgitation; this effect is more pronounced after IV administration. Atropine 0.6 mg IM produces little effect on LOS pressure.

Benzodiazepines

In theory these drugs would appear to be useful as premedicants for pain-free patients, the sedative and amnesic effects being especially useful. In practice there are few such patients, and furthermore, whilst these drugs are normally well absorbed orally their intramuscular injection is painful and absorption can be unpredictable.

Patients with gastric stasis, repetitive vomiting and an acute abdomen should not be given oral premedicants; their absorption would be extremely poor.

Phenothiazines

These are useful drugs for counteracting the emetic effect of opiates, although their duration of anti-emetic action is frequently shorter than the emetic action of opiate drugs. They produce little effect on gastric emptying.

Metoclopramide

This drug has a number of potentially useful effects. It increases gastric emptying, inhibits the chemoreceptor trigger zone and the vomiting centre and is therefore a powerful anti-emetic, and increases the LOS tone thereby decreasing the risk of regurgitation.

- Prevention of regurgitation or vomiting in patients with an acute abdomen can be achieved better by decompressing the bowel with a nasogastric tube than by drugs.

H$_2$ receptor antagonists

The use of the histamine (H$_2$) receptor antagonists (cimetidine, ranitidine) to reduce oxyntic cell histamine secretion and thereby increase gastric pH has become widespread. These drugs do not affect the pH of gastric secretions already present, and therefore need to be given well in advance of surgery in order to increase the overall pH of the stomach contents (*see* p. 271).

The effect that these drugs have on the pH and volume of secretions in patients with an acute abdomen, and thus their role in this situation, is unclear.

Anaesthetic considerations

Regional or general anaesthesia

In practice, emergency intra-abdominal surgery does not lend itself to regional field block techniques for other than the most localized procedures, e.g. gastrostomy, inguinal herniorraphy, etc. The most feasible alternative to general anaesthesia is either intrathecal (spinal) or epidural analgesia. (*see* p. 254)

Advantages of intrathecal/epidural analgesia

- Provides good relaxation of abdominal wall.
- Normally provides contracted bowel.
- Less metabolic and endocrine response to anaesthesia and surgery than with general anaesthesia.
- Well maintained blood flow to bowel favours healing of anastomoses.
- Insertion of catheter acts as route for postoperative analgesia.

Disadvantages of intrathecal/epidural analgesia

- Sympathetic blockade in the presence of large ECF losses and low circulatory volume may produce catastrophic hypotension.
- Bowel distension due to an ileus associated with peritonitis will not be reduced.
- Peritoneal soiling may be enhanced if bowel is perforated.
- Difficulty/failure in achieving adequate blockade especially with upper abdominal surgery.

Induction of anaesthesia

- For minor procedures, anaesthesia with a mask and airway is acceptable provided that the patient has been adequately starved and gastrointestinal motility and function are normal.

- Intra-abdominal surgery requires profound relaxation of the abdominal wall muscle (except in old and debilitated patients); this necessitates controlled ventilation of the lungs to ensure adequate gas exchange. These two factors added to the risk of regurgitation, make endotracheal anaesthesia mandatory.
- A rapid sequence induction, i.e. preoxygenation, IV induction, cricoid pressure, muscular relaxation and endotracheal intubation is recommended.

Intravenous agents

- Drugs that act in one arm–brain circulation time are most appropriate, i.e. thiopentone, methohexitone, etomidate, propofol. There is evidence that thiopentone reduces barrier pressure (barrier pressure (BrP) = lower oesophageal pressure (LOS) — intragastric pressure (IGP); i.e. low BrP = increased risk of regurgitation) but no comparative evidence for the other drugs is available.
- Intravenous atropine causes a significant reduction in barrier pressure (BrP) after 5 min. Therefore this is not a problem if the drug is given at induction.
- In those patients with a large circulatory deficit and/or poor cardiac function, overdosage of induction agent may easily occur due to rapid administration. Assess the dosage and rate of administration accordingly.
- Following short surgical procedures, IV agents associated with a slow and smooth recovery from anaesthesia (e.g. thiopentone [thiopental]) appear to be associated with a lower incidence of vomiting.
- Those agents associated with a high frequency of excitatory effects during or after anaesthesia (ketamine, etomidate) or a rapid recovery (methohexitone [methohexital]) are associated with frequent sickness postoperatively.
- Methohexitone (methohexital) may cause more frequent vomiting during the emergence phase.
- Ketamine is a phenycyclidine derivative available for use IM or IV. Induction is accomplished one to two minutes after IV administration – slower after IM use. The drug has good sedative and analgesic properties, maintains haemodynamic parameters and may produce alveolar hyperventilation. Muscle tone is not reduced, and may be increased. Early suggestions of the preservation of protective airway reflexes have since proved unfounded; ketamine anaesthesia cannot be relied upon to provide effective protection of the airway

from stomach contents. Atropine should be given to reduce
salivation.

Muscle relaxants

- Suxamethonium (succinylcholine) in a dose of 1.5–2 mg/kg
  causes rapid onset of profound muscular relaxation for an
  acceptably short duration, and therefore provides excellent
  intubating conditions. Smaller doses are not advised because
  they may not be completely effective, especially in patients
  with a prolonged circulation time.
- Previously, it was thought that suxamethonium-induced
  fasciculations caused a rise in intragastric pressure (IGP) thus
  decreasing barrier pressure and increasing the tendency to
  reflux (BrP = LOS – IGP). Evidence in man suggests that
  although IGP increases, LOS pressure increases markedly
  causing an overall increase in BrP. The mechanism for the
  increase in LOS pressure is unclear.
- It would appear therefore that, unless specifically contra-
  indicated, suxamethonium is the drug of choice for emergency
  intubation of the patient with an acute abdomen.

Rapid acting nondepolarizing relaxants have been developed
which may be suitable alternatives to suxamethonium when
indicated. Atracurium, fazadinium, alcuronium and vecuronium
will also produce excellent intubation conditions. Atracurium and
vecuronium appear to be devoid of anticholinergic effects;
traction on viscera or the peritoneum may produce a severe bradycardia unless the vagus is blocked by prior atropinization.

Maintenance of anaesthesia

Diethyl ether and cyclopropane constitute a potential risk of explosion and therefore are contraindicated in the presence of
diathermy.

Chloroform has its advocates in some countries, but the
potential hepatoxicity and incidence of postoperative vomiting
render it unpopular. Calibrated vaporizers are not widely
available.

Trichloroethylene causes prolonged postoperative sickness and
delayed recovery from anaesthesia. It cannot be used with soda-
lime because a toxic product may be formed.

There appears to be little to choose between the more modern
agents for anaesthesia of the patient with an acute abdomen. Halothane, enflurane and isoflurane produce good anaesthetic
conditions at nontoxic concentrations.

Halothane has been shown to reduce mesenteric blood flow and gastrointestinal motility. However, comparative data for enflurane is not available. There is some evidence that isoflurane causes splanchnic vasodilatation, but the significance of this is uncertain.

Isoflurane, in common with halothane and enflurane potentiates the effect of nondepolarizing relaxants.

A wide range of narcotic and sedative drugs are available, which are commonly used in 'balanced' techniques consisting of controlled ventilation with O_2 and N_2O, intermittent bolus doses or, more recently, a continuous infusion of an opiate and/or a sedative/hypnotic, and a small increment of added volatile agent.

- For patients undergoing controlled ventilation of the lungs, the maintenance of normocapnia or very mild hypocapnia should be the rule. This minimizes difficulties in re-establishing spontaneous ventilation and prevents the marked decrease in bowel blood flow seen following hypocapnia. The use of the Bain type of co-axial breathing system removes the need for an exogenous source of carbon dioxide, provided that the recommended fresh gas flow is used.

Fluid balance during anaesthesia

There may be a fluid and electrolyte deficit to make good despite IV rehydration pre-operatively. This can be calculated by the following:

Water Deficit
Normal body water $= 0.6 \times$ body wt in kg
Present body water $= \dfrac{\text{normal serum Na}^+ \times \text{normal body water}}{\text{present serum Na}^+}$
$\therefore$ body water deficit = normal body water – present body water

Sodium deficit
Na$^+$ deficit =
normal serum Na$^+$ – present serum Na$^+$ $\times$ 0.2 $\times$ body wt (kg)

Chloride deficit
Cl$^-$ deficit =
normal serum Cl$^-$ – present serum Cl$^-$ $\times$ 0.2 $\times$ body wt (kg)

Potassium deficit
K$^+$ deficit –
normal plasma K$^+$ – present plasma K$^+$ $\times$ 0.4 $\times$ body wt (kg).

Bicarbonate deficit

HCO_3^- required (mmol) = base deficit $\times$ body wt (kg) $\times$ 0.3

- Many of these deficiencies are inter-related, and consideration therefore on an individual basis is unhelpful. In practice, the deficit is often replaced by 500–1000 ml crystalloid; preferably Hartmann's solution or isotonic saline (*see* p. 58).
- *In addition* to this, maintenance requirements during anaesthesia must be provided. A simple regimen consists of 2–4 ml/kg/hr. This regimen, taken *in addition* to replacement of deficit, frequently yields values (for a 70 kg adult) of 700 ml for the first hour of operation, followed by 140–280 ml/hr thereafter.

Alternatively, deficit and maintenance requirements may be replaced at the rate of 10 ml/kg/hr for the first hour of operation, followed by up to 5 ml/kg/hr thereafter. Thus a 70 kg man receives 700 ml/hr for the first hour, followed by up to 350 ml/hr thereafter.

Blood or blood products, and other colloid solutions (gelatine, 5 per cent albumin, etc.) should be used to replenish extensive blood and plasma losses. The debate of crystalloid versus colloid replacement continues unabated. A haematocrit of between 35–40 per cent is a satisfactory balance between ensuring adequate blood oxygen carrying capacity and preventing tissue hypoperfusion due to alteration in blood viscosity.

Where appropriate, central venous or pulmonary capillary wedge pressure will enable adequate volume replacement to be made.

Termination of anaesthesia

Anticholinesterase/anticholinergic combinations have effects on the gastrointestinal tract. Atropine decreases LOS pressure (making postoperative regurgitation more likely) but this effect is antagonized by neostigmine. Neostigmine causes a profound increase in bowel motility and intraluminal pressure, and decreases mesenteric blood flow – effects partially antagonized by atropine. In addition, the durations of action of the two drugs when given together IV are not identical; neostigmine lasts longer.

It may be useful to use a longer acting anticholinergic i.e. glycopyrronium (glycopyrolate) or if possible to avoid neostigmine altogether. Atracurium may be useful in this respect, since its action is terminated by spontaneous (Hoffman) elimination rather than by metabolism and/or excretion. However, if in doubt about residual paralysis reversal agents should always be given (*see* p. 346).

Opiate overdosage may be reversed by intravenous naloxone if necessary. It should be remembered that the duration of naloxone is short.

Following comprehensive oropharyngeal suction, extubation should be performed in the lateral position with a slight head-down tilt. Further suction should be immediately available. Extubation should be performed 'light' when protective airway reflexes have returned; a positive pressure technique, i.e. extubation at the end of a full inspiration, is recommended.

Postoperative considerations

The immediate postoperative management will be influenced by pre-operative factors, the duration and magnitude of surgery, the severity of blood loss, haemodynamic function and metabolic and other factors (*see* Chapter 28).

The sickest patients will be returned to the ICU for a period of supportive IPPV and stabilization. Simple cases may be returned to the recovery room for a short time prior to returning to the ward.

Fluid balance

Appropriate crystalloid replacement should be given:

100 ml/kg/24hr for the first 10 kg body weight
50 ml/kg/24hr for the next 10 kg body weight
25 ml/kg/24hr thereafter

i.e. for 70 kg man approximately 110 ml/hr

The effects of anaesthesia and intra-abdominal surgery are to retain water and Na^+, therefore care must be taken not to over-hydrate the patient.

Central venous lines may be kept open with small volumes of 5 per cent dextrose. Blood or colloid should be given as appropriate. Protein losses may be marked in the early postoperative period.

When postoperative starvation is likely, i.e. following major bowel resections, IV feeding regimens should be started early.

Analgesia

Adequate postoperative analgesia is essential (*see* Chapters 21 and 28).

Regional techniques

Intercostal blockade is useful for high abdominal procedures; however, repeated blocks are uncomfortable for the patient and may be ineffective.

Epidural local analgesia is particularly useful for patients with borderline respiratory function. Catheter placement allows for prolonged administration of local anaesthetics either by intermittent bolus dose or by continuous infusion. Close monitoring of haemodynamic parameters is needed, since sympathetic blockade may produce profound hypotension especially in the presence of even mild hypovolaemia.

Systemic analgesics

Opiate analgesics are useful after abdominal surgery. It would appear that opiate drugs given by any route will delay gastric emptying and cause postoperative intolerance of food and fluids, when compared with regional analgesics.

The extent to which this may be modified by the simultaneous administration of metoclopramide, which of the opiates is least problematic in this respect, and whether the newer more potent anti-inflammatory analgesics will prove any better are all unanswered questions.

The routes available for postoperative opiate administration are as follows:

sublingual (e.g. buprenorphine)
oral – usually inappropriate
IM – nurse administered, either regularly or by patient demand
IV – either patient or physician controlled
epidural – novel but still controversial idea
rectal – rarely used in UK or USA. Hepatic first-pass
   clearance rate may be altered with this route.

Physiotherapy

Chest physiotherapy is important in all patients following high abdominal surgery. Basal collapse of the lungs occurs early in the postoperative period, and physiotherapy with positive pressure breathing should be commenced as soon as possible.

Implications of special conditions

Diabetes

Diabetics undergoing surgery tend to be a high risk group. They are likely to be over the age of 50 years, and have an increased incidence of circulatory and renal disease, and obesity when compared to the nondiabetic. In addition, up to 25 per cent of diabetics on a surgical ward may present as newly discovered cases.

Diabetics are at least as likely to require emergency surgery as the rest of the population. If pre-operative assessment indicates co-existent diabetic coma, precoma or severe metabolic derangement, surgery must be delayed until the metabolic status of the patient has been improved. This is especially true of patients with a surgical acute abdomen. Severe abdominal pain in a diabetic may be caused by ketoacidosis; the pain may disappear with appropriate treatment of the ketoacidosis.

Pre-operative work-up should be carried out with the help of a diabetologist or endocrinologist where appropriate.

Therapy during operation should be directed towards maintaining adequate pre-operative control. An idea of the insulin and glucose likely to be required will be gained from pre-operative requirements.

Insulin, glucose and K^+ may be delivered easily in one of two ways:

(a) 5–20 (normally 10) i.u. insulin + 1–2 g KCl in 500 ml 5 or 10 per cent dextrose.

Deliver over 5 hr, i.e. normally 2 i.u./hr. Adjust according to regular blood glucose measurements.

Or:

(b) 50 i.u. insulin in 50 ml Haemaccel administered via syringe pump (preferably a device capable of giving less than 1 ml/hr.

Give at 0.5–2 i.u. insulin/hr, dependent on blood sugar.

Adjust rate accordingly.

In addition, give 1–2 g KCl in 500 ml 5–10 per cent dextrose over 5 hr.

Insulin should not be added to solutions in glass bottles as it is absorbed onto the glass. The same is true, to a lesser extent, of plastic. A strong solution of insulin in albumin or gelatine minimizes this problem.

Insulin via syringe pump is flexible, and appears to solve the absorption problem. However, pump failure or maladjustment can produce no insulin or profound hypoglycaemia.

Insulin/glucose/K^+ solutions are safe, since turning the infusion on or off stops all three components. They are not as flexible – if insulin dose needs to be adjusted the solution may need to be changed. Absorption still causes a problem.

Postoperatively, therapy should continue until the patient can take food and diabetes can be controlled normally. If fluid restriction is necessary, 20 per cent or stronger glucose solutions may be used, but should be given via a central venous line.

- The pre- and early postoperative monitoring of diabetic control should *always* be carried out by blood sugar estimations; never rely on urinary glucose estimations alone.

Burst abdomen

Wound breakdown occurs usually as a result of infection, although surgical and anaesthetic technique, and the general health of the patient may be influential.

It is notoriously difficult to assess the extent of the problem on superficial examination. A small piece of prolapsed omentum or bowel should be taken as a warning that the whole abdominal incision may need to be re-examined and resutured.

It is essential therefore to treat such cases as emergencies requiring a rapid sequence induction, endotracheal anaesthesia with full muscular relaxation, and appropriate supportive and monitoring facilities.

Acute pancreatitis

This occurs classically in the obese, middle aged or elderly; women are more commonly affected than men.

Trauma, infection, biliary obstruction, alcoholism and local vasculitis have all been postulated as aetiological factors. Many of these have important anaesthetic implications in their own right.

The afflicted patient is in severe and constant abdominal pain. Profuse vomiting and peripheral circulatory shutdown may occur. Glycosuria may occur, due to islet cell damage. Hypoglycaemia may occur resulting in further deterioration of circulatory function and difficulty in reversing nondepolarizing neuromuscular relaxants.

Serum amylase should be measured in order to exclude acute pancreatitis in anyone with atypical and severe abdominal pain. These patients are bad anaesthetic risks no matter what agents or methods are used.

The jaundiced patient

These patients may present for any surgical procedure, but commonly anaesthesia is required for surgery on the hepatobiliary system. The pre-operative state can be assessed more simply by attention to the following:

presence and grading of hepatic coma,
presence of ascites,
the bilirubin concentration,
the serum albumin concentration,
the prothrombin time.

- In the emergency case, anticholinergic premedication is often all that is required. If necessary, small doses of opiates (e.g. pethidine (demerol)) or benzodiazepines may be given by the appropriate route. If analgesic/sedative premedication is used, its effect should be noted carefully.
- Reduction in splanchnic blood flow occurs following regional or general anaesthesia; attention must be paid to good technique, the avoidance of hypotension, hypoxia and venous hypertension and the maintenance of normocapnia during IPPV. Cyclopropane and chloroform should be avoided; other volatile agents including halothane, are acceptable.
- Highly protein (globulin) bound drugs may be required in increased dosage.
- Vitamin K and fresh frozen plasma may be required to counteract coagulation abnormalities.
- Postoperative renal failure following anaesthesia and surgery is a well-documented entity. Suggested aetiological factors include hypoxia, decrease in renal blood flow during anaesthesia, a toxic effect of bilirubin on the kidney and the effect on the kidney of endotoxin from the patient's own bowel flora. This latter appears the most likely.
- Active measures should be taken to prevent renal damage. A urinary catheter should be passed. If the serum bilirubin level is between 20–140 μmol/litre a urinary output of 50 ml/hr should be maintained. To achieve this, 10 per cent mannitol should be used, e.g. 100–500 ml as appropriate. In addition, antibiotics should be given if the serum bilirubin is above 140 μmol/litre. In these patients mannitol will certainly be necessary, and should be continued postoperatively.
- Mannitol (*see* p. 59) appears to be more effective than the other diuretics (e.g. frusemide [furosemide]) and fluid loading in this situation. However, the danger of circulatory overload is real, and central venous pressure monitoring should be used to guard against this.
- Other supportive measures, e.g. a period of postoperative IPPV should be instituted where necessary.

Further reading

Alberti KG, Thomas DJ. The management of diabetes during surgery. *Br. J. Anaesth.* 1979; **51**: 693–710.

Smith G, Hall GM (eds). Symposium on the gastrointestinal tract. *Br. J. Anaesth.* 1984; **56**: 1–101.

Strunin L, Davies H. The liver and anaesthesia. *Canad. Anaesth. Soc. J.* 1983; **30**: 208–21.

Strunin L, Pettingale KW. Renal disease. In: Vickers MD (ed). *Medicine for Anaesthetists, 2nd ed.* Oxford: Blackwell, 1982; 133–53.

10

Orthopaedics

Jeremy N Cashman

Specific problems
    Acrylic cement
    Alcohol intoxication
    Blood loss
    Embolism
    Intravenous regional block (IVRB)
    Patient position
    Tourniquets
Specific conditions
    Femoral neck surgery
    Microsurgical techniques
    Multiple trauma
    Spinal cord injuries

Emergency orthopaedic operations may constitute as much as one third of the emergency work-load in an average hospital. The scope varies from young patients who have suffered relatively minor trauma to victims of major trauma and elderly patients who have sustained fractures of fragile long bones. However, true orthopaedic emergencies which constitute a risk to a limb, and which require urgent surgical intervention are rare; examples include fractures involving blood vessels within a joint, fractures in children (especially supracondylar fractures), severe compound fractures such as those occurring as a result of industrial accidents, blast or gunshot injury, and compartment syndromes requiring urgent fasciotomy. A compartment syndrome is a condition in which high pressure within a closed fascial space reduces the capillary blood perfusion to a level below that needed for tissue viability.

This chapter draws attention to some of the more common problems encountered in orthopaedic surgery and suggests guidelines for their treatment. Specific operations which may present problems for emergency anaesthesia are also discussed.

Specific problems

Acrylic cement

A transient fall in arterial blood pressure associated with the insertion of acrylic cement is frequently observed. In the poor risk elderly patient this can precipitate cardiac arrest. Possible causative factors include:

- Fat or air embolism
- Neurogenic stimuli
- Hypersensitivity to methylmethacrylate monomer.

A greater cardiovascular disturbance has been reported when cement is used for emergency (Thompson's) prosthesis as opposed to elective (total hip) prosthesis. However, the operative mortality is the same whether or not acrylic cement is used to anchor an emergency prosthesis. It is suggested that cement is associated with an increased risk when used in trauma due, amongst other factors, to the hormonal stress response, dehydration and hypovolaemia. General supportive measures of the circulation are usually adequate, paying special attention to maintaining hydration; the patient may be placed in the Trendelenburg position if necessary.

Alcohol intoxication

Acute

In acute haemorrhage there may be loss of the respiratory compensation to metabolic acidosis, resulting in more profound shock. In addition, acute alcohol intoxication is associated with depression of the central nervous, cardiovascular and respiratory systems. Therefore reduced doses of anaesthetic agents should be used. Gluconeogenesis is impaired and hypoglycaemia can occur; a glucose infusion with monitoring of the blood sugar is advised.

Chronic

Alcohol at blood concentrations found in chronic alcoholics has been shown to inhibit platelet aggregation and thromboxane release and thus have a mildly anticoagulating effect. This may explain the lower incidence of thromboembolism in this group of patients. Derangement of clotting can also occur if there is associated liver damage.

- Larger doses of intravenous induction agents and of other highly protein-bound drugs may be required, but the reduction in plasma cholinesterase means that suxamethonium may be associated with a more prolonged action.
- Volatile agents which markedly impair the splanchnic circulation (e.g. cyclopropane), and those drugs which undergo significant hepatic metabolism (e.g. halothane), should be avoided.
- Alcoholic cardiomyopathy may be an added complication.

Blood loss

Whenever possible hypovolaemia should be corrected prior to surgery. The amount of fluid to administer is guided by the systemic pressure, cardiac filling pressure and urine output. A closed fracture of the femur can lose up to 1 litre of blood into the thigh and a severe fracture of the pelvis may lose 2 litres of blood into the retroperitoneal tissue. Whole blood is the fluid of choice, despite some deficiencies of banked blood (*see* Chapter 3). Both the US army in Vietnam and the British army in the Falklands used uncross-matched or limited group compatible blood for battle casualties without problems. However, pending the availability of cross-matched blood, large volumes of crystalloid can safely be used for the initial resuscitation. The administration of 3–4 litres of balanced salt solution in excess of the volume of blood required, is recommended to correct deficits of intravascular and extra-cellular volume. All fluids should be warmed.

Embolism

Air embolism

Air may enter the circulation when the femoral prosthesis is forced into the shaft of the femur. Air enters via open venous plexi in the bone and causes profound haemodynamic collapse. A mill wheel murmur can often be heard through an oesophageal stethoscope, although ultrasound may be more sensitive. The ECG and end-tidal carbon dioxide changes will also be evident.

The patient's lungs should be ventilated with 100 per cent oxygen for some minutes before the insertion of the prosthesis (to remove nitrous oxide from the circulation), and the femoral shaft should be vented. It may be possible to aspirate air from a right atrial line. The patient should be repositioned on the left side if possible.

Fat embolism

Most commonly associated with fractures of the lower limb and pelvis, and characterized by the deposition of fat droplets in the lungs, brain and skin. Has a high mortality. Fat emboli cause a 25 per cent increase in respiratory dead space and a reduction in lung compliance leading to hypoxia and hypercapnia. It is suggested that in emergency hip surgery the medullary cavity should be aspirated before any cement is inserted.

General supportive measures, including oxygen therapy and artificial ventilation should be instituted. Low molecular weight dextran (*see* p. 60) and corticosteroids have proved beneficial in treatment, whilst heparin and clofibrate have also been advocated.

Thromboembolism

The incidence of deep venous thrombosis (DVT) after lower extremity trauma is between 40 and 60 per cent in patients over the age of 40 years, and the incidence of pulmonary embolism is 5–10 per cent of this group. Most of the deaths from thromboembolism occur in patients of 50 years or older (UK Registrar General's figures).

It is disturbing to note that in one study 33 per cent of patients developed fresh thrombus formation despite apparently adequate prophylaxis. Low dose heparin has been shown to have only limited effectiveness in orthopaedic surgery. A dose of 5000 units SC 8-hourly, was inferior to oral anticoagulants, aspirin or dextran. There was no significant difference between warfarin (to a prothrombin ratio of 1.5–2.0 normal), aspirin (600 mg twice daily, commenced pre-operatively) and dextran 40 or 70 (500 ml intra-operatively and 500 ml daily for two to five days post-operatively). However, both dextran and warfarin are associated with greater intra-operative bleeding and postoperative wound haematomas than aspirin. Dextran is also associated with a risk of circulatory overload.

Intravenous regional block (IVRB)

First popularized by August Bier in 1908. Most useful for operations on the upper limb but can also be used for operations on the lower limb. Cuff failure may result in toxic levels of local anaesthetic in the circulation and can precipitate cardiac arrest.

Toxicity has been reported with both lignocaine (lidocaine) and bupivacaine, the latter being particularly difficult to treat due to its high affinity for cardiac tissue. Prilocaine 0.5 per cent is currently the agent of choice. Rapid injection of local anaesthetic or injection of a large volume (especially if the limb has not been completely exsanguinated) can generate sufficiently high venous pressures to exceed the cuff pressure; this problem is compounded the more proximally the injection is made. For all of these reasons brachial plexus block may be preferred (*see* p. 258).

Patient position

Patients often have to be placed in awkward positions. All contact points should be protected with padding. Warming mattresses should be used. The patient should be made immobile, since often quite considerable leverage and traction forces may be exerted during the course of the operation.

Tourniquets

Used to provide a bloodless surgical field. The tourniquet is inflated to a pressure 35–50 mmHg in excess of systolic pressure for the arm and 50–70 mmHg in excess of systolic for the leg. Direct pressure damage to nerves is likely, especially in very thin patients, and these points of contact should be protected with padding.

Safe duration is a function of the absolute amount that the inflation pressure exceeds systolic. A maximum inflation time of 1 hr for the upper limb and 1½ hr for the lower limb is recommended. Tourniquets may not be effective in patients with calcified vessels. They should be avoided in patients with peripheral vascular disease and sickle cell disease.

Specific conditions

Femoral neck surgery

Fracture of the femoral neck is the commonest cause of death from violence over the age of 75 years (UK Registrar General, 1971). The estimated cost of treatment of this one type of fracture in the UK represents nearly one per cent of the total National Health Service (NHS) budget. Although a delay of up to one week after subcapital fracture of the femur does not significantly affect the outcome of surgery, the mortality increases when operation is delayed beyond three days after the injury. Mortality has been reported as varying between 7 and 22 per cent up to six weeks following operation.

The suggestion that mortality after surgical repair of hip fracture may be decreased if regional rather than general anaesthetic techniques are used, remains controversial. In a recent study[1] it was shown that there was a significantly lower mortality by 14 days after surgery in patients who had received spinal anaesthesia, compared to a group who had received a general anaesthetic. However, after two months the mortality rates were similar with either anaesthetic technique. Mortality is higher in males than females, increases with increasing age and in patients with intercurrent medical conditions. In addition these patients are often suffering from hypothermia.

The extremely poor risk patient may be managed by employing a femoral nerve block together with skin infiltration (*see* p. 253).

In the case of subarachnoid anaesthesia employing hyperbaric spinal solutions, the patient will need to be positioned on the side of the fracture for the institution of the block. An alternative is to use an isobaric solution which allows the patient to be positioned with the fracture uppermost for the institution of the block. Scrupulous attention should be paid to maintaining the patient's blood pressure at pre-anaesthetic levels. Prophylactic intramuscular vasopressors (e.g. ephedrine), have been advocated. Additional sedation can be provided by diazepam or ketamine.

Epidural and spinal techniques are associated with a significantly reduced incidence of postoperative thromboembolism in elderly patients as a result of dilatation of the blood vessels in the lower limb. This may explain the apparent initial advantage (in terms of morbidity and mortality), of these techniques. In addition, these techniques attenuate or abolish the 'stress response' to surgery.

Significant and prolonged hypoxia has been shown to occur in elderly patients who have received a general anaesthetic for surgical correction of fracture of femur. This is due to venous admixture to arterial blood and to ventilation–perfusion ($\dot{V}/\dot{Q}$) mismatch, which causes a reduction in functional residual capacity and hence small airways closure. Positive pressure ventilation in the course of anaesthesia will tend to ventilate preferentially the uppermost lung segments which are the least perfused and so exacerbate $\dot{V}/\dot{Q}$ mismatch. Therefore a technique based on spontaneous ventilation would seem to be preferred. Doxapram is not effective in improving the hypoxia occurring after femoral neck surgery, however, it does have very marked analeptic properties, probably reflecting the very light level of anaesthesia employed in these patients.

Microsurgical techniques

Includes nerve and tendon repair and limb/digit replantation. Nerve injuries are classified into three groups:

- Neuropraxia; a minor injury with no loss of axonal continuity.
- Axonotmesis; injury with loss of axonal continuity but no loss of axonal alignment.
- Neurotmesis; injury with loss of both axonal continuity and alignment. This injury requires surgical repair.

Microsurgical operations tend to be very prolonged. Hence special care must be paid to maintaining patient temperature (*viz* high ambient temperature, warmed and humidified anaesthetic gases and warmed intravenous fluids), also care of pressure areas and thromboembolism prophylaxis. Maintaining fluid balance may also be a problem.

In general some form of local or systemic vasodilator therapy will be required since vasodilatation has been shown to enhance survival of revascularized tissues. This can be provided by local anaesthetic blocks; either specific sympathetic blockade or as part of an analgesic block for surgery. Catheter techniques will be needed due to the long duration of surgery.

- Adrenaline (epinephrine) should *not* be employed to prolong the duration of block.

A catheter technique of brachial plexus block suitable for upper limb surgery has been described. Intravenous regional block is useful postoperatively for the prevention of spasm and in this context guanethidine (15–30 mg) may be particularly useful since it induces vasodilatation for up to three days. Specific sympathetic blocks suffer from the disadvantage of being 'single-shot' and thus require repeated injection; there is also a high risk of complications such as intrathecal injection. Systemic vasodilators may alternatively be used, including alpha-adrenergic blocking agents, but their side-effects make them difficult to use.

If general anaesthesia is employed there is the risk of potential organ toxicity resulting from prolonged administration of anaesthestic gases and vapours. Isoflurane appears to be the preferred agent.

Multiple trauma

Also called 'polytrauma'. The most obvious injury may not necessarily be the most life threatening. Thus definitive orthopaedic treatment of fractures may need to be delayed whilst dealing with more physiologically damaging injuries.

Trauma score (American Trauma Society)[2]

This is a numerical grading system for estimating the severity of injury. The scoring system uses the Glasgow Coma Scale (GCS, *see* p. 134) reduced to approximately one-third value, and measurements of cardiopulmonary function. Each indicator is assigned a number (low for impaired function, high for normal function. Summation of the numbers estimates the severity of the injury and total trauma scores may be used to estimate survival (Table 10.1).

Table 10.1 Trauma scores

	GCS scores	Trauma scores
Glasgow	14–15	5
Coma	11–13	4
Scale	8–10	3
(p. 134)	5–7	2
	3–4	1
Respiratory	10–24/min.	4
rate	25–35/min.	3
	>36/min.	2
	1–9 /min.	1
Respiratory	Normal	1
expansion	Retractive/none	0
(use of accessory muscles or intercostal retraction)		
Systolic	>90 mmHg	4
blood	70–89 mmHg	3
pressure	50–69 mmHg	2
(either arm,	0–49 mmHg	1
auscultate or palpate)	No carotid pulse	0
Capillary	Normal (<2 sec)	2
refill	Delayed (>2 sec)	1
	None	0
Total score		1–16

Trauma score	16	15	14	13	12	11	10	9	8	7	6	5	4	3	2	1
Percentage survival	99	98	96	93	87	76	60	42	26	15	8	4	2	1	0	0

- Patients should already be receiving oxygen, and may well have been intubated prior to surgery.
- Tension pneumothorax is a risk and should always be suspected if there is a sudden deterioration in the patient's condition.

If necessary ketamine-suxamethonium can be used for the intubation sequence. Suxamethonium (succinylcholine) is contra-indicated if there is massive tissue damage which can be associated with the release of large amounts of potassium.

- Facilities should be available for immediate tracheostomy (*see* p. 203), especially if there are associated maxillofacial or laryngeal injuries.
- Sedative premedicant drugs should be avoided, but often these patients will have already received a narcotic for analgesia; this will increase the risk of aspiration of gastric contents.

Recent evidence that the administration of naloxone is of bene-fit in non-narcotized, shocked animals, suggests that endorphins and thus perhaps narcotics are detrimental in such circum-stances.

Anaesthesia can be maintained with ketamine either given as repeated intramuscular injections or as an infusion. Alternatively small amounts of an inhalational agent, of which isoflurane is probably the best, can be used. Use 100 per cent oxygen but remember the risk of oxygen toxicity. Acidosis will often reverse with resuscitation, otherwise it should be corrected with bicarbonate. The preponderance of victims of major trauma will be young and thus the CVP is an adequate reflection of the left-sided cardiac filling pressure. Time should not be wasted in insert-ing pulmonary artery catheters. Massive transfusion will often be necessary; it is advisable to filter all blood and to administer calcium and fresh frozen plasma early.

Spinal cord injuries

The annual incidence of spinal cord injury has been reported to be between 8.1 and 16.6 traumatic spinal cord injured cases per million of population. In the UK there are only about 350 new cases a year of injuries to the vertebral column involving the spinal cord or nerve roots. The majority of these occur as a result of road traffic accidents.

- Since the majority of spinal injuries are not admitted directly to a specialist spinal injuries unit the injuries are often not immediately recognized, with subsequent deterioration in neurological function.

The place of early surgery in the management of acute spinal injuries remains controversial. Initial management in the vast majority of cases is conservative, but is abandoned in favour of surgical intervention if there is progression of neurological deficit as indicated by the Yale scale, or if there is marked instability of the fracture site. There is evidence that immediate surgery to stabilize the thoraco–lumbar spine (either by fusion or by fixation such as with Harrington rods), may salvage some otherwise lost neural function. Pneumothorax is a risk in posterior (thoracic) spinal fusion operations. Patients may also require anaesthesia for operative treatment of associated injuries.

Raising the blood pressure to within normal limits may produce a significant improvement in cord recovery.

- Hypotension can occur as a result of blood loss or the 'spinal shock syndrome'.

This syndrome, first described in 1841, may develop in acute injuries to the cervical or upper thoracic regions, usually after a delay of 24 hr. The central sympathetic control is lost and venomotor relaxation leads to bradycardia and hypotension, thus large volumes of fluid and alpha adrenergic agents may be needed to maintain blood pressure.

Intubation should be performed in the 'neutral' position, excessive flexion or extension of the cervical spine should be avoided. A difficult intubation should be anticipated and appropriate precautions taken. Awake intubation is best avoided if there is any likelihood of an associated head injury. As a last resort the technique described by Waters of passing a catheter retrogradely up from the larynx may be employed (*see* p. 78). Suxamethonium (succinylcholine) can be used for intubation since there is no evidence that muscle membrane instability develops within the first few hours following a denervation injury. Massive release of potassium following suxamethonium and leading to cardiac arrest only occurs after at least 24 hr have elapsed. Prior treatment with a small dose of a nondepolarizing relaxant may attenuate the hyperkalaemic response (large doses are required to completely abolish the response).

Sellick's manoeuvre (cricoid pressure) is often difficult to apply in the presence of a cervical injury.

Ventilatory impairment due to associated lung trauma can occur. Cervical cord transection produces intercostal paralysis, but if the lesion is at or above C_4, the diaphragm will also be paralysed. Intermittent positive pressure ventilation may cause a fall in blood pressure as a result of autonomic hyperreflexia, thus an I/E ratio of 1:2 has been recommended.

Other problems include: neurogenic pulmonary oedema, the patient behaves as if poikilothermic, DVT leading to pulmonary embolism (especially with high spinal injury), fat embolism and the problems of massive transfusion.

Finally some success in spinal cord resuscitation has been claimed for the new technique of local spinal cord hypothermia which involves applying cold perfusate at 3°C extradurally to the injured cord through a posterior laminectomy. The practical application is, however, difficult to implement.

Reference

1. McKenzie PJ, Wishart HY, Smith G. Long term outcome after fractured neck of femur. Comparison of subarachnoid and general anaesthesia *Br. J. Anaesth.* 1984; **56**: 581–84.
2. Champion HR, Sacco WJ, Carnazzo AJ, Copes W, Fouty WJ. Trauma score. *Crit. Care Med.* 1981; **9**: 672–6.

Further reading

Bird TM, Strunin L. Anaesthetic considerations for microsurgical repair of limbs. *Canad. Anaesth. Soc. J.* 1984; **31**: 51–60.

Fraser A, Edmonds-Seal J. Spinal cord injuries – a review of the problems facing the anaesthetist. *Anaesthesia* 1982; **37**: 1084–98.

Gallacher TJ, Civetta JM. The multiple trauma patient: assessment and anaesthesia. In: Miller RD, Kirby RR, Ostheimer GW, Saidman LV, Stoelting RK (eds). *Yearbook of Anaesthesia*. Chicago: Yearbook Medical Publishers, 1984; Ch.4: 89–131.

Loach A. (ed). *Anaesthesia for orthopaedic patients*. Current Topics in Anaesthesia – 7. London: Edward Arnold, 1983.

Waters FJM, Nott MR. The hazards of anaesthesia in the injured patient. *Br. J. Anaesth.* 1977; **49**: 707–20.

Weiskopf RB, Fairley HB. Anesthesia for major trauma. *Surg. Clin. of N. Amer.* 1982; **62**: 31–45.

11

Neuroanaesthesia and Head Injury

Robert W McPherson

Evaluation of the head-injured patient
  Airway
  Breathing
  Circulation
  Glasgow Coma Scale (GCS)
Support and resuscitation during diagnostic evaluation
Fluid management
Anaesthetic agents
Haematology
Neurological monitoring
Anaesthesia in patients with possible head injury

Successful resuscitation of patients with head injury is based on simple principles. Cerebral blood flow (CBF) is determined by the perfusion pressure, usually mean arterial blood pressure (MABP) minus intracranial pressure (ICP), and oxygen delivery to the brain is determined by cerebral blood flow × arterial oxygen content. Since many of the parameters of adequate CBF and oxygen delivery to the brain are unknown or changing rapidly, a conservative approach to maximize brain perfusion should be taken (Table 11.1).

Head trauma may cause usual brain compensatory mechanisms such as autoregulation (constant blood flow over wide range of perfusion pressure) to fail, thus blood flow to the brain passively follows the perfusion pressure. Emphasis will be placed on care of patients with acute head injury requiring rapid resuscitation and definitive care such as airway management (tracheal intubation) and surgical decompression.

Preservation of neural function must be of high priority in the trauma patient. Every aspect of resuscitation must be considered with respect to effect on spinal cord and brain preservation. If

Table 11.1 Cerebral physiology

Autoregulation	= Maintenance of constant blood flow over a wide range of perfusion pressure. Normal limits 60–150 mmHg.
Hypoxic response	− Cerebral blood flow increases to maintain oxygen delivery. Arterial oxygen content is more important than Pa_{O_2}.
Carbon dioxide response	− Cerebral blood flow is linearly related to Pa_{CO_2} between 20 and 60 mmHg.
Cerebral perfusion pressure	= Mean arterial blood pressure − intracranial pressure
Cerebral oxygen delivery	= Cerebral blood flow × arterial oxygen content

Arterial oxygen content (ml/dl)

$$= \left(\frac{Hb\ (g/dl)}{100} \times 1.36 \times \frac{\%\ saturation}{100} \right) + \begin{array}{l} dissolved \\ oxygen \end{array}$$

Dissolved oxygen (ml/dl) $= Pa_{O_2}$ (mmHg) $\times\ 0.003$

instituted judiciously, cerebral preservation techniques do not seriously affect the successful resuscitation of other organ systems. The impact of secondary insults on the outcome of neurological injury is unclear, but physiological abnormalities (hypoxia, hypotension) which might contribute to injury are common in multiple trauma victims.

The following management suggestions will be directed at either preserving adequate cerebral perfusion pressure (CPP) or brain oxygen delivery in patients at risk of neurological injury.

Evaluation of the head-injured patient

Airway

The adequacy of spontaneous ventilation should be quickly assessed. If adequate spontaneous ventilation ($Pa_{CO_2} < 40$ mmHg, (5.3 kPa)) can be maintained for even a few minutes, tracheal intubation can be accomplished in a more controlled manner.

- Even if adequate ventilation is present ($Pa_{O_2} > 80$ mmHg, 11 kPa; Pa_{CO_2}, < 40 mmHg 5.3 kPa), absence of airway reflexes requires that the patient be intubated to prevent aspiration of stomach contents.
- Patency of the airway should be assessed using conventional criteria (tracheal retraction in the suprasternal notch, normal tidal volume).

- If facial injuries are present, tracheostomy or cricothyroid-otomy should be considered rather than attempting a difficult or impossible intubation since hypoxia and hypercapnia during such attempts may increase neurological injury.
- The upper airway should be manually cleared without extension of the head on the neck if cervical fracture has not been ruled out by cervical radiography.
- Normal neurological function does not preclude cervical fracture since muscle spasm may have prevented displacement and spinal cord injury.
- An oral airway is preferable to a nasal airway since nasal or basilar skull fractures may prevent the nasal airway from following the normal course and may even allow penetration of the cranial vault.

Breathing

Maintenance of normal Pao$_2$ (>80 mmHg, 11 kPa) and normal Paco$_2$ (<40 mmHg, 5.3 kPa) will minimize further neurological injury. A large number of patients with head injury are hypoxic on arrival at the hospital probably due to aspiration of stomach contents, and arterial blood gases should be immediately assessed. Tracheal intubation offers positive control of the airway both to protect patients from aspiration and for adequate ventilation, and should be considered early in resuscitation.

Several factors optimize the circumstances for intubation.

Exogenous oxygen

Normocapnic or hypocapnic hypoxia is not an indication for rapid intubation, since oxygen by mask will frequently raise Pao$_2$ to normal, thus allowing time for evaluation of the cervical spine for injury. Hypocapnia (Paco$_2$ = 25 mmHg, 3.3 kPa) is useful in decreasing intracranial pressure, and normocapnia is tolerated only until tracheal intubation can be accomplished without injury to the patient.

Manual ventilation of the lungs

- The patient's lungs should be ventilated by mask with oxygen prior to attempted intubation. Although immediate intubation seems attractive in a crisis situation, the time for a difficult intubation (30–60 sec) may be more detrimental than the potential risk of aspiration.
- The Sellick manoeuvre (cricoid pressure) during mask

ventilation minimizes the risk of aspiration of stomach contents (*see* p. 7).
- Prior vomiting, or even evidence of aspiration are not absolute contra-indications to prolonged ventilation by mask. Permanent damage may result from hurried intubation by inexperienced persons in hypoxic patients, and the sequelae of aspiration are much easier to treat.

Pharmacological agents

The choice of pharmacological agents used for intubation of the head-injured patient is controversial and studies are not available documenting the advantages or detrimental effects of any agent or group of agents in such circumstances.

- Short acting barbiturates, e.g. thiopentone (thiopental) blunt both the haemodynamic and intracranial response to intubation.[1] However, barbiturates may produce hypotension, thereby decreasing brain perfusion and usual induction doses (4–5 mg/kg) should be used only in normovolaemic patients.
- Intravenous lignocaine (lidocaine) 1–2 mg/kg is also useful in decreasing or treating the intracranial pressure response to intubation.[1]
- The need for rapid airway control points out the need for rapid skeletal muscle paralysis to facilitate intubation and prevent vascular response to intubation. In addition to facilitating intubation, muscle relaxants prevent increased intra-abdominal and intrathoracic pressure which may markedly elevate ICP during or following intubation (cough).
- Although suxamethonium (succinylcholine) causes rapid muscle paralysis, it may directly increase intracranial pressure.[2] Large doses of pancuronium (0.1 mg/kg) allow rapid intubation but can cause prolonged paralysis thus interfering with serial neurological examinations. Additionally, it may produce increased blood pressure and elevate ICP.
- Short acting neuromuscular blocking agents (atracurium, vecuronium) allow rapid intubation and produce a relatively short period of paralysis (30 min).

Tracheal intubation

The method of intubation must be tailored to the patient's conditions. Oral intubation under direct vision is the most rapid method of intubation. However, extension of the head and neck is required, though frequently not possible due to the temporary collar placed to prevent neck injuries or is avoided due to suspected cervical fracture. Oral intubation without neck extension can be accomplished using the technique described in Table 11.2.

- Blind nasotracheal intubation is useful in spontaneously breathing patients but is only 70 per cent effective. This method requires more time than intubation under direct vision and risks bleeding from the nose and retropharyngeal dissection.
- Fibreoptic nasotracheal intubation is a valuable intubating technique in patients with abnormal airway or who have restricted movement of the neck. However this method requires specialized equipment (fibreoptic bronchoscope) and training, and large amounts of secretions, either gastric or blood, greatly increase the difficulty and length of time to intubation.

Table 11.2   Oral intubation with minimal neck extension

Equipment
1. Curved laryngoscope blade preferable
2. Small endotracheal tube
       7 mm OD for women
       8 mm OD for men
3. Stylette with 120° bend 3 cm from end of tube with tip of stylette at end of tube.
4. Suction
5. Assistant (to hold stylette)

Method of intubation
1. Head should be fixed in neutral position (neck collar or held by assistant).
2. Mask ventilation to ensure adequate oxygenation.
3. Open mouth sufficiently to place blade and displace tongue in caudal direction to visualize tip of epiglottis. This should require *no* neck extension.
4. Place tip of endotracheal tube behind midpoint of tip of epiglottis.
5. Have assistant hold stylette securely and advance tube off stylette into larynx.
6. The 120° angle of the tube (due to stylette) makes it move slightly anteriorly as it advances, which allows the tip of tube to enter the larynx.
7. If the initial attempt is unsuccessful, a smaller endotracheal tube should be used to facilitate entry into the larynx.

Circulation

Systemic injury resulting in blood loss may interact with or hide the haemodynamic consequences of neurological injury, e.g. the vasodilatation following spinal cord transection may be mistaken for blood loss or hypertension with brainstem compression (Cushing's reflex) may be mistaken for patient response to stimulation (pain).

- Aggressive haemodynamic monitoring (arterial catheter, central venous/pulmonary artery catheter) are important tools in stabilizing such patients rapidly.
- In the responsive patient, local anaesthesia should be used to prevent hypertensive responses to stimulation during catheter insertion.
- Early initiation of brain dehydration by osmotic diuretics (mannitol, *see* p. 59 and p. 136) and loop diuretic frusemide (furosomide) may complicate hypovolaemia secondary to blood loss and may make diagnosis of insidious blood loss difficult because of the volume contraction related maintenance of haematocrit.
- A vasoconstrictor (neosynephrine 40 micrograms/ml) should be used to maintain mean arterial blood pressure greater than 80 mmHg in an attempt to maintain cerebral perfusion pressure within acceptable limits.
- Hypertension should be untreated until ICP can be assessed. Indeed, hypertension preserves brain blood flow in the presence of intracranial hypertension.[3] If ICP is monitored and cerebral perfusion pressure is adequate (greater than 60 mmHg), a decrease in MABP may be considered. Conventional hypotensive agents (nitroprusside, nitroglycerin) directly increase ICP and decrease in brain perfusion pressure[4,5] ($\downarrow$ MABP, $\uparrow$ ICP) occurs so these agents should be avoided in patients with closed head injury. β-adrenergic receptor blockade with propranolol (1 mg increments IV) will decrease heart rate and MABP as well as decreasing the amount of other hypotensive agents required to control blood pressure.
- Barbiturates in small doses should be considered to decrease blood pressure since they directly decrease ICP and tend to preserve brain perfusion.[6]
- Drainage of cerebrospinal fluid (CSF) may be used cautiously to lower ICP and preserve CPP exclusive of alterations in MABP. However, ventricular catheter placement may be difficult due to decreased ventricular size in head-injured patients.

- The neurological status by physical examination remains a rapid and accurate method of assessing neurological injury. However, therapeutic agents (barbiturates or neuromuscular blocking agents) should not be withheld in such patients and risk further injury or deterioration.
- Airway difficulties may require the anaesthetist to attend to the patient with head injury prior to the neurosurgeon, therefore observations should be made in all patients concerning extremity movements, posturing, pupillary size and response so that if paralysis is required, baseline data is available.

History

Individuals delivering the patient to the hospital should provide details of the injury to assess the likelihood of associated injury (e.g. presence or absence of seatbelt).

Personal effects and family members may provide information concerning chronic diseases (angina, diabetes) as well as allergies which must be considered in the resuscitation of such patients. It should be remembered that neurological disease (e.g. seizures) may be the cause as well as result of accidents and appropriate history should be obtained.

Glasgow Coma Scale (GCS)

Coma is best defined as inability to obey commands, to speak, or to open the eyes. The degree of coma after severe head injury is the most reliable clinical indication of the severity of brain damage, whether from impact injury or subsequent events. The GCS is an assessment of the patient's responsiveness and can be scored numerically or graphically as time passes (Fig 11.1).[7] It can be used alone or in conjunction with the trauma scoring system (*see* p. 124).

Support and resuscitation during diagnostic evaluation

- Anaesthesia support of the patient with head injury should be continuous from patient arrival in the hospital to definitive treatment. The patient's airway must be secured and the cardiovascular status stabilized prior to movement to diagnostic facilities.
- Electronic monitoring of ECG, arterial pressure and ICP during transport and in the diagnostic areas (radiology suite) allows aggressive treatment during diagnosis.

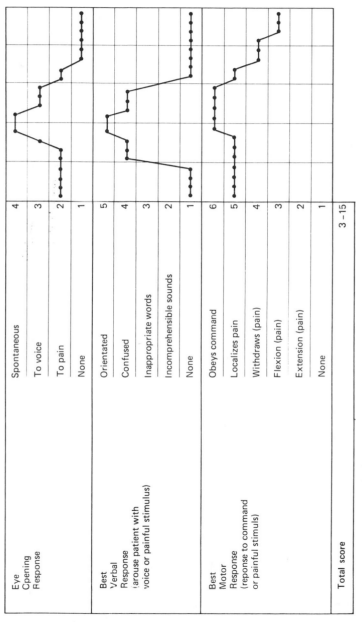

Eye Opening Response	Spontaneous	4
	To voice	3
	To pain	2
	None	1
Best Verbal Response (arouse patient with voice or painful stimulus)	Orientated	5
	Confused	4
	Inappropriate words	3
	Incomprehensible sounds	2
	None	1
Best Motor Response (reponse to command or painful stimuls)	Obeys command	6
	Localizes pain	5
	Withdraws (pain)	4
	Flexion (pain)	3
	Extension (pain)	2
	None	1
Total score		3 – 15

Fig. 11.1 Glasgow Coma Scale.

- Performance of diagnostic studies (CT scan or angiography) in patients who are unco-operative but who have not required paralysis or tracheal intubation is extremely difficult and the patient's unco-operative state frequently leads to suboptimal studies.
- Sedative agents (diazepam, etc) may alter the level of consciousness and lead to hypoventilation and decreased airway reflexes with worsening of the mental status. In such patients, prevention of further neurological injury as well as optimal diagnosis is best obtained by a well-controlled general anaesthetic with endotracheal intubation until the status of the brain has been assessed. Anaesthetic gases and vapours are best avoided initially.

Fluid management

The effects of fluid management on function of the injured brain must be considered during resuscitation. Oxygen delivery to the brain is mainly influenced by oxygen carrying capacity of the blood, and haematocrit (haemoglobin) should be maintained near normal levels. Intracranial hypertension may prevent increases in CBF which normally compensate for lowered oxygen carrying capacity.

- Diuretic therapy should be instituted rapidly to dehydrate the brain. This decreases ICP and increases CBF in the injured brain.
- Small doses of mannitol (0.25 mg/kg) at frequent intervals are as effective as large doses (1 mg/kg) and avoid the increased vascular volume associated with the larger dose.
- The serum osmolarity should be maintained in the range 300–310 mOsm to ensure adequate brain dehydration.
- Frusemide (furosomide) 10 mg is useful in addition to mannitol in shrinking the brain. This is due not only to diuretic effect but also a direct decrease in production of CSF.
- The diuretic effect of contrast media should be considered when planning diuretic therapy.
- The allergic response to contrast media should be anticipated and adequate drugs and resuscitation equipment should be available to all patients undergoing contrast studies (*see* p. 98).

Hyperglycaemia may increase permanent neurological injury following neurological insult.[8] Therefore, glucose containing solutions should be avoided unless hypoglycaemia is demonstrated.

Anaesthetic agents

The use of anaesthetic agents and adjuvants in head-injured patients should be considered for the beneficial effects on the brain in addition to producing anaesthesia.

- Advantageous effects include direct decreases in ICP, decreased or unchanged CBF and decreased cerebral metabolism ($CMRO_2$) so that anaesthetic agents should not necessarily be avoided or the doses minimized in patients with head injury.
- In addition to anaesthetic agents, local anaesthesia will prevent haemodynamic responses to stimulation such as application of the pin-type head holder, and surgical incision.
- Intravenous agents, e.g. thiopentone (thiopental) and fentanyl, appear not to affect cerebral haemodynamics adversely, while anaesthetic gases (N_2O, enflurane, isoflurane) cause a dose-dependent increase in CBF[9] and ICP and may directly decrease CPP. The increased ICP with N_2O can be blunted by prior administration of IV agents.
- Increased ICP due to enflurane and isoflurane may be blunted by prior hyperventilation.[10,11]
- Both hypotension and increased ICP are dose-related effects of anaesthetic gases and therefore high inspired concentrations are best avoided.
- Long-acting sedatives (diazepam, hyoscine) may make accurate neurological assessment after operation difficult and may actually mask the onset of real neurological changes and are best avoided in this group of patients.

Haematology

The oxygen carrying capacity of blood (haemoglobin) should be frequently assessed and maintained near normal (haematocrit 30–35 per cent).

- The oxygen carrying capacity of the blood is more important than PaO_2 in determining oxygen delivery to the brain.[12] A low haematocrit may compromise oxygen delivery to the brain despite high PaO_2. A high haematocrit may lead to sludging in areas of low flow and actually decrease regional oxygen delivery in the brain.
- Disseminated intravascular coagulation should always be suspected in patients with brain injury since brain is a good source of tissue thromboplastin.
- Platelet dysfunction should be considered with abnormal

bleeding and pre-injury consumption of aspirin should be suspected and platelets administered if necessary.

Neurological monitoring

Neurological monitoring (electroencephalogram, evoked potentials) may be useful in the paralysed patient or unresponsive patient to diagnose the extent of neurological injury and to assess the effects of various factors such as surgical positioning and change in blood pressure on neurological function.[13] Additionally, these monitors may be useful in demonstrating spinal cord, peripheral nerve, brachial plexus injury and brainstem injury. Such monitoring can be rapidly established by the teams who have a great deal of monitoring experience. By utilizing needle scalp electrodes and needle stimulating electrodes, such monitoring can be instituted in just a few minutes and give valuable data.

Anaesthesia in patients with possible head injury

Frequently the urgency of other injuries requires surgery/ anaesthesia before complete evaluation of head injury, or in patients whose initial neurological symptoms were minor. Neurological deterioration in the anaesthetized, paralyzed patient is difficult to detect.

- Pupillary signs are valuable signs of deterioration (herniation), but occur *late* in neurological deterioration.
- The use of evoked potentials (brainstem auditory evoked response, somatosensory evoked potential) in such patients may give early indication of neurological deterioration.
- High dose dopamine (> 10 micrograms/kg/min) and trimetaphan may cause pupillary dilation and mask pupillary signs.

Use an anaesthestic technique in the *possible* head-injured patient which is the same as that for a *known* head-injured patient (*see* p. 137).

References

1. Bedford RF, Persing JA, Pobereskin L, Butler A. Lidocaine or thiopental for rapid control of intracranial hypertension? *Anesth. Analg.* 1980; **59**: 435–7.
2. Cottrell JE, Hartring J, Giffin JP, Shurry B. Intracranial and

hemodynamic changes after succinylcholine administration in cats. *Anesth. Analg.* 1983; **62**: 1006–9.

3. Miller JD, Stanek AE, Langfitt TW. A comparison of autoregulation to changes in intracranial and arterial pressure in the same preparation. *Europ. Neurol.* 1973; **6**: 34–8.

4. Cottrell JE, Patel KP, Turndorf H. Intracranial pressure changes induced by sodium nitroprusside in patients with intracranial mass lesions. *J. Neurosurgery* 1978; **48**: 329–31.

5. Rogers MC, Hamburger C, Owen K, Epstein MH. Intracranial pressure in the cat during nitroglycerin induced hypotension. *Anesthesiology* 1979; **51**: 227–9.

6. Shapiro HM, Wyte SR, Loeser J. Barbiturate augmented hypothermia for reduction of persistent intracranial hypertension. *J. Neurosurg.* 1974; **40**: 90–110.

7. Jennett B, Teasdale G. Aspects of coma after severe head injury. *Lancet* 1977; **i**: 878–81.

8. Pulsinelti WA, Waldman S, Raubinson D, Plum F. Moderate hyperglycemia augments ischemic brain damage: A neuropathologic study in the rat. *Neurology* 1982; **32**: 1239–46.

9. Miletich DJ, Irankorvich AD, Alberecht RD, Reiman CR, Rosenberg R, McKissic ED. Absence of autoregulation of cerebral blood flow during halothane and enflurane anesthesia. *Anesth. Analg.* 1976; **55**: 100–109.

10. Adams RW, Gronert GA, Sundt TM, Michenfelder JD. Halothane, hypocapnia and cerebrospinal fluid pressure in neurosurgery. *Anesthesiology* 1972; **37**: 510–17.

11. Adams RW, Cucchiara RF, Gronert GA, Messick JM, Michenfelder JD. Isoflurane and cerebrospinal fluid pressure in neurosurgical patients. *Anesthesiology* 1981; **54**: 97–9.

12. Traystman RJ, Fitzgerald RS, Loscutoff SC. Cerebral circulatory response to arterial hypoxia in normal and chemodenervated dogs. *Circ. Res.* 1978; **42**: 649–57.

13. Sohmer H, Gafni M, Goitein K, Faumesser P. Auditory nerve-brainstem evoked potentials in cats during manipulation of cerebral perfusion pressure. *Electroenceph. Clin. Neurophysiol.* 1983; **55**: 190–200.

Further reading

Barker J. Postoperative care of the neurosurgical patient. *Br. J. Anaesth.* 1976; **48**: 797–804.

McDowall DG, Norman JB (eds). Symposium on neurosurgical anaesthesia. *Br. J. Anaesth.* 1976; **48**: 717–804.

12

Neck Trauma

John P Williams

Resuscitation
  The airway
  Ventilation
  Haemorrhage
  Cervical spine injury
Recognition
  Tracheolaryngeal damage
  Vascular damage
  Neurological injuries
Repair
  Preparations
  Positioning and access
  Monitoring
  Anaesthesia

There is perhaps no other area of the body which is as vulnerable to extrinsic destruction as the neck. Within the confines of this cylindrical structure exist all of the major pathways for life. It is not surprising that this area is involved in numerous types of life-threatening complications following major trauma.[1,2,3] The incidence of neck involvement following major trauma is approximately 10 per cent. Mortality directly attributable to neck injury varies from 4–10 per cent.[4,5]

The basis of sound trauma management is the three Rs:

- resuscitation
- recognition
- repair

Resuscitation

The airway

The routine initial management of any traumatized patient should include establishment of an adequate airway, assessment of ventilatory status and an evaluation of circulatory status. This is particularly true in the neck-injured patient. The airway is of critical import in the care and transport of these patients and it is in this group of patients that the anaesthetist's special knowledge and skills in airway management are crucial.

All neck traumatized individuals should have the benefit of some type of airway protection upon arrival in the emergency department if not already provided in the field. A patient with an apparently innocuous injury may languish in the emergency department until either encroaching oedema or haematoma create the necessity for endotracheal intubation in an emergency setting. This is frequently seen following blunt trauma where hours can elapse before airway obstruction becomes severe enough to require action.

Ventilation

After the provision of an adequate airway, attention must be directed to an assessment of the adequacy of ventilation. The high incidence of both head injury and cervical spinal cord disruption in association with blunt trauma to the neck require the establishment of an adequate minute volume of ventilation; the treatment of associated severe head injuries frequently necessitates hyperventilation.

A normal chest radiograph does not eliminate the possibility of a haemopneumothorax developing later (particularly after the institution of positive pressure ventilation).

Haemorrhage

The most common cause of mortality in penetrating neck injuries is vascular in origin. Thus, control of any obvious sites of bleeding is imperative. This is most effectively accomplished by digital compression and not by blind clipping or clamping. After the initial control of obvious bleeding sites, large bore (14 G or larger) IV catheters should be placed with attention to any sites of possible venous injury (innominate or subclavian).

- If a large open venous injury is present then measures should be taken to prevent the possibility of air embolism.

Cervical spine injury

This is the second most common cause of death in the neck-injured patient.

- All patients with documented or suspected blunt trauma to the neck should be treated as cervical spine fractures.
- All these injuries should be stabilized by use of a cervical collar or sand bags placed on either side of the neck. The latter allow for easy access to the anterior portion of the neck should the need for an emergency tracheostomy arise. Subsequent radiographic examinations in the lateral and antero-posterior plane should be obtained prior to removing these protective devices.

Once these priorities are achieved and the patient is stable, further definitive examinations which might be required may proceed.

Recognition

Tracheolaryngeal damage

The incidence of tracheal or laryngeal damage in neck trauma is fortunately low. Only 24 cases of traumatic rupture of the trachea and 12 cases of traumatic dislocation of the arytenoids were noted in a review of the literature.[1] Although these are uncommon lesions, their incidence appears to be rising with the increasing number of automobile accidents. The mechanism of injury involves a direct antero-posterior blow to the trachea in association with a closed glottis.

Presenting signs and symptoms of injury do not always correlate with severity of the injury and in a small percentage of cases will not be present at all.[6] Suggestive symptoms are dyspnoea, hoarseness, dysphonia or aphonia, and dysphagia.

- The most common presenting sign is subcutaneous or interstitial emphysema although this may be absent in up to 25 per cent of neck injuries.[7] Physical examination frequently reveals loss of the thyroid prominence; crepitations may be heard over the larynx.

Effective and immediate relief of airway obstruction is vital. Although a great deal of controversy still exists concerning the need for emergency tracheostomy in these patients, the following four lesions appear to be absolute indications:[6]

- severe facial trauma in association with upper airway obstruction,
- presence of laryngeal damage with use of accessory muscles of respiration,

- suspected tracheal disruption or separation,
- laryngotracheal separation.

Tracheostomy in these particular situations avoids the possibility of causing further damage to the larynx or trachea and reduces the chances of completing a partial tracheal or tracheolaryngeal separation. Only after the restitution of a patent airway may further examinations to characterize the nature or extent of laryngotracheal damage be undertaken. These include soft tissue radiography, direct or indirect laryngoscopy, tomography or CT scanning.

The type of anaesthetic used for either the placement of the endotracheal tube or tracheostomy is also at the centre of some disagreement. Various types of anaesthetic plan have been devised to cope with this situation[1,2,8,9] and all focus upon specific areas as being the most important.

If none of the four lesions which require emergency tracheostomy are present, awake nasotracheal intubation is preferred. This is most easily accomplished with a combination of 4 per cent lignocaine (lidocaine) spray to the oropharynx and 4 per cent cocaine to the nasal passages.

The reasons for this choice include:

- the risk of disturbing a cervical fracture,
- the presence of a full stomach in all trauma patients,
- lack of need for muscle relaxants,
- maintenance of spontaneous ventilation, and
- the ease and speed with which it can be performed in an emergency situation.

There are at least two major objections to this suggestion. The first is the possibility of provoking coughing and exacerbating bleeding and/or subcutaneous emphysema. Exacerbation of bleeding in neck injuries is important only when the lesion is in Zone 3 (*see* p. 145); exacerbation of subcutaneous emphysema is important only if the airway is unprotected or if there is an associated pneumothorax which can be treated by insertion of a chest drain.

The second objection is the possibility of producing further soft tissue damage.

- Even in the most experienced hands these are often unexpectedly difficult intubations and oral intubation can frequently cause as much soft tissue damage as blind nasal intubation.

If unexpected damage to the trachea or larynx is discovered at the time of surgical exploration, tracheostomy can then be carried out and the appropriate repairs completed. All patients with damage to the neck should have a complete examination of the structure and function of the larynx. The likelihood of completely repairing damage to this organ becomes increasingly remote with delays in diagnosis.[10]

Although exact timing is difficult to predict, the tracheostomy or endotracheal tube should be left in place a minimum of four to seven days to allow for resolution of tissue oedema and haematoma.

Vascular damage

Blunt trauma

The leading cause of morbidity and mortality in the neck-injured patient is the loss of vascular integrity. This is true with both penetrating and blunt trauma, although the mechanisms of injury are different.

Blunt trauma to the neck which initiates serious damage to vascular structures primarily involves damage to arteries and not to major venous structures unless the integrity of the skin is breached.

Blunt trauma to the vascular structures of the neck generally results in a closed injury which may not initially present with signs and symptoms commensurate with the degree of damage. Four mechanisms elicit vascular injuries in blunt trauma:

- hyperextension and contralateral rotation of the head,
- direct blow to the neck,
- blunt intra-oral trauma, and
- basal fracture injuring the intrapetrous portion of the vertebral artery.[11]

The most common cause of this injury in adults is a blow sustained in an automobile accident usually secondary to striking the extended neck on the steering wheel or dashboard. In children, the most common cause is secondary to a fall against the sharp edge of a table or a similar object; intra-oral trauma is also common (i.e. blows to the oropharynx from foreign objects present in the mouth at the time of a fall). Fortunately the incidence of damage is low; accounting for only 3 per cent of all carotid artery injuries.[12]

The onset of symptoms in most cases is delayed and can occur weeks to months after the initial injury. Consequently, the correct diagnosis is entertained in only 6 per cent of cases;[11] the morbidity and mortality from this injury can approach 20–40 per cent.

The diagnosis is generally made with the appearance of transient or permanent unilateral neurological deficits (hemiparesis being the most common, but can also include Horner's syndrome, aphasia and altered state of consciousness). Frequently these injuries occur in association with closed head injuries and the resulting neurological deficit is masked by this injury and accounts for the low rate of diagnosis.

- A high degree of suspicion should be entertained in any patient who has evidence of central neurological damage with a normal CT scan.

Investigations

Management of these injuries entails airway management and investigations for their exact location and nature (i.e. thrombosis, spasm, transection, etc.) by angiography.

- If a central neurological deficit is already present then management should include whatever routine precautions are taken for the closed head injury patient.
- If no deficit is present then management is facilitated by the use of mild sedation and local anaesthesia for angiography. This allows for constant surveillance of the level of consciousness and rapid assessment of the progression of neurological deficits if present.
- If both vessel and skin integrity have been breached, control of bleeding is best accomplished by digital compression and not clips.
- If a venous injury is present then the risk of air embolism exists and precautions such as allowing the patient to remain in the supine position rather than adopting a head-up position become more important. Although the supine position may exacerbate venous bleeding, digital compression is usually sufficient to control it.

Penetrating injuries

All penetrating injuries are open and exsanguination becomes the major consideration. Although the most common vascular injury in the neck is venous, most of the morbidity and mortality within this subgroup is related to *arterial* injuries.

Zone classification

The management and description of arterial injuries in the neck is facilitated by dividing the neck into three zones (Fig. 12.1).[13]

- Zone 1 includes all vessels below the level of the sternal notch.

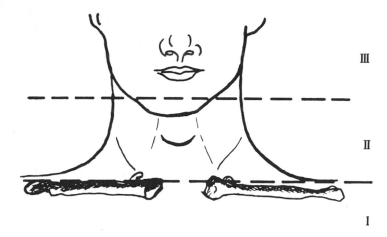

Fig. 12.1 Classification of arterial injuries in the neck.

- Zone 2 extends from the sternal notch to the angle of the mandible.
- Zone 3 extends from the angle of the mandible to the base of the skull.

Control of the airway in this group of patients continues to be of paramount importance. Delayed or slowly accumulating haematomata can obstruct the airway and are best managed electively on initial arrival of the patient in the emergency department; if not, airways problems will arise in the angiography suite. Although caution should exist when intubating patients with injuries in Zone 1, the possibility of increasing the bleeding is of secondary importance to the establishment of an airway.

After initial resuscitation is complete, the nature of vessel injury in Zones 1 and 3 is best clarified by arteriography prior to surgical exploration. This is because proximal and/or distal surgical control of injured vessels in these areas may be difficult to obtain secondary to poor exposure. However, vascular injuries in Zone 2 are best handled by surgical exploration as there is generally good exposure, and proximal and distal surgical control of the vessels is relatively easy to obtain.

Injuries in Zones 1 and 2 may also result in pleural damage; these should be sought both at presentation and again prior to the institution of IPPV as an unsuspected haemopneumothorax is not an infrequent complication.

Neurological injuries

Spinal cord damage

Although there are a number of possible neurological injuries occurring with neck trauma, the most devastating of these is the total or partial transection of the spinal cord. The incidence of this injury is 30–35 per million population in the USA per year with roughly 50 per cent occurring in automobile accidents.[14] In patients presenting with penetrating trauma to the neck, transection of the cord is the second leading cause of mortality.[7] For these reasons, all patients presenting with injuries to the neck should be presumed to have cervical damage until proven otherwise.

Adequate examination of this area should include:

- physical examination to determine sensory and motor levels
- antero-posterior and lateral radiological views of the cervical spine (to include craniocervical and cervicothoracic junctions).

Indications for early or emergent surgery include:

- failure to reduce fracture by closed manipulation
- presence of high unstable fracture
- penetrating wounds or compound fracture
- progressive neurological deficit.[14]

Patients who have sustained complete or partial transection of the spinal cord present with:

- respiratory embarrassment
- hypotension
- and a flaccid paralysis below the level of the lesion.

Initial assessment should include:

- determination of ventilatory and circulatory status
- stabilization of the neck
- thorough neurological examination to determine level of injury and consciousness.

Although ventilation may not be impaired with lesions below C_7, the gradual onset of 'spinal shock' (that is, dysfunction of the spinal cord several levels above the area of permanent section) will frequently lead to ventilatory impairment hours after the initial injury. This represents another group of patients who need airway protection, on an expectant rather than an emergent basis.

Extension of the neck must be avoided in all neck trauma patients with the resultant choice of intubation technique being awake nasotracheal with local anaesthesia.

- If there is sufficient time and expertise available, this is best accomplished using a fibreoptic bronchoscope with the head in traction.

Once the endotracheal tube is in place, further assessment of ventilatory status can be made by measurements of forced vital capacity, negative inspiratory pressure and tidal volume.

Many of these patients will be in shock at the time of initial evaluation. All efforts should be made to determine if and to what degree the hypotension is secondary to a loss of sympathetic tone. Generally those patients with purely neurogenic shock will be bradycardic and hypotensive with systolic pressures in the range 90–100 mmHg. However, 47 per cent of neck injuries occur in association with other major trauma[5] and often both hypovolaemic and neurogenic shock will co-exist. These patients will need anticholinergic and vasopressor drugs as well as fluid to maintain an adequate arterial pressure and cardiac output; at the same time pulmonary oedema must be avoided.

The heart also undergoes acute alterations with this injury and ECG evidence of ST and T wave changes, atrial fibrillation, ventricular tachycardia, multifocal ventricular premature complexes, wandering atrial pacemaker and subendocardial ischaemia may all be noticed.

There are two other common manifestations of spinal cord injury. The first is the sudden cessation of peristalsis at the time of injury which generally lasts 3–5 days in the uncomplicated injury. Nasogastric drainage should be established during this period to avoid serious abdominal distension; this is best placed at the time of surgery after exploration of the neck to avoid causing further soft tissue damage.

The second problem is the complete loss of temperature regulation associated with lesions above C_7. These patients become poikilothermic, i.e. they are extremely dependent upon environmental influences (room temperature, blankets, draping procedures, etc.) to maintain body temperature. The nursing of these patients is best accomplished at 21°C.[14]

There are a host of other possible neurological injuries none of which will be discussed in any detail here. These include injury to the following nerves: vagus, laryngeal, phrenic, spinal accessory, hypoglossal, cervical sympathetic and the brachial plexus. Although damage to the phrenic nerve can be evaluated by observing diaphragmatic motion under fluoroscopy, 75 per cent of individuals have an accessory phrenic nerve. Diagnosis of recurrent or superior laryngeal nerve damage is by visual inspection of vocal cord function and is best made at the time of surgery if conditions permit. High vagal damage is also evaluated in the same fashion but this injury can result in diminution or loss of the cough reflex in the lung on the ipsilateral side.[15]

Repair

Preparations

The preparation of the theatre should include:

- adequate control of room temperature
- availability of at least two blood warmers capable of functioning at high infusion rates
- pre-warmed IV fluids
- the facility to make direct measurement of at least two vascular pressures
- a tracheostomy set
- a fluid-filled warming blanket on the operating table.

Additionally, the operating table should have some form of padding (eggcrate mattress, etc.) to avoid pressure point damage during surgery.

Further preparations should include the availability of large amounts of blood and blood products. Although whole blood is still the preferred product for the massively transfused patient obtaining adequate supplies may be difficult (Chapter 3).

Care must be taken to ensure that no further damage occurs during transfer of the patient from the trolley to the operating table. If the neck is in traction this should be maintained and preferably managed by the neurosurgeon. Often the cervico-thoracic junction cannot be visualized by routine radiography and the patient has no obvious neurological deficit. In this situation a collar is placed to stabilize the neck prior to transfer. If the injury precludes the use of a cervical collar, a board placed behind the patient's neck with sandbags on either side will suffice. Although head elevation will decrease venous bleeding and oedema formation this will also increase the risk of venous air embolism.

Positioning and access

The positioning of any patient for anaesthesia and surgery is dependent upon a number of factors. First is the need for adequate surgical exposure but protection of the obtunded patient is vital. Most surgical repairs involve long, tedious procedures with as many as three different teams of surgeons (thoracic, general, ENT, neurosurgery, plastic, etc.) and their requirements for positioning are often widely disparate. Access to the patient by the anaesthetist is vital at all times. He has to accommodate to the needs of radiography, angiography and changing surgical fields. He needs easy or at least only marginally restricted access to the airway, IV infusion ports, arterial catheter and a neurologically intact extremity.

The use of leg wrappings to increase venous return (particularly useful in the sympathetically denervated patient) will need to be removed to allow for access to the saphenous vein if autogenous grafts are needed to repair arterial damage. Stabilization of the neck during surgery is achieved using bilateral sandbags as described above or continuous cervical traction. The latter also offers the advantage of allowing ready access to the various areas of the neck. The repair and exposure of vascular injuries in Zone 1 frequently necessitates the use of a median sternotomy. This possibility should be kept in mind when positioning ECG electrodes.

Monitoring

Monitoring of these patients is complex.

- Essential monitors include: ECG, temperature, arterial and central venous catheters (choose uninvolved vessels!), oesophageal stethoscope, bladder catheter, neuromuscular stimulator.
- The need for multiple blood sampling to monitor arterial blood-gas tensions makes the direct technique of arterial pressure measurement the one of choice.
- Placement of a central venous line may be very difficult; the femoral or antecubital approach may be used depending on the site of injury.
- A neuromuscular stimulator is important when the incidence of unsuspected neurological injuries is high. This allows the anaesthetist to titrate neuromuscular blockade against surgical requirements to evaluate nerve integrity.

Other optional monitoring devices which are helpful are: capnography, evoked potentials from the spinal cord, EEG or compressed spectral array, pulmonary artery catheter, and facilities for rapid measurements of serum electrolytes, osmolality and colloid oncotic pressure. Oncotic pressure measurement is becoming a standard in most centres in the USA which handle large volumes of trauma patients.

- Rapid blood transfusion is associated with changes in serum K^+ concentration.
- CVP is an unreliable indicator of left ventricular filling in the

massively transfused patient secondary to an increase in pulmonary vascular resistance.
• Instead of measuring cardiac output directly it is often better to follow the urine output, central venous oxygen saturation, arterial pressure and heart rate as indicators of adequate volume replacement and cardiac output.

Anaesthesia

There is no single anaesthetic technique which is to be preferred over all others; rather, there are certain objectives which must be met in order to produce a successful result.

The use of sedatives or tranquillizers prior to institution of a patent airway is to be condemned. The restless, anxious patient in this situation is usually hypoxic and hypercarbic secondary to ventilatory impairment from the variety of causes already described. Once the airway is secured they may be appropriate choices but these patients need constant surveillance after administering these agents. The combination of sedatives and tranquillizers with alcohol can result in significant depression of ventilation. However, the use of the benzodiazepines (e.g. lorazepam) can be particularly helpful *intra-operatively* in producing an amnesic patient with little or no cardiovascular depression.[16]

The choice of IV induction agents is still open to question. Although etomidate might appear to be the agent of choice because of good cardiovascular stability, the associated high incidence of aberrant muscular activity may make its use dangerous in the patient with an unstable neck fracture. Etomidate also causes adrenal supression although this is probably not of clinical significance in single doses.

Ketamine has been the standard induction agent in the trauma patient for many years. This does not mean that it can be used with impunity, however, as it can cause direct myocardial depression. This is especially important in a patient with maximal sympathetic tone already present where any decrease in myocardial drive can be detrimental. Ketamine also produces postoperative hallucinations. Both these effects are particularly troublesome in the patient with spinal cord trauma who may already be suffering from a de-afferentation syndrome (i.e. the removal of all external stimuli to the body resulting in hallucinations) and is disconnected from central sympathetic nervous system. Hallucinations from ketamine can be minimized by the administration of a benzodiazepine drug.

The use of thiopentone (thiopental) in the traumatized patient was well documented at Pearl Harbour in 1941. Even though the fatalities recorded at that time were the result of overdosage, the deadly interaction of thiopentone and hypovolaemia remains true. Thiopentone still offers a viable alternative in the normovolaemic patient requiring IV induction; a 'quick tilt' test just prior to induction will help establish the adequacy of volume replacement in most patients.

Inhalation anaesthesia has a special place in the management of the neck trauma patient. It has been recommended in the evaluation of patients with laryngeal and tracheal damage, particularly children[1,2] although others have said that it should be avoided for induction.[8] The most reasonable course is to take a middle of the road approach, i.e. an inhalation induction when there exists a mild obstruction and the evaluation of laryngeal function is indicated. The possibility of the full stomach must always be kept in mind and the left lateral position with head-down tilt should be used during induction (*see* p. 8).

The need for the avoidance of irritation and coughing on induction dictates the use of halothane rather than one of the ethers. One further problem exists with the use of the inhalation anaesthetics which is the discrepancy in time between the onset of unconsciousness and amnesia, and cardiovascular depression. The same warning expressed concerning thiopentone (thiopental) is true for all the inhalation anaesthetics as well. Although isoflurane seems to affect cardiovascular stability less than other inhalation agents, it is a potent vasodilator: not the ideal agent for a hypovolaemic patient. Isoflurane is also extremely pungent and is not the agent of choice for pure inhalation induction of anaesthesia.

The use of muscle relaxants in this group of patients is particularly dangerous. Many of these patients while awake have marginal airway patency and the use of relaxants to facilitate intubation will often deprive the patient of both airway and ventilation. In patients with laryngeal and tracheal injuries, the maintenance of spontaneous ventilation will decrease the degree of subcutaneous and interstitial emphysema. Further, their use in the neck-injured patient prior to definitive stabilization of a compound or highly unstable neck fracture may result in worsening of that lesion.[14] This is secondary to the loss of support from muscular spasm in the surrounding tissue. If surgical relaxation is absolutely necessary, however, then a short acting nondepolarizing agent is to be preferred.

Opiates, in common with sedatives, must be used with extreme caution prior to the institution of a patent airway. Although they represent an extremely useful group of drugs as a whole, they are not without drawbacks. Most of the potent synthetic opiates (fentanyl, sufentanil, alfentanil) have little or no effect on the cardiovascular system. However, the reverse is true for the respiratory system. These agents are potent ventilatory depressants and are potentiated by the presence of alcohol. Therefore, every patient with neck trauma should be carefully supervised after administration of an opiate. There is no 'best' opiate in these situations. The decision depends on the degree of cardiovascular stability, expected duration of surgery, duration of action of the opiate and the need for postoperative sedation and/or analgesia. A high dose fentanyl technique is popular for this purpose; however, this is by no means the only choice and, appropriately utilized, methadone, papaveretum, morphine, and diamorphine (heroin) offer viable alternatives.

Conclusions

The management of the neck-injured patient is not straightforward in any sense. It involves an extraordinary amount of planning, preparation, information, co-operation, and experience in both the anaesthetic and surgical teams. There must be a tremendous amount of latitude given to both groups if the patient is to receive optimum care. In short: if the three R's are followed (resuscitation, recognition and repair); the ABCs of resuscitation remembered; the specific injuries outlined; and the intra-operative management a synthesis of the preceding tenets; a satisfactory outcome should be the result.

References

1. Seed RF. Traumatic injury to the larynx and trachea. *Anaesthesia* 1971; **26**: 55–65.
2. Clarke RSJ. Trauma to face and neck. In: *Anaesthesia for Eye, Ear, Nose and Throat Surgery*. Edinburgh: Churchill-Livingstone, 1975; 78–93.
3. Duncan JAT. A case of severely cut throat. *Br. J. Anaesth.* 1975; **47**: 1327–9.
4. Fogelman MJ, Stewart RD. Penetrating wounds of the neck. *Am. J. Surg.* 1956; **91**: 581–96.
5. Stone HH, Callahan GS. Soft tissue injuries of the neck. *Surg. Gynec. Obstet.* 1963; **117**: 745–52.
6. Balkany TJ, Jafek BW, Rutherford RB. The management of neck injuries. In: *The Management of Trauma, 3rd ed*. Philadelphia: W. B. Saunders, 1979; 342–60.
7. McKenna J, Jacob HJ. Trauma to the larynx. In: Walt AJ, Wilson RF (eds). *Management of Trauma: Pitfalls and practice*. Philadelphia: Lea and Febiger, 1975; 294–302.

8. Ellis FR. The management of cut throat. *Anaesthesia* 1966; **21**: 253-7.
9. Donlon JV (Jr). Anesthesia for eye, ear, nose, and throat surgery. In: Miller RD (ed). *Anesthesia*. New York: Churchill-Livingstone, 1981; 1265-1361.
10. McKenna J, Jacob HJ. Injuries to the neck. In: *Management of Trauma: Pitfalls and practice*. Philadelphia: Lea and Febiger, 1975; 294-302.
11. Maurer PK, Plassche W, Green RM. Blunt trauma to the carotid artery with transient deficit and early repair. *Surg. Neurol.* 1984; **21**: 110-2.
12. Vamada S, Kindt GW, Youmans JR. Carotid artery occlusion due to nonpenetrating injury. *J. Trauma* 1967; **7**: 333-42.
13. Committee on Trauma, American College of Surgeons. Neck. In: *Early Care of the Injured Patient, 3rd ed.* Philadelphia: W. B. Saunders, 1982; 222-34.
14. Kopaniky DR, Frost EAM. Management of spinal cord trauma. In: *Clinical Anesthesia in Neurosurgery*. Boston: Butterworths, 1984; 375-95.
15. Klassen KP, Morton DR, Curtis GM. The clinical physiology of the human bronchi. III. The effect of vagus section on the cough reflex, bronchial caliber, and clearance of bronchial secretions. *Surgery* 1951; **29**: 483-90.
16. Katz J, Butler BD, Hills BA, Johnson P. Safety of lorazepam in hypovolemic shock. *Anesthesiology* 1983; **59**: A96.

Further reading

Jones RF, Terrell JC, Salyer KE. Penetrating wounds of the neck: an analysis of 274 cases. *J. Trauma* 1967; **7**: 228-33.

13

Facio-maxillary, Ear, Nose and Throat Problems

John R Wedley

Facio-maxillary emergencies
    General problems
    Specific problems
    Operations
    Choice of anaesthetic technique
    Recovery
Ear, nose and throat emergencies
    General problems
    Specific problems
    Operations
    Choice of anaesthetic technique
    Recovery

The operative field involves the upper airway. There may therefore be difficulties in obtaining and maintaining an adequate airway before, during and after surgery.

Facio-maxillary emergencies

General problems

Haemorrhage

Facio-maxillary trauma almost inevitably leads to haemorrhage into the airway.

The full stomach

Much of this blood may be swallowed presenting the risk of subsequent vomiting, regurgitation and aspiration during induction of anaesthesia. Blood in the stomach further delays gastric emptying (*see* p. 6).

Shock

Gastric emptying may also be delayed in shock which may well be unsuspected where haemorrhage has been covert and the blood aspirated or swallowed.

- Assess and correct any circulatory failure. Postpone surgery for 24 hr if possible. Replace blood volume. Immediate surgery may be necessary if there is upper airway obstruction which cannot be cleared or continued major bleeding.
- Pass a wide-bore stomach tube pre-operatively and aspirate as much gastric contents as possible.
- Premedicate with atropine plus metoclopramide or domperidone to increase gastric motility and raise cardiac sphincter tone.
- Position carefully during induction to minimize aspiration.
- Ensure the presence of efficient suction.
- Consider awake oral intubation.
- Inhalation anaesthesia is safer than intravenous induction.
- The use of muscle relaxants for intubation increases the risk of aspiration. They can be lethal if intubation proves impossible.
- Shock leads to the unpredictable absorption of drugs given IM or subcutaneously pre-operatively.
- Uncorrected shock can lead to complete circulatory collapse upon induction.

Specific problems

Airway obstruction

Obstruction of the upper airway may occur in the pre- or post-operative period.

- Severe soft tissue injury may cause gross swelling and oedema of the lips, tongue and pharynx.
- Pain and swelling may cause spasm of the jaw muscles.
- The upper airway may be obstructed by the presence of saliva, vomit, blood, loose teeth, fragments of bone, and in the postoperative period swabs and pharyngeal packs.
- Persistent oedema, distortion of the airway and wiring the upper and lower jaws together may cause problems in the first 24 hr postoperatively.

Difficult intubation

Oral intubation may be impossible due to inability or limitation of mouth opening. This may be due to pain and swelling or mechanical obstruction where a fracture has interfered with the function of the temporomandibular joint. Local anaesthetic injection into the temporomandibular joint may relax masseter spasm due to pain. Limitation of jaw movement due to pain usually resolves once general anaesthesia is established.

- It may be difficult to visualize the larynx due to distortion of the upper airway. A gum elastic bougie or flexible stilette protruding one inch beyond the tip of the endotracheal tube may facilitate intubation (*see* p. 73).
- Awake blind nasal intubation and tracheostomy under local anaesthesia must be considered.
- Intubation using a flexible bronchoscope should only be attempted if the anaesthetist is skilled and experienced in this technique. This is not the time to practice something new.

Head injury

- Full neurological examination should be carried out pre-operatively. This is both clinically and medicolegally important. Bleeding from the external auditory canal should be looked for specifically.
- Regular pre-operative observations should be recorded of level of consciousness and rate, rhythm and depth of ventilation.
- Airway obstruction and inadequate ventilation will lead to carbon dioxide retention and a rise in intracranial pressure (*see* p. 129).

Cervical cord damage

It has been estimated that approximately two per cent of patients with facio-maxillary trauma have some degree of cervical cord damage (*see* p. 147).

- Pre-operative cervical spine x-ray and assessment of cervical spine stability should be made.
- If instability is suspected the head should be moved as little as possible and can be stabilized in a cervical collar and by the use of sandbags.
- Extension of the neck must be avoided (*see* pp. 126 and 147).

Operations

Zygomatic fractures

- A kink resistant reinforced or 'armoured' endotracheal tube should be used.

- Intubation should be oral. There is a danger that the fixation wire may penetrate a nasal tube making extubation impossible.
- The tube should be secured at the contralateral side of the mouth.

Fractures of the middle third (maxilla)

Intubation should be oral. The nasal airway can be evaluated once the patient is asleep.

Mandibular fractures

- Haematoma and oedema may obstruct the airway. It may be impossible to open the mouth. A clear airway must be secured prior to induction of anaesthesia. Blind nasal intubation or elective tracheostomy may be required.
- The jaws may be wired together postoperatively.

Choice of anaesthetic technique

Pre-operative assessment should include flexion of the neck (suspect cervical cord damage: care! *see*   p. 147), opening of the mouth, movement of the tongue, vocalization, stridor, the patency of the nostrils and a search for and removal of any loose teeth, crowns, bridgework or bone fragments.

- Do not use intravenous induction or muscle relaxant if there is any doubt about the patency of the airway or ability to control ventilation with a face-mask.

If the airway is compromised in any way, gaseous induction with halothane and oxygen is preferred. The superior aspect of the epiglottis is supplied by the glossopharyngeal nerve. It is possible therefore, gently, to inspect the airway using a Macintosh laryngoscope either prior to the induction of anaesthesia or before using a muscle relaxant without the attendant risk of laryngospasm.

Once anaesthesia is established and the airway is secure the choice of anaesthetic agent and whether or not to use a muscle relaxant or allow spontaneous ventilation is somewhat arbitrary. However, a technique which allows a rapid return of consciousness and control of laryngeal reflexes is preferable and one which also provides some analgesia in the immediate postoperative period is desirable. A modified neurolept-analgesic technique is, therefore, suitable.

Recovery

In the postoperative period oedema and distortion of the airway still present a hazard and in addition the jaws may be wired together. The airway must be carefully protected for the first 24 hr and the patient closely observed.

- The patient must not be extubated until he is awake or an adequate nasopharyngeal airway can be guaranteed.
- Where nasotracheal intubation has been employed the partially withdrawn endotracheal tube can be employed as a nasopharyngeal airway in the postoperative period.

It is best if the optimum position of the tube is determined at the time of induction of anaesthesia. If suitable manufacturers' markings are not provided, this position is best re-obtained by noting the length of tube remaining outside the nose. Marking the tube with ink is unreliable as the marks can be wiped off during passage through the nose.

When the tube has been withdrawn to the correct position its position can be marked by transfixing the tube with a safety pin at the point where it exits from the nostril. Care should be taken not to occlude the lumen to the passage of a suction catheter. The nasopharyngeal airway can be useful for suction but care must be taken to suck out its whole length or the tip will become blocked with a plug of blood and mucus and so obstruct rather than maintain the airway. The nasopharyngeal airway should be kept in place until the patient can maintain his own airway.

- Humidified air with added oxygen should be administered.
- When the jaws are wired together wire cutters and a diagram of the position of the wires must be kept at the bedside. The nurses should be instructed how to cut the wires if the patient vomits and the airway cannot be sucked clear.

It may be safer to leave the endotracheal tube *in situ* for about 36 hr after major surgery as oedema around the airway continues to increase for this length of time; adequate analgesia and IPPV can be provided in the ICU.

Ear, nose and throat emergencies

General problems

As in facio-maxillary surgery haemorrhage can lead to shock and swallowed blood may exacerbate the problem of the full stomach. As ENT emergencies are more likely to involve children who invariably swallow blood in the upper airway and who have smaller blood volume, these problems are likely to be more acute.

Specific problems

The problems of an obstructed airway and difficult intubation are again the same as those found in facio-maxillary emergencies and once again are greater in children who have a smaller diameter and more vulnerable upper airway.

Airway obstruction and difficult intubation

- Trismus (spasm of the muscles of the jaw) may be provoked by inflammation (peritonsillar abcess), tumour or irradiation. Early passage of a nasopharyngeal tube will remove any respiratory obstruction. Do not cause a nose bleed; use a local vasoconstrictor (*see* p. 74).
- Oedema of the pharynx, glottis or epiglottis may obstruct the airway (particularly in children with laryngotracheitis or epiglottitis). The epiglottis may become impacted into the airway and require disimpaction under direct vision using a laryngoscope. Swelling of the aryepiglottic folds may produce a one–way valve effect allowing expiration but impeding inspiration. Spasm of the vestibular ligament may occur with oedema of its overlying mucous membrane which together make up the vestibular fold (false cord). Spasm of the vocal ligament may occur with oedema of its overlying mucous membrane which together make up the vocal fold (true cord).

Oral intubation with halothane/oxygen anaesthesia, emergency tracheostomy or emergency cricothyroidotomy may be required. *In extremis* cricothyroid puncture with transtracheal insufflation may be necessary (note: a standard 15 mm taper, size 3.5 mm endotracheal tube connector can be fitted to any Luer-fitting cannula) (*see* p. 17).

Operations

Fractured nasal bones

In experienced hands minor manipulations can sometimes be carried out under intravenous anaesthesia in the head-down position.

- This is a trap for the unwary and inexperienced. Profound haemorrhage can occur in the middle of the procedure. It is safer to use cuffed orotracheal intubation with a throat pack to prevent aspiration of blood.

Post-tonsillectomy haemorrhage

- Beware – this is a very dangerous condition.

The patient, usually a child, will have covert blood loss and be in circulatory shock. The stomach will be full of blood clot and circulatory collapse may occur on induction of anaesthesia.

- Resuscitate with IV fluids and order an emergency supply of blood before inducing anaesthesia.
- Induce anaesthesia by inhalation with the patient head down lying on his left side. (The tongue does not then get in the way of the laryngoscope blade as it would with a patient on his right side).
- Nasotracheal intubation is contra-indicated after adenoidectomy; intubation will be more rapid in the accustomed position so turn the patient on his back and intubate orally (use cricoid pressure, *see* p. 7).
- It is almost impossible to empty the stomach through a gastric tube. Therefore, postoperative vomiting will occur; position the patient to avoid aspiration and have efficient suction apparatus immediately to hand.

Peritonsillar abscess

If there is no respiratory obstruction light general anaesthesia in the head-down position may be given for incision of the abscess.

- If respiratory obstruction is present it is safer to incise the abscess under topical anaesthesia with lignocaine (lidocaine) or cocaine.
- Ensure adequate suction and head-down position.
- Emergency tracheostomy may be required.

Laryngoscopy/bronchoscopy for inhaled foreign body

In adults a foreign body passing the vocal cords will lodge in the bronchial tree; in children it may lodge in the narrow sub-glottic part of the trachea and emergency tracheostomy or cricothyroidotomy with transtracheal ventilation may be required.

Where there is no upper airway obstruction the use of a Sander's[5] insufflator attached to the bronchoscope or laryngoscope may force the foreign body further down the airway. This danger is greatest in children. The safest technique is deep halothane and oxygen anaesthesia with the patient breathing spontaneously.

Injuries to the larynx and trachea

Tubes may be passed into holes in the larynx and trachea. They can be changed to orotracheal tubes once anaesthesia is established (*see* p. 142)

- A rigid bronchoscope may be used to provide an artificial airway in a trachea which is collapsing.

Emergency tracheostomy (*see* p. 203)

- Inhalation anaesthesia is safer as a partial obstruction may become total when muscle relaxation occurs.
- Have a large selection of tube sizes available.
- A gum–elastic bougie may be used as a guide to railroad a tube down a partially obstructed trachea.
- The low density of helium enables it to flow through an orifice three times faster than air. When mixed with 20 per cent oxygen it may enable more oxygen to reach the alveoli through a narrow tube.

Middle-ear emergencies

All middle-ear surgery can be performed electively. Myringotomy to release pus from the middle ear can be performed under local anaesthesia in adults and light general anaesthesia in young children.

Choice of anaesthetic technique

As with facio-maxillary surgery once anaesthesia is established with an adequate airway the choice of anaesthetic agent is somewhat arbitrary. Hypotensive anaesthesia is used for some ENT operations (usually middle-ear surgery) but is contra-indicated when any element of hypovolaemia may be present. Very small doses of anaesthetic agents are required in shocked patients. Intravenous agents are especially dangerous – remember Pearl Harbor (mortality from barbiturate anaesthesia in the 1930s, 1:800; mortality from barbiturate anaesthesia at Pearl Harbor, 1:80).

Recovery

- Where partial airway obstruction was present prior to induction, carbon dioxide retention may maintain the blood pressure. Relief of respiratory obstruction and return of

arterial carbon dioxide tension to normal may produce a profound fall in blood pressure.
- Following tracheostomy a tracheal obturator and tracheal dilating forceps must be kept by the patient and a spare tracheostomy tube of the same size and type. It can be extremely difficult to replace a tracheostomy tube in the immediate postoperative period.

References

1. Baraka A. Bronchoscopic removal of inhaled foreign bodies in children. *Br. J. Anaesth.* 1974; **46:** 124.
2. Lee ST. Ventilating laryngoscope for inhalation anaesthesia and augmented ventilation during laryngoscopic procedures. *Br. J. Anaesth.* 1972; **44:** 874.
3. Seed RF. Traumatic injury to the larynx and trachea. *Anaesthesia* 1971; **26:** 56.
4. Smith RB, Myers EN, Sherman, H. Transtracheal ventilation in paediatric patients. *Br. J. Anaesth.* 1974; **46:** 313.
5. Sanders RD. Two ventilating attachments for bronchoscopes. *Del. Med. J.* 1967; **39:** 170.

Further reading

Stoddart JC. *Trauma and the Anaesthetist.* Ballière Tindall: London, 1984.

14

Dental Problems

Ann M Skelly

Acute toothache
Dento-alveolar trauma
Bleeding
Local analgesia
   Intravenous benzodiazepines (diazepam and midazolam)
   Inhalation sedation
General anaesthesia
   Assessment and planning of general anaesthesia
   Anaesthetic technique
Other problems
   Infections and trauma
   Foreign bodies

The practice of dentistry has changed dramatically in character in the past 30 years. Before this time, the bulk of treatment consisted of the extraction of painful teeth as necessary and finally the clearance of all remaining teeth and roots and the provision of full dentures. Particularly in the United Kingdom and the USA, general anaesthesia was routinely used for these procedures.

Such use now represents a very small part of general dental practice. Factors which have contributed to this change include the introduction and widespread use of antibiotics, effective local analgesics and ultra high speed cutting instruments, so that infections can be treated and complex restorative work undertaken using local analgesia.

General anaesthesia is required, however, for certain dental emergencies. Whilst anaesthetists in training programmes in hospitals associated with dental schools or busy oral surgical units may receive comprehensive training in the techniques of dental anaesthesia, many will gain their first experience of these in the management of an emergency.

Emergency dental treatment may be required in the following circumstances:

- Acute toothache
- Dento–alveolar trauma
- Bleeding

Acute toothache

This may be due to inflammation of the dental pulp (pulpitis) or to abscess formation. The treatment required may be:

- removal of decay and obtundent dressing,
- removal of pulp tissue and dressing,
- drainage of pus through tooth,
- incision of soft tissue abscess, or
- extraction of tooth.

Dento-alveolar trauma

This results mainly from road traffic accidents and civil injuries among adults (frequently associated with the use of alcohol), and from home or playground accidents in the case of children.

The treatment required may be:

- Tooth fractures – dressing
  removal of pulp and dressing
  removal of fragments or remains of teeth
  splinting
- Alveolar bone fractures – splinting
  intermaxillary fixation
- Soft tissue injuries – debridement of wounds
  removal of teeth and foreign material
  suturing

Bleeding

This may persist after surgery, necessitating suturing of sockets.

Local analgesia

All of the above procedures can be performed using local analgesia, either immediately or after a period of antibiotic and analgesic therapy. This is the method of choice whenever it is possible. Soft tissue abscesses can be incised under topical ethyl chloride analgesia.

Usually appropriate infiltrations and nerve blocks are given by the dental surgeon. Special syringes and needles are used with commercially prepared cartridges of local analgesics usually containing a vasoconstrictor. These include:

Lignocaine (lidocaine) 2 per cent with adrenaline (epinephrine) 1:80 000 or 1:100 000

Prilocaine 3 per cent with felypressin 0.03 i.u./ml

Mepivacaine 3 per cent

The use of local analgesia may be impossible in the following circumstances

- Where patients are unable or unwilling to co-operate: e.g. very young children, mentally or physically handicapped individuals, and excessively anxious patients.
- Where local analgesia is ineffective or contra-indicated: e.g. in the presence of local infection, in patients with bleeding disorders (haemophilia, Von Willebrand's disease etc), and true allergies to components of local analgesia solutions.

Where local analgesia alone is not possible, treatment may be facilitated by the use of conscious sedation techniques. The anaesthetist may on occasion be called upon to provide such sedation.

Intravenous benzodiazepines (diazepam and midazolam)

These may enable treatment to be carried out under local analgesia on highly anxious patients or can be used to cover particularly unpleasant or stressful procedures in co-operative individuals. For example, intermaxillary wiring can be successfully accomplished where jaw fractures are dento-alveolar only, or easily reduced and stabilized. These drugs do not, however, produce reliable sedation in young children and teenagers and are therefore not useful in these cases. In addition they cannot be used for painful procedures where local analgesia is prohibited or ineffective.

Inhalation sedation

Inhalation sedation with low concentrations of nitrous oxide (Relative Analgesia) is very useful for the anxious but reasonably co-operative adult or child. This technique has the added advantage of conferring a degree of analgesia and may be used therefore where local analgesia is not complete or without analgesia. This may be invaluable in the emergency relief of pain for patients with bleeding disorders in whom obtundent dressings may be needed pending definitive surgical treatment such as extractions after factor replacement therapy.

Concentrations of between 20 and 40 per cent nitrous oxide in oxygen commonly provide excellent sedation but higher concentrations may be required if the nitrous oxide is the sole analgesic used. In an emergency this can be delivered from any standard anaesthetic machine but many dental units are equipped with special machines limiting the maximum concentration of nitrous oxide used to 70 per cent.

General anaesthesia

Where general anaesthesia is required for emergency dental treatment the following factors are very important and the anaesthetist should not agree to providing general anaesthesia without their consideration.

Assessment and planning for general anaesthesia

Many of these patients can be treated on an outpatient or day-case basis. Where facilities are available this is the most satisfactory system. The anaesthetic and operation time will frequently be very short and the majority of patients will be fit and well aside from their dental problems.

General physical status

- Normally outpatient anaesthesia should only be considered for ASA class I and II patients. The strict interpretation of class II may, however, be modified by circumstances – some of which are discussed below.

Age of the patient

Many patients will be young children. They are often distressed and in pain, and both they and their parents may be short of sleep. They require treating in the most expeditious and considerate manner and preferably as outpatients.

Exceptions to the strict ASA I and II clause may be made for these children and indeed to adults for short procedures.

It has been suggested that outpatient anaesthesia need not be denied to patients with such conditions as bronchial asthma, mild congenital heart disease, diabetes or epilepsy providing that they are well controlled. In these circumstances general anaesthesia should only be undertaken by a very experienced anaesthetist working with an experienced dental surgeon and facilities for overnight hospital admission must be available in case of problems. It should be remembered that the dental condition may affect the underlying disease; e.g. acute infection can upset diabetic control and trauma and anxiety may precipitate an exacerbation of asthma or epilepsy.

Immediate condition of the patient

The following factors may affect the planning of treatment:

Pain
Relief must be effected as soon as possible within the confines of safety.

Fever and dehydration
A combination of the effects of pyrexia and prolonged abstinence from fluids (due either to toothache or instructions to fast prior to attending for general anaesthesia) may result in patients and in particular in children who are markedly dehydrated. This may cause problems in finding a suitable venepuncture site. It is unlikely that dehydration will be severe enough to require IV fluid replacement although this may occasionally be the case with spreading fascial space infections. In these cases admission and rehydration is essential.

If general anaesthesia cannot be carried out immediately for dehydrated children, it is often better to give a long glucose drink and electively delay anaesthesia for at least 4 hr.

Swelling and trismus
Buccal swelling may render the use of a face-mask difficult and painful but does not usually impede airway control unless it is associated with much limitation of opening. Lingual space swelling can both involve the pharynx directly affecting the patency of the airway and is more commonly a cause of trismus. Pre-anaesthetic examination of any dental patient must include a careful inspection of swelling and the degree of trismus.

Where it seems likely that airway maintenance will be severely compromised, the anaesthetic should be postponed until the swelling has been reduced by antibiotic therapy; if necessary by intravenous infusion.

In those cases where surgical intervention is considered essential to establish drainage of pus, an anaesthetic must only be given by an experienced anaesthetist.

- In these cases awake intubation can be used or the trachea intubated either with deep inhalational anaesthesia (e.g. halothane) under direct vision or by blind nasal intubation (*see* p. 74); no intravenous drugs are given.

Analgesics and alcohol

Patients who require emergency dental treatment may have taken large quantities of analgesics. Alcohol is also commonly used to achieve both analgesia and sufficient courage to attend for treatment.

- Alcohol should be borne in mind when such patients are examined and the possibility of potentiation of anaesthetic agents considered. The risk of gastric regurgitation may be increased in patients who have consumed alcohol and must always be considered in cases of trauma.

Anaesthetic technique

Premedication

It is not usual to premedicate any dental outpatients and in the emergency situation this is certainly the case. Whilst a number of these patients may be highly anxious and some authorities recommend the use of oral benzodiazepines (*see* p. 105), their effect may be unpredictable and they may merely delay recovery. Anticholinergics should be avoided. Drying agents are not usually required and atropine may cause undesirable tachycardias especially in conjunction with high levels of endogenous catecholamines.

Induction of anaesthesia

Where possible this should be by IV injection, methohexitone (methohexital) being the drug of first choice. Intravenous induction may be impossible for young children or for adults with needle phobias.

Inhalational induction with halothane is the usual alternative to the use of IV agents. The use of either enflurane or isoflurane has been shown to reduce the incidence of arrhythmias which are commonly associated with dental manipulations but they are probably not suitable for inhalational induction in the emergency case as induction may be less smooth.

Position

Traditionally dental anaesthetics have been given with the patient sitting upright in the dental chair, and in the nonintubated patient some consider that airway control is easier in this position. In view of the potential risk of hypotension and the hazard of inhalation of vomit or blood by the upright patient the supine position is preferable. In modern dental chairs it is possible to elevate the legs above hip level and have the back set at a slightly upward tilt. From a practical point of view it must be remembered that many children and some anxious adults will not submit readily to being laid flat and induction may have to be carried out in the sitting position or on a parent's lap, and the appropriate position established once consciousness is lost.

Tracheal intubation

This will usually be required for procedures lasting more than about 10 min, where airway control is anticipated to be difficult or where the site or nature of the operative treatment makes it impossible in the presence of a face or nose mask (e.g. for surgery in the region of the upper incisor teeth).

Nasotracheal intubation is commonly used for dentistry to allow for maximum access by the surgeon. Spraying the nose with a solution of 0.5 per cent phenylephrine will reduce the risk of epistaxis. Atropine or glycopyrronium (glycopyrrolate) may be required in the unpremedicated patient before a muscle relaxant is used, particularly in children as they are very liable to bradycardia.

If intubation is used there must be facilities for an adequate stay in the recovery area and overnight admission if necessary. Under these conditions even small children may be intubated on a day-stay basis and discharged only when any risk of obstructive laryngeal oedema is considered to have passed.

Packing

A throat pack must be placed around any endotracheal tube by the anaesthetist. In the nonintubated patient, the oral cavity must be adequately isolated from the oropharynx both to avoid escape of fresh gases and to protect the airway against the inhalation of saliva, blood, pus or teeth. Packing is usually carried out by the surgeon using gauze strips or preformed commercially made packs. Efficient suction is of course essential.

It is the responsibility of the anaesthetist to maintain airway control at all times and surgery must not proceed in the presence of inadequate packing or persistent obstruction. Maintenance of an adequate airway can be difficult and the presence of a pack can considerably limit operative access for the dentist so that team co-operation is essential. The operator can often improve airway patency by holding the mandible forward and the anaesthetist can provide counter pressure against extractions to the top of the head or the angle of the mandible. Where airway maintenance proves difficult this may sometimes be overcome by the use of a naso-pharyngeal tube.

- It is important to ensure at the end of the anaesthetic that the mandible is in the correct position as dislocation forward is common and may be difficult to reduce once muscle tone is restored.

Monitoring

Opinions vary as to the amount of monitoring that is required but an electrocardiogram should be considered a minimum requirement.

Recovery

Even after extremely short anaesthetics, patients should not normally be discharged until at least an hour has elapsed, and as mentioned previously any patient who has been intubated must stay for at least 3 hr.

Other problems

Infections and trauma

The anaesthetist may be called upon to provide assistance in airway control for patients with dental or facio-maxillary infections or trauma in the emergency department.

Bilateral spreading fascial space infection (Ludwig's angina) or acute postsurgical bleeding may result in airway loss and intubation or even cricothyroidotomy or tracheostomy may be required urgently.

Similarly, acute airway loss can occur due to loss of tongue control in the case of bilateral parasymphyseal fractures of the mandible or the impaction of middle third (Le Fort II and III) fractures (*see* p. 158) if consciousness is lost.

Foreign bodies

Dental problems may also affect the management of anaesthetics given for other purposes.

Dentures, loose teeth or crowns may be broken or dislodged into the pharynx during intubation.

- If there is any likelihood that foreign bodies may have entered the lungs a chest radiograph is mandatory and must be taken at the earliest opportunity. If the object is indeed lodged within the lungs appropriate antibiotic therapy must be started and arrangements made for its removal. Lung abscess is a feared complication.

If teeth are broken or crowns removed, arrangements should be made for these to be dealt with as soon as possible. In hospitals with dental departments it is usual to arrange for this to be carried out on site if the patient so wishes. In all such cases the patient must be informed of the mishap and adequate notes made for medico-legal purposes.

Trismus, limitation of mouth opening or oddly placed over-erupted teeth can make endotracheal intubation difficult in otherwise routine cases. Careful pre-anaesthetic examination allows for such difficulties to be anticipated and planned for in advance.

Further reading

Coplans MP, Green RA (eds). *Anaesthesia and Sedation in Dentistry* (Monographs in Anaesthesiology – 12). Amsterdam: Elsevier, 1983.

15

Ophthalmic Emergencies

John H Cook

Minor emergencies
Major emergencies
    Local anaesthesia
    General anaesthesia
Postoperative pain

Ophthalmic emergencies can be classified as minor or major, the latter being subdivided into those where the globe is not perforated and those when it is either perforated or is to be opened during the course of surgery.

The factor that separates anaesthesia for ophthalmic surgery from that for other branches of surgery is the intraocular pressure and its control at any time that the globe is open. Anything which in a normal eye would cause a rise in intraocular pressure may cause the contents of the eye to be extruded while the corneoscleral coat is breached.

In clinical practice any patient presenting with an ophthalmic injury should be assessed to exclude other injuries. However, in this chapter it will be assumed that non-ophthalmic injuries have been excluded.

Minor emergencies

Minor ophthalmic injuries such as cuts of the soft tissues round the orbit or foreign bodies on the cornea are relatively common and can usually be dealt with satisfactorily under local anaesthesia.

Cuts of the lids can be cleaned and sutured after infiltrating the site with 1 per cent lignocaine (lidocaine). The eyelids are very vascular and hence always heal well, but bleeding can be troublesome at the time of repair. This can be reduced by using lignocaine solution containing adrenaline (epinephrine) 1:400 000.

Superficial foreign bodies of the cornea or conjunctiva can be removed and conjunctival lacerations repaired after instilling local anaesthetic drops such as 1 per cent amethocaine into the conjunctival sac. All local anaesthetics produce some degree of toxicity to the cornea but this is particularly marked with cocaine. Before the introduction of antiviral agents this effect was commonly used in carbolizing dendritic ulcers. Instillation of cocaine loosened the corneal epithelium and made it easier to remove. However, in treating a corneal abrasion it is best to avoid repeated instillation of a local anaesthetic agent as this will delay healing. Pain can usually be adequately controlled by instillation of a mydriatic such as 1 per cent atropine drops, and, having applied antibiotic eye ointment, closing the eye for 24–48 hr.

Babies and young children may need a general anaesthetic for treatment of minor ophthalmic injuries in order to keep them still. Any inhalation anaesthetic will suffice, halothane being perfectly satisfactory. If the patient has been starved it may not be necessary to intubate; removal of the face mask will allow one or two minutes for the procedure and this is commonly all that is needed. Alternatively the breathing circuit can be attached to a special oral airway (e.g. Charles' airway) sealed in place with strong adhesive tape.

Major emergencies

Major emergencies can be treated under local or general anaesthesia but the latter is the better choice wherever possible. This is because general anaesthesia relieves the patient from the necessity of keeping still for what can be a long anxious time and guarantees the surgeon an immobile patient, which is especially important if the operating microscope is used.

Local anaesthesia

This may be administered as follows:

- Amethocaine 1 per cent eye drops are instilled into the conjunctival sac every 5 min for ½ hr.
- A retrobulbar injection of 1.5 ml of 0.5 per cent bupivacaine is given. This is to anaesthetize the part of the eye not reached by the topical amethocaine, particularly the iris and ciliary body. It is important not to use adrenaline as the central retinal artery is an end-artery.
- If surgery to the lids is needed or if lid retraction sutures are going to be placed, then local anaesthetic solution is infiltrated at the necessary sites.

- If a superior rectus stabilizing suture is to be used then a bleb of local anaesthetic solution is injected into its tendon.

This completes the induction of analgesia but in order to avoid the orbicularis oculi muscle 'squeezing' the eye, akinesia is achieved with a facial nerve block.

Problems of local anaesthesia

- Patient co-operation is required. LA is best avoided with patients who do not understand the language, are deaf, or who have any other impediment to communication.
- The first instillation of amethocaine causes a stinging sensation. This can cause squeezing of the lids which can be detrimental to a perforated eye.
- A retrobulbar haemorrhage is a recognized complication of a retrobulbar injection; there are many veins in the orbit. By the time this complication has been recognized, there will already be increased pressure behind the eye. If the eye is already open this can be disastrous. If it is to be opened there is increased risk of loss of ocular contents. Although elective surgery is always postponed for a few weeks after a retrobulbar haemorrhage in the emergency situation postponement may not be possible and the risk to the eye is increased.

The patient may be helped to tolerate the procedure under local anaesthesia by being sedated. Drugs ranging from a small dose of a benzodiazepine (diazepam) to the lytic cocktail (pethidine [demerol], promethazine and chlorpromazine), have been used for this purpose. Depending on the level of sedation, the patient's ability to co-operate can be lost and he may move without realizing what he is doing. It is easy to move the head unintentionally while supporting the chin which may be necessary to avoid airway obstruction. The technique of local anaesthesia plus heavy sedation can be the worst compromise of all.

General anaesthesia

There are no specific problems for major ophthalmic emergencies (such as repair of the lachrymal apparatus) so long as the globe of the eye is intact and will not be opened during surgery. Any standard emergency technique will suffice provided that the trachea is intubated.

- If there is any doubt as to whether or not the globe is

perforated anaesthesia should be conducted as for a perforating eye injury.

Anaesthesia for a perforating eye injury

It is often possible to postpone emergency surgery for a patient with a full stomach who has small perforating eye injury. This will be of some help in reducing the risk of pulmonary aspiration occuring during subsequent anaesthesia in a patient with no other injuries. In such cases the administration of metoclopramide (10 mg IM or IV) to assist gastric emptying is of value; however, administration of narcotics will negate this effect and gastric emptying will be delayed.

- Intraocular pressure (IOP) must not be allowed to rise during anaesthesia for fear of expulsion of the contents of the globe through the perforation.

The following points are important in any anaesthetic technique.

- Avoid anything that causes a rise in CVP such as coughing, straining or bucking on the endotracheal tube; any such increases in CVP are directly transmitted to the veins of the eye and orbit. Avoid a head-down tilt for the same reason.
- Do not press on the eye (take care with face-mask).
- Do not use ketamine as it raises IOP.
- Suxamethonium (succinylcholine) produces a rise in IOP. The use of 'pretreatment' with a small dose of a nondepolarizing neuromuscular blocking drug does not help and in fact can compound problems with intubation (*see* below).

IOP may be reduced by:

- Hyperventilation to reduce $P\text{aco}_2$.
- Relaxation of the extraocular muscles by use of a nondepolarizing neuromuscular blocking drug.
- Use of a volatile anaesthetic agent, e.g. halothane, enflurane, isoflurane.
- Mannitol (50 g IV slowly) should be considered to increase the tonicity of plasma (*see* p. 59).

The choice of anaesthetic technique for tracheal intubation is controversial. Suxamethonium (succinylcholine) is known to increase IOP and therefore methods to avoid the use of this drug have obvious appeal; on the other hand, the nondepolarizing neuromuscular blocking agents do not act as swiftly and therefore the patient is potentially at danger from pulmonary aspiration for a slightly longer time and there is also the possibility of a serious situation developing if tracheal intubation proves impossible.

Provided that assessment of the patient leaves no doubt about the feasibility of tracheal intubation, and the anaesthetist is experienced, the following technique is suggested in the presence of a full stomach.

- Use atropine as a premedicant (anti-sialogogue and vagolytic action).
- Preoxygenation is essential but difficult because it is important not to press on the eye with the face-mask.
- Vecuronium 0.2 mg/kg is given into a fast running IV infusion.
- Cricoid pressure is applied (*see* p. 7) as paralysis begins to take effect as judged by the development of ptosis; strangely enough patients feel that they are going to sleep.
- Immediately this sign appears a generous predetermined dose of thiopentone (thiopental) (8 mg/kg) is given quickly provided that the patient's cardiovascular status is satisfactory. The trachea can be intubated without reaction by the patient with a cuffed reinforced (nonkinking) endotracheal tube in about 90 sec from the time the relaxant has been given; the overall time to intubation is therefore hardly longer than the rapid sequence intubation time using suxamethonium (succinylcholine).

Vecuronium is to be preferred to atracurium because histamine release is not a problem even in high dose. Both drugs in high dosage have an onset time which is faster than conventional non-depolarizing neuromuscular drugs, e.g. tubocurarine, alcuronium or pancuronium; however, although atracurium releases less histamine than tubocurarine this effect is a potential problem when atracurium is used in doses > 0.6 mg/kg which would be necessary with this technique.

The problem remains that laryngoscopy and intubation of the trachea are both procedures that provoke large rises in IOP and arterial pressure even if suxamethonium is not used. For this reason it has been suggested that this pressor response can be attenuated by giving an IV bolus of 2 mg/kg lignocaine (lidocaine) and that in these circumstances suxamethonium may be used although there are as many supporters as opponents regarding the effectiveness of this.[1,2,3] Some argue that even without the use of a lignocaine (lidocaine) bolus a rapid sequence intubation technique using 'pretreatment' with tubocurarine 3–6 mg or gallamine 10–15 mg followed by thiopentone (thiopental) and suxamethonium (succinylcholine) does not clinically result in extrusion of the contents of the globe through the perforation.[4] If this approach is thought to be of over-riding importance, e.g. from the patient's survival point of view, a large dose of suxamethonium (2 mg/kg) should be used so as to give the best possible chance of a swift and atraumatic intubation. A large dose of suxamethonium (succinylcholine) *per se* does not result in a less deleterious effect on the eye in terms of rises in IOP as has been suggested.[5]

- IPPV is established with oxygen and nitrous oxide; anaesthesia is supplemented with halothane (0.5 per cent), enflurane (1 per cent) or isoflurane (0.75 per cent).
- At some stage during anaesthesia a large bore stomach tube (*see* p. 12) is passed to remove any gas and fluid to minimize postoperative retching and vomiting and the risk of pulmonary aspiration during recovery.
- At the conclusion of surgery the patient is turned onto his side with the operated eye uppermost, any secretions in the pharynx gently aspirated, residual neuromuscular block antagonized, the gaseous anaesthetic withdrawn and 100 per cent oxygen substituted. Extubation is a matter of delicate judgement: there is less likelihood of coughing and laryngeal spasm if the patient is 'deep' rather than 'light' – the main requirement is that the anaesthetist is able to avoid any of the potential problems which may arise at this stage, e.g. apnoea, laryngospasm or vomiting, without compromising the injured eye or the life of the patient.

Oculocardiac reflex

The oculocardiac reflex is initiated by manipulating the eye and especially by traction on the extraocular muscles. An ECG monitor is mandatory when administering general anaesthesia for eye surgery. Bradycardia or multiple extrasystoles may develop: surgical traction on the extraocular muscles should be immediately released. Bradycardia usually responds to IV atropine, and multiple extrasystoles to a small dose of a β-adrenergic receptor antagonist, e.g. 3–5 mg IV metoprolol.

Postoperative pain

A painful eye after operation is often less severe than might be anticipated and responds to mild analgesics, e.g. paracetamol. In patients where opiates are indicated nausea and vomiting may be reduced by the use of antiemetic drugs.

References

1. Murphy DF. Anesthesia and intraocular pressure. *Anesth. Analg.* 1985; **64**: 520–30.

2. Smith RB, Babiusk M, Leano N. The effect of lidocaine on succinylcholine–induced rise in intraocular pressure. *Canad. Anaesth. Soc. J.* 1979; **26**: 482–9.
3. Drenger B, Péer J, BenEzra D, Katzenelson R, Davidson JT. The effect of intravenous lidocaine on the increase in intraocular pressure induced by tracheal intubation. *Anesth. Analg.* 1985; **64**: 1211–13.
4. Libonati MM, Leahy JJ, Ellison N. The use of succinylcholine in open eye surgery. *Anesthesiology* 1985; **62**: 637–40.
5. Cook JH. The effect of suxamethonium on intraocular pressure. *Anaesthesia* 1981; **36**: 359–65.

Further reading

Smith GB. *Ophthalmic Anaesthesia*. London: Edward Arnold, 1983.
Smith RB (ed). Anesthesia in ophthalmology. *International Anesthesiology Clinics* 1973; **13** (2).
Spence AA, Norman J (eds). Symposium on anaesthesia and the eye. *Br. J. Anaesth.* 1980; **52**: 641–703.

16

Major Vascular Surgery

Charles Beattie

Pre-operative preparation
Monitoring and case preparation
   Hypothermia
   Vasoactive drugs
Anaesthesia
   Renal function
Aortic cross-clamp
   Suprarenal cross-clamp
Aortic clamp release
Postoperative care

The term 'major vascular surgery,' herein refers to procedures which require cross-clamping of the aorta, usually for repair of aneurysms or for replacement of a vascular segment due to aorto-occlusive disease. Most of the physiological and pharmacological principles are also applicable to penetrating wounds involving the aorta. Special anaesthetic considerations are required even in elective cases because:

- these patients have a high incidence of ancillary disease, mostly cardiovascular (cerebral, coronary, renal)
- they will be subjected to multiple stresses in the peri-operative period some of which are unique to this procedure.

In this review practical clinical aspects of management with an emphasis on emergency situations involving leaking or ruptured aortic aneurysms are outlined. Problems associated with high aortic cross-clamp (above the renal arteries) are emphasized since these cases offer the most serious anaesthetic challenge.

Pre-operative preparation

Patients for major vascular surgery may be encountered with a wide range of presentations. The clinical spectrum includes at worst an individual with a ruptured aneurysm who is hypotensive and may require surgical intervention in the emergency room including abdominal or thoracic clamping of the aorta. At the other extreme is a patient for elective repair of a known aortic aneurysm or with aortic occlusive disease suffering only claudication. Even patients in this latter group, however, are extremely high risk for peri-operative morbidity.

If the surgery is imminent but not urgent, it should be preceeded by a medical work-up which focuses on pulmonary dysfunction and cardiovascular disease.[1,2]

- Often correction of coronary or cerebral lesions is indicated prior to aortic repair.[3] The association of these disease states is quite high and their presence should be assumed even in symptom free individuals.[4]

The patient with a leaking aneurysm is usually a treated hypertensive who presents with alarmingly high blood pressure which may be quite difficult to control. Whereas prompt institution of a nitroprusside infusion is the primary treatment, pure vasodilatation is often insufficient. The patient will respond with an increase in heart rate and may increase cardiac output. (Elevated shear forces in this state could conceivably be injurious in the presence of aortic dissection.) Early institution of the β-adrenoceptor blocker propranolol is desirable unless contra-indicated (heart block, bronchospasm). It should be administered in sufficient doses IV with, of course, continuous arterial pressure and electrocardiographic monitoring. It is sometimes necessary to give large cumulative doses (up to 10 mg) from multiple increments ($\sim$ 1 mg bolus). Continuous infusion of verapamil (300–400 micrograms/min) is a newer alternative which might serve several useful purposes (vasodilatation, negative chronotropy and inotropy) at once. When blood pressure has been stabilized the operation may be planned and may proceed in an orderly fashion.

Aneurysmal rupture constitutes a medical/surgical emergency with features identical to blunt or penetrating aortic vascular injuries. The patient will probably be in shock and be receiving resuscitative ministrations (mast trousers, IV fluids, central line placement, etc.) from other medical personnel when first encountered by the anaesthetist. Oxygen supplementation is often overlooked by surgical and emergency room physicians if the patient is breathing well and if so it should be instituted. To intubate or not to intubate the trachea prior to arrival in the operating room is frequently a difficult judgement (airway protection *vs.* overstimulation). Fluid administration should be vigorous as appropriate but volume overloading is best avoided. Dilutional anaemia, coagulopathy, congestive heart failure and hypothermia are all real dangers in the poorly monitored period before operation. If possible an anaesthetist should be dispatched to participate in the patient's early care while others prepare the operating room for his arrival (Table 16.1).

Monitoring and case preparation

- Continuous intravascular measurement of arterial pressure via an indwelling arterial cannula and central pressure from an intrathoracic cannula are considered to be routine for any cross-clamp procedure.
- Two leads of ECG including inferior and lateral are continuously monitored.
- Intravenous access for the rapid administration of large fluid volumes is necessary and includes at minimum two large bore (14 G) peripheral lines.
- The issue of whether or not to place a pulmonary artery catheter is based upon the degree of cardiovascular and pulmonary dysfunction which the patient displays pre-operatively, the urgency of the procedure, and the level of the aortic cross-clamp which will be necessary during surgery.

We use flow-directed pulmonary artery catheters in virtually all patients who are to receive cross-clamps above the renal

Table 16.1   Pre-operative patient preparation (compare urgent situation with the elective)

Elective	1. Pulmonary and cardiovascular work-up.
	2. Coronary artery bypass graft or carotid endarterectomy if indicated.
	3. Optimize medications.
Leaking aneurysm	1. Vigorous blood pressure control with continuous infusion vasodilator. Add β-adrenergic receptor blocking drug in sufficient dose to control HR and/or CO.
	2. Proceed forthrightly but calmly when stable.
Ruptured aneurysm	1. Resuscitation with blood, fluids, multiple IV access, O_2, airway protection.
	2. Possible cross-clamp in emergency room.
	3. High mortality.

arteries. In addition, any evidence of significant coronary artery disease or ventricular dysfunction dictates placement of a pulmonary artery catheter for infrarenal cases as well.

The minimal monitoring of arterial pressure and central venous pressure are reserved for those patients receiving infrarenal cross-clamps and who are otherwise relatively healthy individuals.

- Under no circumstances should surgery for a patient in shock be delayed for the insertion of invasive monitoring devices. These may be placed while the case is underway.

Hypothermia

Hypothermia is a major problem due to exposure of intra-abdominal contents and large fluid requirements. Patients who have received fluid resuscitation in the emergency room may be profoundly hypothermic upon arrival in the operating room.

- All intravenous fluids, including those given during induction, should be administered through blood warmers. A heated humidifier should be inserted into the breathing system. In addition, the room temperature is increased as much as possible, commensurate with reasonable comfort for the operating personnel.

Vasoactive drugs

Continuous infusion sets for vasoactive agents are prepared pre-operatively including at least an infusion of a vasodilator, usually nitroprusside. Nitroglycerin is an acceptable alternative and depending upon the situation both infusions may be set up beforehand. Dopamine is probably the inotrope of choice by virtue of its renal vasodilating and renal tubule effects. Other vasoactive agents that may be useful during the procedure include α-agonists such as phenylephrine which are used for vasoconstriction.

- Whether or not these multiple infusions are prepared, syringes of these agents should be available for bolus administration (sodium nitroprusside 40–100 micrograms/ml, phenylephrine 50–100 micrograms/ml, calcium chloride 1 mmol/ml), together with routine drugs, (*see* p. 19).

It is important to arrange infusions such that the delivery rate can be rapidly changed in response to abrupt intra-operative haemodynamic alterations. Responsive arrangements are of two types. A multiple lumen catheter may be placed centrally which has four or five separate ports for the various infusions to be introduced. An alternative method uses a carrier system whereby an array of stopcocks are put in series and turned on as needed while a carrier fluid runs briskly (75-125 ml/hr) through a central line. This latter arrangement is quite convenient and is possible because the commonly used agents are compatible.

Anaesthesia

Obviously, the techniques of anaesthetic induction will vary widely depending upon the urgency of the situation. In elective cases the anaesthetic agents are chosen according to personal experience of the anaesthetist in conjunction with any specific requirements of the patient's history or status. Generally our preference is a balanced technique with a narcotic base (usually fentanyl) supplemented with nitrous oxide and an inhalational agent as necessary or tolerated. Induction should consist of slow incremental doses or continuous infusions of the drugs of choice. For the moribund patient, intubation with a muscle relaxant but no sedation is appropriate. If the patient is responsive and marginally stable then some form of analgesia and sedation are required but must be chosen carefully.

- Agents which are direct myocardial depressants or vasodilators should be avoided (thiopentone).
- Drugs such as ketamine (2-3 mg/kg), etomidate (0.3-0.5 mg/kg) or fentanyl (25-50 micrograms/kg) or some combination of these (in reduced dosages) offers the best cardiovascular stability in our experience.
- It should be anticipated, however, that patients in poor condition may be dependent on maximal central sympathetic discharge. These patients may develop sudden hypotension secondary to reduction in sympathetic tone attendant upon induction of anaesthesia regardless of the agent used. Simultaneous delivery of vasopressors may be necessary.

Blood should be available in the room and hanging in blood administration sets early in the case as surgery is beginning. This early availability of blood (even in elective cases) is a precaution against the ever present possibility of major bleeding secondary to a surgical mishap.

- In the case of aneurysm rupture the blood requirements are prodigious and outstrip the blood bank's ability to supply cross-matched material. Type specific blood is really quite safe and there should be no hesitation about using it.

Occasionally it is even necessary to use universal donor blood.
- Coagulopathy should be anticipated and the blood bank notified to prepare fresh frozen plasma and platelets.
- During rapid administration of banked blood serious problems of hypocalcaemia, hypo- or hyperkalemia and hypothermia may develop.
- Hypotension occuring in the face of adequate filling pressures should be treated with $CaCl_2$ (5 mEq; 2.5 mmol Ca^{2+}) over about 5 min (*see* p. 20).
- Frequent determinations of serum K^+ and blood-gas status should be obtained.
- Peaked T waves (not necessarily seen in all leads) or a widened QRS complex are indications for initiating treatment for hyperkalaemia (bicarbonate, $CaCl_2$, insulin/glucose: 12.5 units/25 g). Hypokalaemia may present as arrhythmias. Hypothermia can be life threatening as cardiac output decreases approximately 10 per cent/$^\circ$C and rewarming is difficult.

There is usually a small amount of continuous bleeding that persists throughout the case especially after the administration of heparin prior to cross-clamp.

- Attempt to stay somewhat ahead of the estimated surgical blood loss again as a defensive posture against the event of major rapid blood loss. Utilization of a blood scavenging cell saver is probably advisable in these cases.

Renal function

Renal function is a major concern immediately following the stabilization of intravascular volume. There are multiple factors involved in this consideration:

- The aneurysm may involve the renal arteries.
- Periods of hypotension and/or cross-clamping above the renal vessels dispose to ischaemia.
- These patients have a high incidence of renal dysfunction before operation.

The issue of diuretic administration for purposes of renal protection has been debated for some time. It is generally agreed that mannitol administration prior to suprarenal aortic cross-clamp exerts a protective effect tending to prevent ischaemic injury to the kidneys. Recent speculation as to the mechanism for this protection involves the scavenging of free radicals, thereby attenuating reperfusion injury. Less clear is the mechanism whereby infrarenal cross-clamping may change the distribution of renal blood flow and cause alteration in renal function in the peri-operative period. Studies have shown minimal problems with renal dysfunction postoperatively if adequate circulating volume has been maintained during surgery. This has lead to some counsel against the administration of diuretics prior to infrarenal cross-clamp.

- We recommend administering diuretics including mannitol (25 g) and frusemide (furosemide) (20 mg) to establish a brisk urine output of up to 4 ml/kg/hr.

The rationale for this is that urine output is used as a rough index of renal perfusion and overall kidney function.

During the operative procedure surgical manipulation of the renal arteries, veins, and ureters may alter renal perfuson or urine flow. At urine outputs of only 1 ml/kg/hr it is possible for large lag times to exist between the actual production of urine by the kidney and appearance of urine in the collection bag.

Urine tends to accumulate in the bladder and then be expressed in bolus amounts which may be very misleading as to the true renal function which that urine production represents. Administration of diuretics to initate a brisk flow is analogous to increasing the gain or amplification of a measuring device to obtain greater sensitivity.

Because of the above recommendations we have been able to provide immediate feedback to the surgical team on several occasions involving emboli to the kidney or interruption of the ureters. In addition to this consideration, it is occasionally necessary for the surgeon to convert an infrarenal to a suprarenal cross-clamp due to technical difficulties with the graft anastomosis. Under these circumstances, prior administration of mannitol may indeed prove to be protective to the kidney.

Aortic cross-clamp

Haemodynamic changes upon application of an aortic cross-clamp are only partially predictable and may be surprisingly complex depending upon the level of the cross-clamp and the patient's pre-existing circulatory state. Cross-clamps below the renal arteries usually have minimal effects on any of the usually measured cardiovascular parameters with the exception of a slight increase in measured systemic vascular resistance (SVR) and a small increase in arterial pressure. Even these changes may be nil in those individuals with aorto occlusive disease who have poor 'run off' pre-operatively.

Suprarenal cross-clamp

The most obvious and expected change in the systemic haemodynamic profile after cross-clamping the aorta above the renal arteries is an increase in after-load and a concomitant increase in the arterial pressure.

- The normal cardiovascular response to an increase in after-load is an increase in the left ventricular pre-load (PCWP) in an attempt to maintain cardiac output.[6]
- The combination of increase in after-load and increase in pre-load can cause a serious increase in left ventricular wall tension (through the La Place relationship).
- Subendocardial ischaemia is a real possibility under these circumstances especially in the face of pre-existing coronary disease or left ventricular hypertrophy.

These changes may be blunted or perhaps eliminated by the administration of vasodilators.

- Administer a bolus of the vasodilator of choice (either nitrogycerin or nitroprusside) immediately prior to cross-clamping. The cross-clamp is then applied slowly as the effect of the dilator appears on the arterial trace.

It is not possible to predict exactly what dose of bolus administration will be necessary. It is useful to start with small doses of 40–100 micrograms nitroprusside and perhaps a little more (100–200 micrograms) nitroglycerin with immediate increases to double or triple these doses as necessary to control the blood pressure.

After the application of the cross-clamp and the initial control by bolus vasodilator it is almost always necessary to maintain the blood pressure by a continuous infusion of drug. The purpose of the vasodilator is actually two-fold. In addition to controlling the blood pressure, systemic vasodilatation during cross-clamp allows the administration of large amounts of fluid (1.5–3 litres) which is desirable to provide a buffer against hypotension when the clamp is released (*see* p. 188).

Some interesting questions arise as to assessment of the haemodynamic state during aortic cross-clamp. Profound decreases may be observed in both the left ventricular stroke work index (LVSWI) and the cardiac index (CI) during cross-clamping even if filling pressures have been returned with the use of vasodilators to values observed before the clamp was applied. This could be interpreted as myocardial depression, but other factors are important.

- A significant portion of the body is no longer being perfused, especially for high aortic cross-clamps which may exclude not only the renal vessels but the splanchnic circulation as well.

Thus, the system behaves as if the heart is too large for the amount of body it has to perfuse. It is probably reasonable to accept a 20–40 per cent decline in these parameters without undue concern as to their interpretation as left ventricular dysfunction.

- Check the lateral and inferior ECG leads carefully during the cross-clamp period for ischaemia.
- Any residual elevation of filling pressures should be viewed with caution.

If these occur it may be beneficial to institute a continuous infusion of nitroglycerin unless, of course, it is already in use. In this case consideration should be given to the administration of verapamil as that has been shown to influence ischaemic changes when nitroglycerin has failed;[7] verapamil has a long duration of action and prolongs atrioventricular node conduction time as well as having a negative inotropic effect.

Aortic clamp release

The haemodynamic changes during declamping are the reverse of those seen during application of the clamp, namely, a sometimes precipitous decline in arterial pressure and computed SVR. Cardiac output usually increases but may decrease depending on a number of factors.

The decrease in SVR is due to opening of the closed vascular beds along with a presumed reactive hyperaemia occurring in the previously ischaemic tissues. Other mechanisms for the hypotension have been postulated including the release of myocardial depressant factors and a wash-out of acid metabolites from the reperfused tissues.

The acidosis which occurs when high aortic cross-clamps are released can be quite profound and is a combination of metabolic and respiratory components. The respiratory acidosis is secondary to release of CO_2 from peripheral tissues. The relative amount of respiratory *vs.* metabolic acidosis varies between patients. This matter is not necessarily trivial as the treatment for the respiratory component would be hyperventilation whereas the administration of bicarbonate is appropriate to treat the metabolic component.

Hypotension following release of the aortic clamp is treated as follows:

- When the surgeon is 1–2 min from being ready to remove the cross-clamp administration of the vasodilator drugs is stopped. As their effect diminishes, vascular tone returns and the arterial pressure and filling pressures begin to rise.

- As the cross-clamp is slowly released small bolus doses of vasopressors, commonly phenylephrine (40–100 micrograms), are administered to prevent a dangerous decline in arterial pressure.
- Communication with the surgeon and timing in these manoeuvres is crucial.
- It is often necessary to re-apply the just released cross-clamp to correct anastomotic bleeding. If this occurs just as a vasopressor bolus reaches the vasculature, alarming hypertension may ensue.
- If cardiovascular support is required on a continuous basis a low dose of dopamine (<2.5 micrograms/kg/min) is infused since return of renal function (demonstrated by urine output) is always of primary concern.
- Blood gases and pH should be measured shortly after removal of the cross-clamp to assess any degree of acidosis.

In complicated surgical procedures involving supracoeliac cross-clamp there will be multiple removals and re-applications of the clamp as the surgeon works his way down the vascular tree anastomosing the major vascular run-offs. Thus, the above sequence of preparation for cross-clamp removal must be repeated several times. As the clamp is moved more and more distally there are several vascular vessel-to-graft anastomoses which are then exposed to the systemic arterial pressure. These anastomoses must be protected from 'blow out' due to hypertension.

- The possibility of anastomotic bleeding secondary to hypertension exists from the termination of the case through transport and into the postoperative period.

Postoperative care

All patients should be transported from the operating room to the ICU accompanied by an anaesthetist prepared to administer either bolus or continuous infusion of vasodilator drugs as well as a full complement of resuscitation drugs. We do not routinely administer long-acting narcotics prior to leaving the operating room unless the patient's pre-operative pulmonary status or multiple transfusions indicates that prolonged ventilation will be required.

There are several causes of postoperative instability.

- In spite of adequate volume administration during the procedure, third space losses continue well into the hours immediately after operation and patients may continue to require prodigious amounts of fluid to maintain haemodynamic stability.
- Coagulopathies may continue or develop anew.
- Hypothermia may persist and require heating blankets for treatment.
- Electrolytes and blood gases should be watched carefully with frequent determinations of complete haemodynamic profiles to continue optimum control.
- Patients who have experienced ruptured aneurysms or prolonged suprarenal cross-clamps or both are prime candidates for renal failure.
- Knowledge of all haemodynamic parameters is necessary to provide adequate therapy while avoiding overload.

Summary

Ruptured aortic aneurysm carries an extraordinarily high incidence of mortality. However, complete recovery of patients transported to the operating theatre in full arrest with CPR in progress or who had been treated with a thoracic cross-clamp in the emergency room is possible.

With adequate preparation, attention to detail, and aggressive, skilful haemodynamic manipulation, high cross-clamp surgery in the controlled situation may be successfully performed on severely compromised patients.

References

1. Boucher CA, Brewster DC, Darling RC, Odada RD, Strauss HW, Pohost GM. Determination of cardiac risk by dipyridamole–thallium imaging before peripheral vascular surgery. *New Engl. J. Med.* 1985; **312**: 389–94.
2. Hertzer NR, Beven EG, Young JR, O'Hara PJ, Ruschaupt WF III, Graor RA, De Wolfe VG, Maljovec LC, Coronary artery disease in peripheral vascular surgery patients. *Ann. Surg.* 1984; **199**: 223–33.
3. McCollum CH, Garcia–Rinaldi R, et al. Myocardiac revascularization prior to subsequent major surgery in patients with coronary artery disease. *Surgery* 1977; **81**: 302–4.
4. Tomatis LA, Fierens E, Verbrugge CP. Evaluation of surgical

risk in peripheral vascular disease by coronary arteriography. *Surgery* 1972; **71**: 429–35.

5. Carlson DE, Karp RB, Kouchoukos NT. Aneurysms of the descending aorta. *Ann. Thorac. Surg.* 1983; **35**: 68–9.

6. Ross J. Afterload mismatch and preload reserve. A conceptual framework for the analysis of ventricular function. *Prog. Cardiovasc. Dis.* 1976; **18**.

7. Humphrey LS, Blanck TJJ. Intraoperative use of verapamil for nitroglycerin-refractory myocardial ischemia. *Anesth. Analg.* 1985; **64**: 68–71.

17

Cardiac and Thoracic Emergencies

James C Schauble

Resuscitation
Trauma to chest and intrathoracic structures
  Blunt chest trauma
  Penetrating trauma
Infectious processes
  Empyema
  Lung abscess
  Tracheostomy
High technology

The anaesthetist must be swift and certain during provision of care to patients with emergency conditions of the chest wall and its contents; it is essential that the anaesthetist should function as a team member and maintain clear communication so that if, e.g. the left subclavian artery is to be clamped the anaesthetist will not insert a catheter in the left radial artery for monitoring of blood pressure.

Resuscitation

In many emergency conditions of the heart and lungs, resuscitation is the first priority. Heavily traumatized patients require little anaesthesia; for example, cautious IV administration of diazepam, 2.5 mg every 15 min may be perfectly adequate in the critically ill patient to confer hypnosis and amnesia. The administration of narcotics, e.g. morphine, may be attended by peripheral vasodilatation and may be disastrous in hypovolaemic patients dependent upon vasoconstriction for maintenance of blood pressure. Intravenous administration of narcotics is particularly hazardous for patients who have pericardial tamponade. In general, mixtures of diazepam and narcotics, or inhalational agents and narcotics, are poorly tolerated by severely ill patients. Neuromuscular blocking agents which release histamine e.g. tubocurarine and metocurine should be avoided.

Replacement of massive blood loss is best accomplished with whole blood. The frequent fractionation of blood into components is not without drawbacks, e.g. the increased viscosity of packed red blood cells makes quick administration difficult. At present, effort is being made in the United States to reduce the expensive use of fresh frozen plasma because it offers no intrinsic advantage as an expander of intravascular volume and incurs risk of transmission of viral disease; the bleeding associated with massive transfusion is usually due to reduction of platelets rather than of plasma coagulation factors.

In many of the emergency conditions of the chest, the use of high inspired concentrations of oxygen is indicated. Nitrous oxide may be a particularly mischievous agent to use because of its demonstrated depression of cardiac function in the presence of narcotics[1] and because of its effect in expanding air containing spaces in the body.[2]

It is important not to confuse partial pressure of oxygen, PaO_2 and oxygen content of blood. In the presence of anaemia, PaO_2 may be high with inadequate delivery of oxygen to the tissues nonetheless.

The importance of monitoring of arterial blood gases in critical situations cannot be overemphasized. Adequacy of oxygenation and of ventilation must be assessed on the basis of actual measurement of PaO_2 and $PaCO_2$ respectively. The measurement of pH provides valuable insight into both respiratory and metabolic processes when assessed in relationship to $PaCO_2$.

Trauma to chest and intrathoracic structures

Prominent among the factors which relate to mortality after chest trauma are the age of the patient and the presence of associated injuries. Most of the deaths in patients with flail chest occur in patients with shock, three or more associated injuries, head injury, or more than seven fractured ribs.[3] Young patients (< 30 yr) survive such injuries; on the contrary, patients over 70 years of age with flail chest and these associated risk factors have a mortality rate of almost 90 per cent regardless of the kind of treatment employed.

The American College of Surgeons has in recent years organized an approach to advanced trauma life support[4] with priorities of care which reflect the causes of mortality. In the case of chest trauma it has been shown that the combination of shock and respiratory failure is particularly lethal with a mortality of 73 per cent, ten times that of shock alone; no patient with a combination of shock and respiratory failure over 45 years-of-age survived.[5]

The foregoing helps delineate the priorities in surgical and anaesthesia care of a patient with chest trauma. Many of these patients will be the victims of motor vehicle accidents. If respiratory insufficiency is produced by lung contusion or multiple rib fractures or both, ventilation of the lungs (IPPV) through an endotracheal tube is required. Minimal sedation should be employed since there is usually a need to conduct continuing evaluation of neurological and other potential injuries (*see* p. 123). The possibility of pulmonary aspiration of gastric contents must always be considered.

Endotracheal intubation and ventilator support are best used early if Pa_{O_2} falls below 70 mmHg despite supplemental inspired oxygen or if Pa_{CO_2} rises above 55 mmHg with a respiratory rate greater than 30/min. Patients with flail chest injuries and shock not receiving IPPV until gross respiratory failure was present experienced 95 per cent mortality.[3]

- Patients with chest wall trauma must be carefully observed as flail chest secondary to anterior rib fracture or costochondral separation may increase with time though scarcely apparent on admission. Both the work of breathing and oxygen consumption is elevated in such patients.[6]
- The rapid development of severe air hunger, pneumothorax and pneumomediastinum, and particularly of massive subcutaneous emphysema suggests the possibility of a tear of the trachea or a major bronchus.
- The patient should be taken to the operating theatre as quickly as possible and after sedation with a minimal amount of diazepam or ketamine, should be intubated with a long oral endotracheal tube.
- Once the surgeon opens the chest wall, the air leak may be enormous.
- The ability of the anaesthetist to advance the long endotracheal tube into the uninjured mainstem bronchus may be lifesaving (the surgeon's finger may assist in directing the tube). A double-lumen endobronchial tube can be used but the anaesthetist needs great skill since improper placement of this tube may be rapidly lethal.

Blunt chest trauma

- Blunt chest trauma always entails the possibility of

pneumothorax which may be overlooked if attention is primarily focused on associated major abdominal injuries. Tension pneumothorax may be rapidly lethal due to the displacement of mediastinal structures producing impairment of venous return and cardiac output.

The usual physical signs of a pneumothorax are well known. Less widely recognized is the wheezing heard on auscultation of patients with a tension pneumothorax; this may be confusing and passed over as asthmatic bronchospasm. Tension pneumothorax is a great dissembler and must always be considered in the differential diagnosis of shock.

• If there is any reasonable doubt as to the possibility of tension pneumothorax, thoracentesis should be performed immediately by the anaesthetist or other team member.
• The possibility of pneumothorax in association with chest trauma contra-indicates the use of nitrous oxide given the ability of this gas to expand air containing spaces rapidly.

Blunt trauma may include contusion of the myocardium with progression to infarction. Changes in both the anterolateral and inferior walls of the ventricle, should be looked for in the ECG, e.g. leads V_5 and aVF. Should ischaemic ECG changes develop during noncardiac surgery for trauma, treatment is directed toward control of elevated rate pressure product, (i.e. heart rate × systolic arterial pressure), particularly of elevated heart rate,[7] and the use of glyceryl trinitrate (nitroglycerin) for relief of elevated cardiac intraventricular pressure; glyceryl trinitrate (nitroglycerin) should be avoided if there is intracranial injury as it may increase intracranial pressure. Nonspecific ST segment changes in the ECG are common in trauma patients and not diagnostic of infarction or contusion.

Severe blunt trauma to the chest may result in rupture of the descending thoracic aorta at the level of the ligamentum arteriosum. The adventitia of the aorta and the surrounding parietal pleura may contain the bleeding so that the patient survives. At times the pressure in the distal aorta is markedly decreased and pulses diminished. If massive bleeding does not cause immediate demise, surgical repair should be attended with good result.

The lesion is best defined angiographically before operation.

• Hypertension should be avoided. The advantages of a double-lumen endobronchial tube may not outweigh the difficulties in controlling hypertension as this tube is inserted.
• Urine output must be carefully monitored as with all procedures where there is cross-clamping of the aorta,

maintaining urine output as far as possible with appropriate administration of mannitol and frusemide (furosemide) in large doses if necessary.
• In older patients with the possibility of left ventricular disease, a balloon flotation pulmonary artery catheter is useful in assessing vasodilator therapy to keep pulmonary venous pressures in the normal range during the period of the high aortic cross-clamp.

A major problem for the anaesthetist in assuring adequate oxygenation of the patient relates to initial attempts at resuscitation of a traumatized or exsanguinating patient.

• Patients who have been hypoxic and hypotensive and subsequently resuscitated with large volumes of crystalloid may develop degrees of venous admixture equivalent to a right-to-left shunt of as much as a quarter of the cardiac output.
• Control of ventilation with an inspired concentration of 100 per cent oxygen should be established as an initial step and arterial blood gases monitored closely.
• Therapy includes positive end-expiratory pressure (PEEP) and administration of diuretics if there is adequate circulatory stability.
• In the trauma patient, cardiac failure may not be easily distinguished from pulmonary oedema developing at low pulmonary venous pressure unless a pulmonary artery catheter is used to measure the pulmonary artery occluded pressure (pulmonary capillary wedge pressure).

Penetrating trauma

Injury may be limited to the lung following a stab wound or small calibre gunshot wound. A small pneumothorax may be treated by needle aspiration. The anaesthetist should be wary of using PEEP; chest tube drainage of the pneumothorax is advisable. Haemothorax or haemopneumothorax may be treated with chest tube drainage, particularly when the wound is limited to the lung with bleeding at relatively low pulmonary artery pressures. Decision to undertake thoracotomy is based on an assessment of rate and total volume of bleeding. If the patient is undergoing laparotomy or other surgery following chest tube drainage of intrathoracic bleeding, the chest tube drainage must be closely monitored; a decrease or cessation of drainage may be due to a clot in the tubing. This caution concerning occlusion of drainage tubing applies in the case of haemopneumothorax where there is the additional risk of tension pneumothorax should the drainage tube not function.

- The possibility of pericardial tamponade must always be considered when there is a penetrating chest wound with possible injury of intrapericardial structures and especially in penetrating wounds of the upper abdomen whenever clinical findings of elevated central venous pressure (CVP) and hypotension are present.
- The value of measuring CVP, pulmonary artery and pulmonary artery occluded pressures, which all tend to be at the same elevated level in diastole ('pressure plateau'), has been demonstrated.[8] As tamponade develops, cardiac output slowly declines until the volume of blood within the pericardial sac increases to a level at which there is usually a further sudden decrease in the output of the heart.[7] It is because of this relationship that needle aspiration of relatively small volumes of blood from the pericardial cavity may dramatically improve the patient's condition.
- Be alert that tamponade does not insidiously develop when the primary focus of surgical attention is elsewhere; pericardial tamponade must be considered in any differential diagnosis of markedly elevated CVP.
- Emphasis on pharmacological treatment of this condition is misdirected and the primary therapy is removal of blood from the pericardial sac and control of bleeding.
- Patients usually come to surgery since pericardiocentesis is considered an interim therapy; the patients do not tolerate narcotics or vasodilators well if there is significant tamponade.

Oesophagus

Acute obstruction of the oesophagus is seen in patients who classically ingest a large bolus of meat which lodges in mid-oesophagus (at about the level of the crossing of the aorta) or in the lower oesophagus. The patient may be unable to swallow even saliva. Oesophagoscopy is usually undertaken although at times chymopapain may be administered in small sips of water with good result.

- If general anaesthesia for oesophagoscopy is elected in these patients, it should be induced after awake endotracheal intubation or alternatively with rapid sequence induction of general anaesthesia and cricoid pressure since the obstructing bolus in the oesophagus does not reliably prevent aspiration of gastric contents.

- It is imperative that patients undergoing oesophagoscopy, particularly with a rigid oesophagoscope, should not move during light general anesthesia as the oesophagus may be perforated.

Two pathological conditions of the oesophagus which may bring patients to the operating theatre as an emergency are the Mallory–Weiss lesion and bleeding oesophageal varices secondary to portal hypertension. Both conditions frequently involve an exercise in massive restoration of intravascular volume.

The Mallory–Weiss lesion is induced by emesis and comprises a tear of the gastric mucosa and submucosa crossing the oesophago-gastric junction into the oesophagus without perforation of these organs, but often with massive bleeding. Induction of general anaesthesia requires care to avoid aspiration of blood and gastric contents. Choice of anaesthetic is then appropriate to the hae-modynamically unstable patient.

Patients with oesophageal varices present with a multiplicity of problems.

- Again, there must be protection against aspiration during induction of general anaesthesia.
- If a thoraco-abdominal incision is employed, there may be massive release of ascites compounding the requirements for intravascular volume resuscitation.
- These patients frequently have elevated pulmonary venous admixture and require high inspired oxygen concentrations. The haemodynamic pattern is usually that of high cardiac output with low systemic vascular resistance and attendant low normal arterial pressures despite adequate restoration of intravascular volume.
- Care should be taken to maintain urine output, particularly in jaundiced patients, since oliguria has a particularly ominous prognosis for renal function in the patient with bilirubinaemia.
- It is rare that a patient in this category is a candidate for extubation at the end of the surgical procedure and postopera-tive ventilator support should be anticipated.
- Small doses of narcotics and diazepam often serve adequately for purposes of hypnosis and amnesia.
- Halothane should be avoided as these patients are candidates for increasing liver failure (the agent and the anaesthetist may receive unfair blame).

In 1724, Boerhaave described a patient with rupture of the distal oesophagus following vigorous and repeated emesis. When this so-called 'spontaneous rupture of the oesophagus' occurs, there is extravasation of gastric and oesophageal contents into the mediastinum. If the patient has delayed seeking medical attention there will be well established mediastinitis. This condition is quite different from the Mallory–Weiss lesion. Induction of anaesthesia is not so urgent and appropriate IV fluid can be given prior to induction. The haemodynamic picture may be one of sepsis with high cardiac output, peripheral vasodilatation and relatively low arterial pressure. As a rule, a double-lumen endobronchial tube is not particularly helpful since a low thoracotomy incision is used.

Aorta

Problems relating to the anaesthetic management of patients with blunt trauma and disruption of the aorta have already been noted. Patients with penetrating wounds of the aorta rarely reach the operating theatre and present as problems in volume resuscitation and management of high aortic cross-clamp. They require little anaesthesia.

One of the most interesting challenges of emergency thoracic anaesthesia is posed by the patient with acute dissecting aortic aneurysm. These lesions are usually seen in patients with well established, severe systemic arterial hypertension or with the medial cystic necrosis of the aorta associated with Marfan's syndrome.

- The critical point in the care of these patients is the control of arterial pressure and avoidance of hypertension.
- This is one of the few occasions when vigorous reconstitution of intravascular volume may be inappropriate since it may reinstate the patient's usual hypertension. Unless the dissection has involved the right innominate artery, a right radial arterial catheter should be inserted with careful local anaesthesia. A balloon flotation catheter should be introduced via the internal jugular vein and floated into the pulmonary artery; with sedation and careful local anaesthesia, the introduction of the catheter will not change haemodynamic parameters.

A double-lumen endobronchial tube is useful only if the surgeon intends to use a left thoracotomy incision. The disadvantage of the double-lumen tube is that it is more difficult to place and the longer period of laryngoscopy and the subsequent manipulation of the tube is more apt to be attended by hypertension than is the quick introduction of a simple single-lumen endotracheal tube. Successful intubation without hypertension can reliably be accomplished following administration of fentanyl 50 micrograms/kg of body weight as a bolus via a central venous line followed by suxamethonium (succinylcholine). The fentanyl and suxamethonium produce a bradycardia which is advantageous since hypertension is much more difficult to control if the pulse rate is elevated.

A vasodilator such as nitroprusside administered as a bolus through a central line at the time of sternotomy and particularly when the pericardium is opened may be of value. Surges in blood pressure are common at these times. Treatment should err in a direction of hypotension rather than hypertension.

When the aneurysm is approached through a left thoracotomy incision, a double-lumen endotracheal tube is useful. Usually aneurysms to be approached in this way are not particularly unstable and prone to free rupture or rupture into the pericardial sac.

- Nevertheless, hypertension should be avoided. General anaesthesia supplemented by careful topical anaesthesia of the tracheobronchial tree is used for introduction of a double-lumen endobronchial tube. The one-lung ventilation thus permitted facilitates surgical exposure and avoids trauma and bleeding into the lung when the patient is heparinized.
- If partial cardiopulmonary bypass or a Gott shunt is used, the pressure in the distal aorta may be below the approximately 50 mmHg mean pressure needed to maintain urinary output; this situation is best monitored via a small catheter inserted in the femoral artery.
- Close co-operation between the members of the anaesthesia and surgical teams (and perfusionist during cardiopulmonary bypass) are necessary to avoid excessive afterload of the left ventricle during cross-clamp and yet provide adequate perfusion pressure in the aorta distal to the lower cross-clamp.

The heart

The most common emergency cardiac surgery performed is re-exploration for bleeding. Such patients often have some degree of cardiac tamponade and may be rushed with great urgency into the operating theatre. Usually they are intubated and require only a neuromuscular blocking agent and a minimum of hypnotic agent.

- In the presence of tamponade, administration of a narcotic with subsequent peripheral vasodilatation may be productive of remarkable hypotension and occasionally of cardiac arrest. Once the tamponade is relieved, improvement in cardiac function is often dramatic.

• Prior to reopening the incision, the patient should be transfused to maintain high ventricular filling pressures. The period of time during skin preparation and draping should be kept at a minimum, particularly if chest tubes draining the mediastinum are removed during the preparation since development of tamponade may then be accelerated.

Patients with valve lesions who most often present as an acute emergency are those with aortic or mitral valvular regurgitation. Patients with aortic regurgitation, particularly those with bacterial endocarditis, will present with increasing and refractory left heart failure. Cardiac anaesthetists generally are quite happy with low pulse rates in the range of 50–60 beats/min for their patients, but this does not apply to the patient with aortic regurgitation because the diastolic pressure falls so low as to compromise coronary flow during the long diastolic period attending bradycardia.

After the prosthetic aortic valve is in place and cardiopulmonary bypass discontinued, cardiac output is usually good. Pulse pressure may still be widened and this probably reflects changes in the Windkessel function of the aorta and is often less apparent as the postoperative period continues.

A balloon flotation pulmonary artery catheter is useful in assessing the degree of failure and its management during anaesthesia prior to valve replacement and in measuring cardiac output and haemodynamic function after bypass.

Patients with mitral valvular regurgitation are not uncommonly seen as emergencies following myocardial infarction or consequent to persisting myocardial ischaemia and papillary muscle dysfunction. Both the lateral and inferior aspects of the heart should be monitored with appropriate ECG leads as is true of all patients with coronary artery disease. A pulmonary balloon flotation catheter is strongly indicated in these patients for the adjustment of the interrelated after-load and pre-load of the left ventricle. Elevation of systemic arterial pressure to a critical level (varying from patient to patient but relatively constant in a given patient) may produce an abrupt and marked increase of 10–15 mmHg in the level of pulmonary artery occluded pressure as the valve becomes markedly regurgitant, and reduction of arterial pressure below the critical level may reduce this elevated pre-load dramatically as the valve becomes more competent. Many cardiac anaesthetists use large doses of fentanyl (bolus or infusion) as the principal component of the anaesthetic management of these patients. Active intervention in controlling rate (fentanyl, β-adrenoceptor blocking agent, calcium channel blocking agent, neostigmine), pre-load (nitroglycerin), and after-load (hydralazine, nitroprusside, nitroglycerin) often dramatically improves these patients prior to bypass and reduces the level of oxygen consumption of the myocardium.

Many of these patients have a poor overall level of left ventricular function and it should be anticipated that following mitral valve replacement and coronary artery bypass there may be little immediate improvement in ventricular function. Judicious pharmacological management of the loading conditions of the heart and possible use of inotropic agents must be anticipated.

Infectious processes

Empyema

The availability of potent antibiotics reduces the frequency of purulent pleural effusion and that with which suppurative infections of the lung progress to empyema (the presence of pus in the pleural cavity). A principal concern for the anaesthetist must be the frequent association of empyema with a bronchopleural fistula.

- Incautious induction of general anaesthesia in a patient with empyema and bronchopleural fistula may lead to massive dissemination of purulent material throughout the tracheobronchial tree.
- If the empyema consists of purulent fluid, chest tube drainage may be established as initial emergency therapy with local anaesthesia and minimal sedation.
- If the empyema cavity appears to be circumscribed by adherence of surrounding lung to the parietal pleura, local anaesthesia is again adequate for the rib resection and large tube drainage of the empyema cavity which are indicated as an initial step.

If these patients come to thoracotomy, the possibility of persistent bronchopleural fistula must be kept in mind; a double-lumen endobronchial tube should be used with the bronchial lumen introduced into the bronchus of the noninvolved lung.

An unfortunate emergency seen following pneumonectomy and occasionally lobectomy, is the breakdown of a bronchial suture line with opening of a bronchopleural fistula into the space formerly occupied by the resected lung.

- A large air leak may result in a tension pneumothorax, particularly if positive pressure ventilation is initiated, and at this juncture appropriate drainage of the pneumothorax must be established immediately.

During anaesthesia an endobronchial tube is enormously useful in these patients. To assure precise placement of the double-lumen tube, a fibreoptic bronchoscope introduced into the bronchial lumen of the tube is used to guide placement of this lumen into the stem bronchus of the previously unoperated lung.

- The dangers involved in induction of anaesthesia for the patient with a bronchopleural fistula relate to ensuring adequate ventilation and to the avoidance of aspiration of contaminated material into previously normal lung.

With patience and skill the double-lumen tube may be introduced with topical anaesthesia and minimal sedation, or as an alternative, the patient may be permitted to breathe spontaneously during induction of anaesthesia with an inhalational agent.

- Premature use of a neuromuscular blocking agent may be disastrous and is best deferred if at all possible until the double-lumen endotracheal tube is ascertained to be correctly in place.

Lung abscess

Patients presenting for emergency pulmonary resection for lung abscess are unusual since the advent of potent antibiotic therapy; they are at risk of aspiration of infected material throughout the tracheobronchial tree.

- A double-lumen endobronchial tube should be employed and placed with the aid of a fibreoptic bronchoscope. Choice of double-lumen tube should permit placing the bronchial lumen in the bronchus of the unaffected lung.
- The patient's position during induction of anaesthesia should be such that gravity will not facilitate drainage of infected material from the abscess into the tracheobronchial tree.

Tracheostomy

The anaesthetist attending a patient undergoing tracheostomy should be aware that this operation is often too lightly regarded as simplicity itself.

- This operation is not infrequently difficult and attended by

bleeding and difficult access to the airway.
- If at all possible, an endotracheal tube should be introduced before the tracheostomy is undertaken.

The role of neuromuscular blocking agents can be debated; they should not be employed prematurely so that the patient's ability to breathe spontaneously is lost before an airway can be assured. With an endotracheal tube in place, neuromuscular blockade should be established for infants; if they cough and strain on the tracheostomy tube as it is placed, they are prone to develop bilateral pneumothorax.

- As the tracheostomy is accomplished, the endotracheal tube should be withdrawn only a short distance, still leaving it within the trachea, until problems of sizing of tracheostomy tube and secure introduction within the lumen of the trachea are resolved.

High technology

It has been already noted that in patients with major cardiac and thoracic problems, particularly trauma patients, priority must be given to assurance of an adequate airway, adequate venous access, support of oxygenation and ventilation, and restoration of intravascular volume. What then is the role of high technology in these patients and indeed what constitutes high technology? A few years ago the analysis of arterial blood gases was considered to be 'high technology' and the anaesthetist with responsibility for care of the seriously ill patient was unlikely to resort to the measurement of arterial blood gases in emergency situations. Today, equipment has improved (blood gas analysers may be found within many operating room suites), skill in cannulating the radial artery is common, and arterial blood gas analysis and arterial pressure monitoring are widely used.

Balloon flotation pulmonary artery catheters

The anaesthetist should consider that the use of the balloon flotation pulmonary artery catheter is now evolving as did the use of arterial blood gases. The morbidity associated with the use of this technique is small and is essentially that of the procedure necessary to gain venous access. The real difficulties in using this technology are in assuring that equipment is calibrated (in the emergency setting, calibrated in advance and on standby), that a single anaesthetist is not attempting to handle all aspects of intricate care, and that the anaesthetist understands the meaning of the physiological measurements and numbers obtained. Appropriate selection from the many therapeutic possibilities open to the anaesthetist during care for the patient with sepsis or trauma or major disease cannot be made in the absence of adequate assessment of pulmonary and haemodynamic function.

Pulmonary artery catheters provide measurement of right atrial pressure (filling pressure of the right ventricle), pulmonary artery occluded or wedge pressure (filling pressure of the left ventricle) and of cardiac output. Reliance on central venous or right atrial pressure measurement as an indication of adequacy of intravascular volume presumes a normally functioning right ventricle which is not pumping into high pulmonary artery pressures, i.e. a high right ventricular after-load, or that is compromised by tamponade. These assumptions do not hold for the diseased right ventricle and certainly do not hold for the normal left ventricle under stress or for the diseased left ventricle. It has been demonstrated that the Starling curve of the left ventricle is critically dependent on aortic pressure[10] and that attempts to guess the pre-load of the left ventricle or the level of left ventricular performance from clinical findings are very often in error.[11]

The balloon flotation catheter provides information which makes it possible to sort out these haemodynamic interrelationships and devise early and appropriate therapy. In assessing the use of inotropic agents, it must be recalled that there are dose dependent differences in the effects of each of these agents.[12] Often it is desired to use inotropic agents to maximize *flow*, i.e. cardiac output; and this cannot be done without actual measurement.

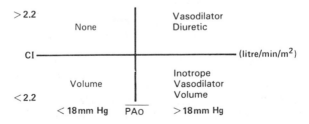

Fig. 17.1 Subsets of haemodynamic function and appropriate therapy. CI = cardiac index (litre/min/m^2); $\overline{PAo}$ = mean pulmonary artery occluded (mean 'wedge') pressure. The horizontal bar distinguishes CI as greater or less than 2.2 litre/min/m^2 body surface area; the vertical bar distinguishes $\overline{PAo}$ as less or greater than 18 mmHg.

Assessment of the effects of inotropic agents on the basis of arterial blood pressure is uncertain at best and the optimal use of these agents requires the use of balloon flotation catheter for the measurement of ventricular filling pressures and cardiac output. Appropriate therapy for subsets of haemodynamic function, determined in relation to cardiac index and filling pressure of the left ventricle, is shown in Figure 17.1. It should be recognized that these subsets cannot be distinguished on the basis of arterial blood pressure alone nor the appropriate therapy chosen. Figure 17.1 also makes the point that inotropic agents are appropriate only when there is a background of ventricular failure[13] with the exception of low dose dopamine infusion used for effect on renal blood flow.

References

1. Lappas DG, Buckley MJ, Laver MB, Daggett WM, Lowenstein E. Left ventricle performance and pulmonary circulation following addition of nitrous oxide to morphine during coronary-artery surgery. *Anesthesiology* 1975; **43**: 61-9.
2. Eger EI, Saidman LJ. Hazards of nitrous oxide anesthesia in bowel obstruction and pneumothorax. *Anesthesiology* 1965; **26**: 61-6.
3. Sankaran S, Wilson RF: Factors affecting prognosis in patients with flail chest. *J. Thor. Cardiovasc. Surg.* 1970; **60**: 402-10.
4. *The Advanced Trauma Life Support Course Manual.* Committee on Trauma of the American College of Surgeons, 1981.
5. Wilson RF, Gibson DB, Antonenko D. Shock and acute respiratory failure after chest trauma. *J. Trauma* 1977; **17**: 697-705.
6. Garzon AA, Gouvin A, Selzer B, Chin CJ, Karlson KG. Severe blunt chest trauma. *Am. J. Thor. Surg.* 1966; **2**: 629-39.
7. Loeh HS, Saudye A, Croke RP, Talano JV, Klodnycky MC, Gunnar RM. Effects of pharmacologically induced hypertension on myocardial ischemia and coronary hemodynamics in patients with fixed coronary obstruction. *Circulation* 1978; **57**: 41-6.
8. Weeks KR, Chatterjee K, Block S, Matloff J and Swan HJC. Bedside hemodynamic monitoring. *J. Thor. Cardiovasc. Surg.* 1976; **71**: 250-52.
9. Reddy PS, Curtiss EJ, O'Toole JD, Shaver JA. Cardiac

tamponade. Hemodynamic observations in man. *Circulation* 1978; **58**: 265–72.

10. Sonnenblick EH, Downing SE. Afterload as a primary determinant of cardiac performance. *Am. J. Physiol.* 1963; **204**: 604–10.

11. Conners AF Jr, McCaffree DR, Gray BA. Evaluation of right-heart catheterization in the critically ill patient without acute myocardial infarction. *New Engl. J. Med.* 1983; **308**: 263–7.

12. Bendixen HH, Osgood PF, Hall KV, Laver MB. Dose-dependent differences in catecholamine action on heart and periphery. *J. Pharm. Exp. Therap.* 1964; **145**: 299–306.

13. Kirk ES, LeJemtt TH, Nelson GR, Sonnenblick EH. Mechanism of beneficial effects of vasodilators and inotropic stimulation in the experimental failing ischemic heart. *Am. J. Med.* 1978; **65**: 189–96.

Further reading

Branthwaite MA. *Anaesthesia for Cardiac Surgery and Allied Procedures, 2nd ed.* Oxford: Blackwell, 1980.

Chung DC. *Anaesthesia in Patients with Ischaemic Heart Disease.* Current Topics in Anaesthesia-6. London: Edward Arnold, 1982.

Kaplan JA (ed). *Cardiac Anesthesia.* New York: Grune & Stratton, 1979.

Opie LH. *Drugs and the Heart.* London: Lancet, 1980.

Russell WJ. *Central Venous Pressure. Its clinical use and role in cardiovascular dynamics.* London: Butterworths, 1974.

18

Emergency Anaesthesia in Severe Burns

Shirley Firn

Pathophysiology
Resuscitation
   Resuscitation plan
   Estimation of size of burn
   Analgesia and sedation
   Transfusion plan
   Treatment of burn wound
   Assessment of adequacy of resuscitation
Anaesthesia
   Pre-anaesthetic assessment
   Premedication
   Induction
   Intubation
   Muscle relaxants
   Maintenance of anaesthesia
   Monitoring techniques
   Important management points
   Blood loss and replacement
Pulmonary complications
   Inhalation injury
      Criteria for diagnosis
      Complications
      Management
   Carbon monoxide poisoning
   Cyanide poisoning

Emergency anaesthesia for a severely burned patient can be a medical minefield. It requires an experienced anaesthetist to circumvent all the problems presented by this group of very ill patients with gross metabolic upset, who are possibly emotionally disturbed as a result of their injuries or whose psychological state may have lead to the burn injury in the first place. Anaesthesia should not be carried out by unsupervised junior anaesthetists. The risks of anaesthesia can be reduced to acceptable levels only by meticulous attention to the patient's general management and a careful general anaesthetic administered by a skilled anaesthetist using a suitable technique.

Pathophysiology

- A burn, even a localized one, is a very serious injury, which produces many systemic ramifications. Skin is destroyed with consequent upset in thermal regulation, fluid and electrolyte homeostasis and the loss of protection against bacterial invasion.
- A burn patient often looks deceptively well in the early stages, but life threatening pathophysiological changes commence within the first half-hour after severe burning and require urgent effective treatment if a fatal outcome is to be avoided.
- Cardiac output is reduced.
- Burn oedema at the site of the injury begins within minutes. Without treatment the patient with a 50 per cent burn or more of the body surface area (BSA) can loose one third of his total blood volume in 3–4 hr, resulting in the occurrence of *burn shock*. Burn oedema fluid is essentially plasma with a slightly reduced protein content.
- Fluid is lost from the vascular compartment into the burn wound and sequestrated in extravascular space, resulting in haemoconcentration.
- Increased ADH secretion decreases urine output.
- All burned patients are hypermetabolic. The increase in metabolic rate reaches a maximum in a few days after injury and persists for weeks or months, depending on the extent of the injury. The patient's core temperature rises. This metabolic response to thermal injury may be caused by alteration in hypothalmic function resulting in increased catecholamine production[1] and is probably maintained by transference of the large heat load using the latent heat of evaporation of water from the burned surface. When more than 40 per cent total body surface is burned, metabolic rate is decreased in a warmer environment (25–33°C ambient temperature).[1] Covering the burn wound with dressings or grafts, thus reducing evaporative losses also helps to reduce metabolic rate.[2]
- The increased heat production in the burned patient occurs due to the utilization of the body stores of energy rich materials. Fasting blood sugar rises, the hyperglycaemia is related

to the extent of the injury and the increase in catecholamine excretion. Gluconeogenesis occurs from the breakdown of skeletal muscle protein into amino acids, especially alanine plus lactate and pyruvate.

- Urine cortisol levels are increased in all patients (up to 10 times upper limit of normal and maximum in severe burns by the second post-burn day). Urine cortisol levels may indicate the rate of cortisol synthesis.[3] They correlate with the excretion of magnesium and creatinine (end products of muscle metabolism). Cortisol promotes potassium release from cells because muscle protein is catabolized.

- The negative nitrogen balance produced is related to the extent of the injury. Sepsis induces acute protein malnutrition, which further reduces the patient's resistance to infection.

- Adipose tissue is another source of gluconeogenesis. Triglyceride lipolysis produces free fatty acids for oxidative and ketogenic purposes and glycerol for gluconeogenesis.

- Insulin/glucagon ratio is lowered and glucagon production predominates.

- Sympathetic activity only returns to normal with closure of the burn wound. Normal relationship between insulin, catecholamines and glucagon returns, associated with weight stabilization and weight gain.

Resuscitation

The aim is to prevent burn shock and correct as far as possible deranged physiology. It requires the infusion of adequate amounts of fluids of the correct quality and at the correct rate. The optimum sodium load requirement is approximately 0.5 mmol/kg/per cent BSA burn. Total volume can be reduced by the use of colloid or hypertonic salt solution. Moderate hypernatraemia is the aim.

Volume and composition of the fluid used varies widely according to the various recommended formulae, depending upon which side of the Atlantic the patient is being treated. A typical UK resuscitation plan is given below.

Resuscitation plan

Ensure a clear airway

Criteria for early intubation include

- Severe burns of face and neck.

- Stridor or hoarse voice.
- Carbon monoxide poisoning.

Ascertain time of accident

- Resuscitation period is based on time of accident *not* admission.

Set up a reliable infusion

- Preferably in the arm (even cut through burnt skin).
- Use a large cannula and secure it well.
- Take blood for haemoglobin (Hb), haematocrit (Hct), urea and electrolytes, blood group and cross matching, before connecting up the infusion.

Catheterize the bladder

- Attach a drainage bag with a short length of tubing.

Weigh the patient

- Reduce value by 20 per cent for fat patient when calculating fluid requirements.

Estimation of size of burn

- Use Wallace's Rules of Nines[4] or Lund and Browder[5] charts (Fig. 18.1).

Analgesia and sedation

- Intravenous morphine injected slowly (dose 0.1–0.2 mg/kg body weight; concentration 1 mg/ml).
- Continue sedation six-hourly with chlorpromazine (dose 0.5 mg/kg; concentration 5 mg/kg); this also produces peripheral vasodilatation.

Transfusion plan

Equal volumes of fluid are given in six successive periods of 4, 4, 4, 6, 6, and 12 hr.

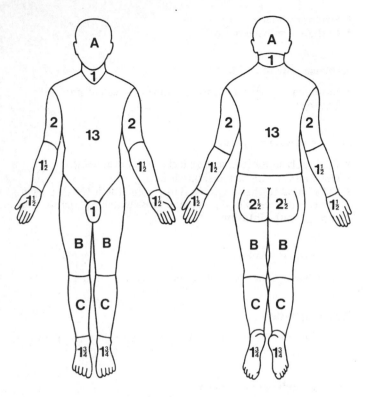

Age in years	0	1	5	10	15	Adult
A = $\frac{1}{2}$ of head	$9\frac{1}{2}$	$8\frac{1}{2}$	$6\frac{1}{2}$	$5\frac{1}{2}$	$4\frac{1}{4}$	$3\frac{1}{2}$
B = $\frac{1}{2}$ of one thigh	$2\frac{3}{4}$	$3\frac{1}{4}$	4	$4\frac{1}{4}$	$4\frac{1}{2}$	$4\frac{3}{4}$
C = $\frac{1}{2}$ of one leg	$2\frac{1}{2}$	$2\frac{1}{2}$	$2\frac{3}{4}$	3	$3\frac{1}{4}$	$3\frac{1}{2}$

Fig. 18.1 Lund and Browder charts. Relative percentage of areas affected by growth.

- *Calculation of expected plasma requirement* for the first 4 hr post-burn period.

$$\text{Volume} = \frac{\text{Total \% area burn} \times \text{weight in kg}}{2} \text{ ml}$$

- *Calculation of actual volume of plasma deficit* assuming no red cell loss.

$$\text{Deficit} = \text{Blood volume} - \left(\frac{\text{Blood volume} \times \text{normal Hct}}{\text{observed Hct}} \right)$$

This second calculation becomes important if the start of resuscitation is delayed for several hours by providing a cross check for the first. These formulae were originally intended as guidelines for freeze dried plasma, which is no longer available. It seems likely that the substitute Human Albumin Solution (HAS) 4.5 per cent previously known as Human Plasma Protein Fraction (HPPF) may be required in larger volumes, but the size of this increase has not yet been formulated on a scientific basis (*see* p. 35)

An assessment of the adequacy of resuscitation is made after 1 hr and at the end of each resuscitation period, to allow for adjustments.

- *Whole Blood Requirement*

For deep burns of more than 10 per cent, the requirement is 1 per cent of patient's normal blood volume for each 1 per cent of burn.

With burns of 10–25 per cent blood is given in the sixth period; with burns of more than 25 per cent it is given in the second and sixth periods, replacing an equivalent volume of plasma (except where changes in Hct are particularly important). Estimated Blood Volumes:

> Neonates 85–90 ml/kg
> Infants 80–85 ml/kg
> Children 80 ml/kg
> Adults 75 ml/kg

- *Metabolic Water Requirement* varies with age and weight and is assessed from appropriate tables, e.g.
    > up to 2 yr 30 ml/hr in first 24 hr
    > 20 kg or 5 yr 40 ml/hr in first 24 hr
    > 40 kg or 12 yr 70 ml/hr in first 24 hr
    > 60 kg or 16 yr 90 ml/hr in first 24 hr
    > 70 kg adult 100 ml/hr in first 24 hr

The requirement is given either as oral fluids or 5 per cent dextrose IV. Fluid requirements in a military situation are given on p. 227.

Treatment of burn wound

- Clean burns with cetrimide and chlorhexidine mixture (Savlon) then isotonic saline (0.9 per cent).
- Divide constricting eschar.
- Decide on exposure or dressing of wound. Type of dressing may affect resuscitation programme, e.g. silver nitrate (popular in the USA) leaches large amounts of electrolytes out of the body water. Flamazine cream (silver sulphadiazine) is commonly used in the UK.
- Decide the need for systemic antibiotics.

Assessment of adequacy of resuscitation

- Clinical examination i.e. pulse, respiratory rate, peripheral venous filling, blood pressure (if possible).
- Skin and core temperature (maximum difference 2–4°C).
- Venous Hct at end of each resuscitation period (desired Hct in small children 35 per cent, women 40 per cent and men 45 per cent).
- Hourly urine volume and osmolarity (detects early signs of renal failure).

No single parameter is used. Each is judged in relation to the others and the fluid volume and composition adjusted accordingly. On-line invasive monitoring is considered by many to be unnecessary or even hazardous in most burned patients, increasing the risk of septicaemia.

Anaesthesia

In general, general anaesthesia should only be carried out once the initial resuscitation is completed. Hypovolaemia should be avoided as these patients compensate poorly for relatively minor changes in blood volume. Factors militating against successful anaesthesia and surgery are:

- high percentage BSA burn
- extremes of age
- pre-existing disease
- fluid or electrolyte imbalance
- head injuries
- internal or skeletal injuries

- septicaemia
- pulmonary problems

Deferral of the procedure or variation of technique may be necessary. Anaesthesia may be required early in the burn illness for emergency skin grafting, e.g. of eyelids to protect the corneas or early tangential excision of devitalized tissue, with skin grafting in areas such as the hands to preserve good function.

Pre-anaesthetic assessment

May be difficult but must be done carefully in an attempt to highlight possible anaesthetic complications.

- Physical examination is difficult and auscultation of the chest in a severely burned patient swathed in bandages may be impossible.
- Chest radiographs are notoriously unhelpful in predicting which patients may develop respiratory complications, but may detect areas of collapse or consolidation.
- ECG may be technically very difficult or impossible.
- Knowledge of the aetiology of the burn is helpful: *super-heated steam or irritant gases* may produce respiratory complications; *mains electrical burns* are 'full thickness' with damage to nerves and blood vessels caused by passage of the electrical current; *high tension electricity* produces entry and exit wounds, with extensive muscle damage between the two. This can include myocardium, if the current has passed across the chest. Muscle damage releases myoglobin which is excreted in the urine and early renal failure may occur. Urgent excision of dead muscle or amputation of charred limbs may be required to prevent this and to remove a possible site of Gram-negative or clostridial infection, within hours of admission, even before resuscitation is completed.
- Request up to date Hb, Hct, full blood count, urea and electrolytes.

Premedication

Oral route preserves valuable intramuscular sites.

- Children up to about 30 kg in weight: trimeprazine syrup forte (6 mg/ml) in dose of 1 mg/kg at least 1.5 hr pre-operatively.
- Children 30–35 kg: diazepam syrup in a dose of 2 mg 1 hr pre-operatively.

- Children over 35 kg: diazepam 5 mg or lorazepam 1 mg tablet 1 hr pre-operatively.
- Adults: diazepam 10 mg or lorazepam 2 mg 1 hr pre-operatively. If necessary diazepam or lorazepam can be given in same dose IM.

Induction

If possible have a reliable infusion *in situ* prior to induction and certainly before surgery.

Inhalation induction is useful in small children, with a mixture of 30 per cent oxygen, 60 per cent nitrous oxide and 10 per cent cyclopropane, with later addition of enflurane, increasing 0.5 per cent every five breaths. Cyclopropane is discontinued when 1.5 per cent enflurane is reached. Children can be intubated on a concentration of 4 per cent enflurane. This can be achieved even in the presence of facial burns with the mask held in gentle contact with the face. Enflurane or isoflurane may be used in countries where cyclopropane is unavailable.

In older children and adults minimal sleep doses of thiopentone (thiopental) are used; alternatives include etomidate and propofol if the patient has a history of asthma or allergies, or diazemuls in very debilitated or unstable patients, titrated slowly intravenously.

Intubation

All patients with major burns require intubation.

Face and neck burns make fixation of the endotracheal tube difficult, but intubation is necessary to secure the airway. The tube can be tied in place using a soft bandage, provided the burnt areas are covered with sterile 'Sofratulle' and then padded with a thin layer of polyurethane foam. Intubation may be difficult and even very careful introduction of the laryngoscope may cause bleeding from burned lips.

Muscle relaxants

- Suxamethonium (succinylcholine) is contra-indicated. Cardiac arrest can occur due to transient hyperkalaemia.[6]
- Nondepolarizing muscle relaxants are the drugs of choice for intubation and maintenance of anaesthesia, but they are required in increased doses in patients with more than 25 per cent burns. In adults a 3–5-fold increase in total dose and serum concentration of tubocurarine is required to produce the same degree of muscle twitch suppression compared to healthy subjects.[7]

Burned children require three times the dose of metacurine (dimethyl tubocurarine) and twice the plasma concentration compared to the non-burned to produce identical degrees of neuromuscular blockade.[8]

- Reversal of neuromuscular blockade poses no problems, even though the serum concentrations would produce 100 per cent twitch depression in normal subjects.[7, 8] This may be due to a fundamental change at the neuromuscular junction in burned subjects, e.g. an additional barrier such as metabolites of burned tissue at the motor end-plate.

Maintenance of anaesthesia

Oxygen and nitrous oxide with IPPV. Additional analgesia can be produced by a low concentration of enflurane (1 per cent or less). The dosage of enflurane is easily controlled and the effects do not persist and depress the patient in the postoperative phase.

Monitoring techniques

Even normal minimal monitoring may be difficult. Placement of a sphygmomanometer cuff may be impossible and even finding an accessible pulse to palpate difficult.

- ECG should always be possible, even in the most severely burned patients by the use of sterile needle electrodes.
- Blood loss needs very careful monitoring, especially in children.
- Monitor skin and core temperature.
- Watch for signs of inadequate peripheral perfusion.

Important management points

- Skin grafting operations may be prolonged.
- Several changes of position may be required. All handling must be gentle. Avoid postures likely to cause hypotension. Transfer from bed to table in anaesthetic room and from table to bed at the end of surgery.
- Planned surgery may have to be curtailed if patient's condition deteriorates.
- Theatre temperature should be high and all irrigant fluids warmed. If the patient's temperature falls, postoperative vasoconstriction and hypoxaemia increases energy demands and delays return of consciousness and resumption of feeding.
- Incidence of nausea and vomiting can be reduced by careful choice of postoperative medication.

Blood loss and replacement

- Massive blood loss can occur in a short time, due to oozing following curettage of granulating burns and/or donor sites.
- Pre-operative anaemia may be present.
- Blood is also lost postoperatively into the dressings.
- Very septic patients require more blood than the amount lost.
- Estimation of blood loss by gravimetric or colorimetric methods may give a 50 per cent underestimate in children.
- Hb content of stored blood is uncertain, therefore use freshest blood available.
- Warm all blood transfused using blood warming coils. Selective cardiac cooling tends to occur with massive transfusions.

Pulmonary complications

The time scale for the development of respiratory complications in severe burns overlaps with the period in which emergency surgery may be required. Patients with a bad prognosis based on age and percentage burn often develop pulmonary complications. Pulmonary complications cause or contribute to the death of most patients who die after thermal injury. More efficient management of burn shock and sepsis has unmasked the high incidence and mortality of pulmonary complications. The extent of the burn and the history, e.g. enclosed space, may be more important predictors of pulmonary complications than facial burns[9].

Inhalation injury

This occurs at three levels:

- Upper airway (larynx, vocal cords) producing airway obstruction (60 per cent).
- Major airways (tracheobronchial tree) producing infection (35 per cent).
- Parenchymal (terminal bronchi and alveoli) giving rise to impaired gaseous exchange (5 per cent).

The first two can be diagnosed by fibreoptic bronchoscopy, with the aid of topical anaesthesia of the nasal and pharyngeal mucosa after pre-oxygenation.

Criteria for diagnosis

- Oedema, erythema or ulceration of the laryngeal or tracheal mucosa.

- Carbon particles in the tracheobronchial tree.
- Xenon[133] lung scanning can diagnose parenchymal injury.[10]

Complications

May occur in three time phases.

1st phase (within minutes or hours of the burn injury).

Respiratory distress or insufficiency can occur with severe injury of the proximal or distal airways, due to bronchospasm and/or extensive alveolar damage and is usually lethal.

Very little direct thermal injury occurs below the larynx, due to reflex closure of the vocal cords, but products of combustion are very toxic to the airways and alveoli.

2nd phase (twenty-four to 48 hr post burn).

Oedema of upper airways and loss of protective ciliary action. Hoarseness or stridor indicate impending obstruction. Cyanosis is due to hypoxaemia.

Tachypnoea produces hypocarbia and respiratory alkalosis. Lung compliance is reduced and airway resistance increases; surfactant is lost.

3rd phase (late complications after 3rd post-burn day).

Bacterial pneumonia associated with profuse bronchorrhoea.

Management

- Warm moist air.
- Vigorous physiotherapy.
- A nasotracheal tube is used to splint the air passages, till the oedema subsides (usually 4th post-burn day). It also allows frequent suction. Wheezing and bronchospasm are treated with systemic and nebulized bronchodilators. Respiratory insufficiency, if severe, is treated with IPPV with volume cycling and positive end-expiratory pressure (PEEP), or constant positive airway pressure (CPAP) with spontaneous ventilation.

Tracheostomy in general is now avoided, due to the associated complications which give rise to a high mortality in severely burned patients (50–86 per cent or even almost 100 per cent in some paediatric series).[11] Tracheostomy opens up the tracheobronchial tree to direct infection from the burn wound.

Pneumonias are treated with appropriate systemic antibiotics. Steroids have been shown to increase mortality.[12]

Carbon monoxide poisoning

Carbon monoxide is a toxic product of combustion. Its chemical affinity for Hb is about 240 times greater than oxygen and its dissociation is slow (half-life of 4 hr). The presence of carboxyhaemoglobin (COHb) shifts the oxygen dissociation curve to the left and oxygen is not released, unless the oxygen tension in the tissues is dangerously low, giving rise to tissue hypoxia and eventually cerebral oedema. The Po_2 can remain near normal but oxygen saturation falls rapidly.

Measurements

* Serial arterial blood gases; uncompensated metabolic acidosis in the initial measurement is a bad prognostic sign.
* COHb levels. Easy measurement: Clarke[13] has suggested the use of a nomogram based on the COHb concentration on admission and time after removal from exposure, to obtain an approximate COHb value at exposure, to help identify patients likely to require intensive respiratory therapy. Other patients are managed with high flow oxygen therapy. Concentration of COHb reduces by 50 per cent for each 40 min of treatment.

Cyanide poisoning

Can be caused by the fumes from modern furnishing materials. Cyanide interferes with oxygen utilization at cellular level.

Whole blood cyanide level measurements are difficult and less useful than COHb levels, because of the faster decay (half-life about 1 hr) after removal from exposure. It has been suggested that COHb levels combined with history of exposure might be sufficient to predict necessity of cyanide antidote treatment.[13]

References

1. Wilmore DW, Long JM, Mason AD, Skreen RW, Pruitt BA. Catecholamines; mediators of the hypermetabolic response to thermal injury. *Ann. Surg.* 1974; **180**: 653–69.
2. Coombes EJ, Batstone GF. Urine cortisol levels after burn injury. *Burns* 1982; **8**: 333–7.
3. Caldwell FT, Bowser BH, Crabtree JH. The effect of occlu-

sive dressings on the energy metabolism of severely burned children. *Ann. Surg.* 1981; **193**: 579–91.

4. Barclay TL, Wallace AB. Fluid replacement in burned patients. *Lancet* 1954; **i**: 98–100.

5. Lund C, Browder MC. The estimation of areas of burns. *Surg. Gynec. Obstet.* 1944; **79**: 352–8.

6. Gronert GA, Theye RA. Pathophysiology of hyperkalaemia induced by succinylcholine. *Anesthesiology* 1975; **43**: 89–99.

7. Martyn JAJ, Szyfelbein SK, Ali HH, Matteo RS, Savarese JJ. Increased *d*-tubocurarine requirement following major thermal injury. *Anesthesiology* 1980; **52**: 352–5.

8. Martyn JAJ, Goudsouzian NG, Matteo RS, Liu LMP, Szyfelbein SK, Kaplan RA. Metocurine requirements and plasma concentrations in burned paediatric patients. *Br. J. Anaesth.* 1983; **55**: 263–8.

9. Achauer BM, Allyn PA, Furnas DW, Bartlett RH. Pulmonary complications of burns. *Ann. Surg.* 1973; **177**: 311–14.

10. Moylan JA, Wilmore DW, Mouton DE, Pruitt BA. Early diagnosis of inhalation injury using Xenon[133] lung scan. *Ann. Surg.* 1972; **176**: 477–84.

11. Eckhauser FE, Billote J, Burke JF, Quinby WC. Tracheostomy complicating massive burn injury. *Amer. J. Surg.* 1974; **127**: 418–23.

12. Moylan JA, Chan CK. Inhalation injury; and increasing problem. *Ann. Surg.* 1978; **188**: 34–7.

13. Clarke CJ. Measurement of toxic combustion products in fire survivors. In: Howie CM, Brown J, Adams AP (eds). Modern trends in burns care. *J. Roy. Soc. Med.* 1982; **75(suppl. 1)**: 40–44.

Further reading

Howie CM, Brown J, Adams AP (eds). Modern trends in burns care. *J. Roy. Soc. Med.* 1982; **75(suppl. 1)**: 1–51.

Settle JAD. *Burns – the first 48 hours*. Romford, England, Smith & Nephew Pharmaceuticals Ltd, 1986.

19

Military Conflicts and Civil Disasters

Malcolm C Thompson

Military conflicts
Problems of military anaesthesia with multiple casualties
    Related to the environment
    Related to the casualty
Pre-operative considerations
    Documentation
    Triage
    Resuscitation
    Analgesia
    Full stomach
Choice of anaesthetic technique
    Inhalational methods
    Total intravenous anaesthesia
    Regional anaesthesia
Induction of anaesthesia
    Rapid sequence induction
    Induction agents
Maintenance of anaesthesia
    Volatile agents
    Oxygen
    Muscle relaxants
    Analgesics
Ventilators
    Self-inflating bag
    Powered mechanical ventilators
Recovery from anaesthesia
Civil disasters
Sequence of events and arrangements
Role of the anaesthetist
    On site
    In the accident and emergency department
    In the intensive care unit (ICU)
    In the operating theatre

Military conflicts

Military anaesthesia, as with the surgery it accompanies, is at a considerable disadvantage in the front line situation. Much of modern anaesthesia is reliant on sophisticated equipment, drugs and techniques. In isolated areas, the anaesthetist cannot work with his familiar Boyle's machine, supplied with piped gases. There are no large drug cupboards, cardiovascular or respiratory monitors, or sophisticated recovery facilities with postoperative IPPV.

Problems of military anaesthesia with multiple casualties

Related to the environment

- The surgical unit will be located away from an organized permanent hospital. The area may be unfamiliar and the environment may be hostile. Enemy action may result in a chemical or nuclear threat.
- The supply of drugs, blood, IV fluids, compressed gases and equipment will be limited and uncertain. The stocks of these articles can be rapidly exhausted, and the anaesthetist is then reliant on re-supply or improvisation.
- Locally available drugs and apparatus may be unfamiliar.
- There may be a paucity of water and mains electricity resulting in poor lighting and heating, a lack of suitable surgical scrubbing facilities, and no power for electrically driven equipment.
- Ancillary services, such as pathology and radiology, will be simple if present at all.
- Altitude and climate can affect personnel, casualties and drugs.

Related to the casualty

Evacuation to the surgical unit

- Difficult terrain may lead to problems in location and evacuation. The time interval between injury and receiving the casualty can be prolonged.
- Potent IM analgesics may have been administered, possibly on more than one occasion. This can lead to respiratory depression during resuscitation when increased muscle blood

flow liberates the poorly absorbed analgesic from the injection site.

Receiving the casualties

- Unexpected arrival in batches may lead to delay before resuscitation and surgery is commenced.
- There will be many grades of injury and illness. The types of problems that could be expected include:
  - gun shot wounds (GSWs), both high and low velocity; to the head and neck, chest, abdomen and limbs. High velocity missile wounds are noted for a massive amount of tissue destruction.
  - shrapnel wounds
  - burns
  - blast injury, both internal and external
  - trauma not resulting from enemy action, such as road accident injury
  - chemical and radiation injury
  - medical problems, such as dysentery
  - psychiatric problems

Pre-operative considerations

Documentation

This is usually started at aid posts forward of the surgical unit. It needs to be full and accurate, because the casualties will pass through several surgical units before treatment is complete.

Triage

- Triage is the sorting of casualties, and the allocation of them to specific groups. The numbering of the groups relates to the urgency of the required surgery. This process ensures that the most urgent cases receive their treatment first. There is then a descending order of precedence. A casualty who is later deteriorating can be re-allocated to a group with a higher precedence at any time following admission to the surgical unit.
- The processing of casualties through a surgical unit is accelerated by triage. Different grades of injury can be allocated to areas most appropriate to their treatment, e.g. minor treatment area.

Resuscitation

Control of the airway

- The presence of adequate alveolar ventilation is a prerequisite for successful resuscitation. The airway and mechanics of ventilation can be compromised in:
    - head injuries with obtunded consciousness
    - maxillo-facial injuries
    - neck injuries, especially with tracheal involvement
    - chest injuries, crushing or penetrating
    - lung injuries, blast or inhalational
    - neuromuscular blockade due to chemical agents
- The airway should be secured by artificial means if the prone or semiprone position, with support of the jaw and extension of the head on the neck, is inadequate in preventing respiratory obstruction. The methods used include:
    - naso- or oropharyngeal airways
    - tongue suture in maxillo-facial injuries
    - endotracheal intubation
    - cricothyroidotomy (*see* p. 72)
    - tracheostomy (*see* p. 162)

Insertion of chest drains (*see* p. 71)

Arrest of bleeding

Correction of hypovolaemia

Prior to the induction of anaesthesia hypovolaemia should be corrected as fully as possible in the time available. This time depends on the individual injuries of the casualty and the flow of casualties. A compromise has sometimes to be made between adequacy of blood replacement and the necessity to proceed with surgery to stop further blood loss. Hypovolaemia can be due to:

- *Blood loss*: blood for transfusion may not be readily available on the battlefield. A compromise has then to be made when replacing lost blood. Electrolyte solutions and colloids will perform some of the physiological functions of blood for varying lengths of time, but will not carry oxygen (*see* p. 59). Figure 19.1 indicates a possible plan of action when the supply of blood is limited. Human Albumin Solution 4.5%, fresh frozen plasma and platelets would not normally be available. British Army soldiers are blood grouped on joining and carry their blood group engraved on their identity discs. If

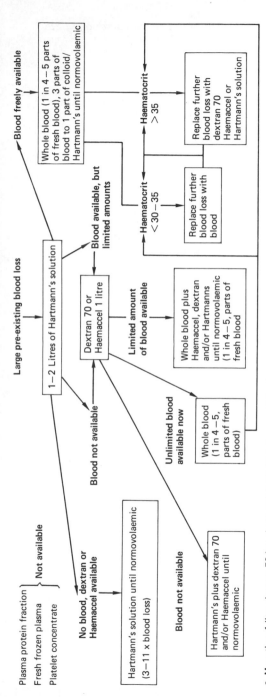

Fig. 19.1 Front line blood replacement.

- More than 1 litre dextran 70 in a short period results in increased bleeding.
- Dextran 70 and Haemaccel cause anaphylactoid reactions. The incidence is probably higher with Haemaccel.
- A haematocrit of 30–35 per cent is ideal. A haematocrit of 20 per cent (Hb 6.0) can still result in normal oxygen delivery to tissues in the normovolaemic and resting state.
- 0.9 percent sodium chloride solution can replace Hartmann's solution, but results in excess Cl⁻ being given.
- Less than one-third of the volume of Hartmann's given is retained in the vascular space.
- One part of fresh blood to 4–5 parts of older blood and colloid, is ideally given to maintain adequate labile clotting factors.
- Warming of cold intravenous fluids, and the filtering of old blood should be performed where possible.

injured they receive group compatible, uncross-matched blood.
- *Burns*. The British Army Formula for fluid replacement following burns is (compare, *see* p. 211)
    Colloid: Dextran or plasma: Rate 120 ml per 1 per cent BSA burn in 48 hr. Divide total: half in first 8 hr from time of burning: quarter in next 16 hr; quarter in next 24 hr.
    Blood: 50 ml for each 1 per cent whole skin loss during the early phase of treatment.
    Electrolyte solution either orally or IV calculated on a volume of 50 ml/kg body weight/24 hr.
- *Dehydration.*

Analgesia

- Opiates are available for IM injection by fellow soldiers (the Buddy aid system) at the place of wounding. Reduced tissue perfusion from shock can reduce absorption until resuscitation commences. Multiple injections of opiate can then be rapidly absorbed and cause respiratory depression. At the surgical unit opiate analgesia is given intravenously in small doses.
- Splintage of injured limbs.
- Nerve blocks have only a limited place. Injuries will often involve regions not amenable to nerve blocks or multiple areas, which would require large volumes of local anaesthetic to perform several nerve blocks.
- Ketamine in subanaesthetic doses. The suggested initial dose would be 0.5 mg/kg IV or 1.0 mg/kg IM.
- Entonox if available.

Full stomach (*see* p. 6)

Choice of anaesthetic technique

Inhalational methods

At present this is the method of choice for most anaesthetics given in the field. The supply of cylinder gas is uncertain, so draw-over apparatus employing air as the carrier gas is used. The British Army uses the Tri-service anaesthetic apparatus. This is comprised of two Oxford Miniature draw-over vaporizers (OMVs) in series, a length of wide-bore tubing acting as an oxygen reservoir and similar tubing connecting to a self-inflating bag. This apparatus fulfils the requirements of a military anaesthetic system, namely it is

- simple,
- robust,
- light and easily portable,
- easy to maintain and clean,
- versatile, able to function with any available volatile agent,
- resistant to extremes of heat and cold,
- easy to use,
- inexpensive and standardized.

Halothane and trichloroethylene are usually used, but the following agents can be administered with the Tri-service anaesthetic apparatus: enflurane, isoflurane, methoxyflurane, chloroform and diethyl ether. One or 4 litres/min of oxygen can be added from a compressed oxygen source, via a purpose designed reduction valve. Drawbacks lie in the small capacity of the OMV reservoirs, lack of temperature compensation, inability to give 100 per cent oxygen and the need for a ventilator to free the anaesthetist from the task of ventilating the patient's lungs by hand.

Total intravenous anaesthesia

Ketamine alone can be used for procedures of short duration not requiring muscular relaxation or endotracheal intubation. More major procedures would require the use of endotracheal intubation, muscle relaxation, IPPV and ketamine by infusion or intermittent bolus. Benzodiazepines should be given in conjunction, to prevent the psychological recovery problems associated with ketamine.

Regional anaesthesia

- *Specific nerve blocks*; use in front-line anaesthesia is limited. Multiple or extensively injured areas are not suitable for regional blockade. The long induction time also limits their usefulness.
- *Spinal and epidural anaesthesia*; the use of this method of anaesthesia in the field is controversial. Sterile conditions and a normovolaemic patient are required. In past conflicts there have been deaths when spinal anaesthesia has been used in shocked casualties.
- *Intravenous regional anaesthesia* (*see* p. 254).

Induction of anaesthesia

Rapid sequence induction

The majority of general anaesthetics at a front-line field surgical unit commence with a rapid sequence induction, i.e. pre-oxygenation, induction agent, cricoid pressure, suxamethonium bromide, tracheal intubation, ventilation of the lungs.

Induction agents

- *Thiopentone* (*thiopental*): a potent myocardial depressant and peripheral vasodilator. These properties are dangerous in the hypovolaemic casualty. Slow administration by skilled personnel is essential.
- *Ketamine*: advocated for use in acute trauma and hypovolaemic shock. By decreasing re-uptake of endogenous catecholamines ketamine increases pulse rate and blood pressure. Myocardial work and oxygen consumption are increased and in the situation of a patient with a maximally sympathetically stimulated cardiovascular system plus severe shock the overall effect can be myocardial depression.
- *Etomidate*: known to be cardiostable in the normovolaemic, normotensive subject. Although it is too early to recommend use in shocked human subjects, animal studies suggest that it might have a place as an induction agent following severe trauma.
- *Relaxants on induction*: the primary muscle relaxant used on induction of anaesthesia would be suxamethonium bromide. Suxamethonium chloride (succinylcholine) in solution requires refrigerated storage, which would be unavailable in the field.

Maintenance of anaesthesia

Volatile agents

- Halothane is the primary agent used in the Tri-service anaesthetic apparatus. It can be used in both spontaneous and controlled ventilation. In the latter it gives good hypnosis and muscle relaxation, without appreciable cardiovascular depression, when used in low concentration (0.5 per cent).
- Trichloroethylene when supplementing halothane provides the analgesia for a more balanced anaesthetic. In low concentrations (0.25 per cent) it does not appreciably prolong awakening.

- Enflurane, methoxyflurane, isoflurane, diethyl ether (in two OMV vaporizers in series), and chloroform can all be administered from the same OMV vaporizers as used for halothane and trichloroethylene. The concentration scale is readily changed for the use of a new agent.

Oxygen

Oxygen can be added at either 1 or 4 litres/min into the reservoir tubing of the Tri-service anaesthetic apparatus. The former is used during maintenance and the latter during pre-oxygenation, induction and reversal. Supplies of oxygen will be limited, so a compromise has to be made between what ideally should be given, and what can be given.

Muscle relaxants

- *Alcuronium*: a good relaxant for use in the field. Has acceptable storage characteristics. Does not cause large falls in blood pressure when used with halothane.
- *Pancuronium*: a good relaxant for shocked casualties, but requires refrigeration for prolonged storage.
- *Vecuronium*: a cardiostable drug with acceptable storage characteristics for field use.
- *Tubocurarine* can be used in the stable normovolaemic casualty, but is not recommended for use in conjunction with halothane in the shocked patient.

Analgesics

Adjuncts, such as papaveretum, morphine or pethidine (demerol) can be effectively employed to supplement anaesthesia, and to provide immediate postoperative analgesia.

Ventilators

Self-inflating bag

The Laerdal bag is included in the Tri-service anaesthetic apparatus. It does cause blistering on the hands when squeezed for prolonged periods, and it hinders the anaesthetist when he wishes to perform other tasks, such as changing infusions or drawing up drugs.

Powered mechanical ventilators

If these are used for controlled ventilation, then allowance must be made for their transportation, power supply and maintenance. Power supply is a particular problem in the field. The Penlon–Oxford, the East–Radcliffe P3 and RP4, and the Cape TC50 can all be used with the Tri-service anaesthetic apparatus. The Penlon–Oxford needs a compressed air or oxygen source of power whilst the East–Radcliffe ventilators can be powered manually or electrically with an AC or DC current. The Cape TC50 is mains electricity or generator powered.

Recovery from anaesthesia

Recovery facilities in the field are limited both in the number of staff and in the equipment available. Techniques of anaesthesia used should be associated with rapid recovery of consciousness and reflexes. Light general anaesthesia with muscle relaxation and IPPV, followed by the use of doxapram or naloxone, as indicated, is an acceptable method. Extubation can be delayed to allow a secure airway, when recovery room supervision is less than ideal. The lateral position should be used where possible. Either IM or IV analgesia can be given.

Civil disasters

In recent years many and varying incidents have resulted in large numbers of persons being killed or injured. Air, train and coach crashes, fires in buildings, explosions in factories, and urban terrorist activities have all caused multiple casualties in single incidents. Such an incident becomes a major accident or disaster when, because of the number of casualties the normal response of the emergency services, as in a small and limited accident, is not adequate.

The various aspects of responding to such a situation are enveloped in the local major accident plan. This plan is evolved after discussion and exercises by the local hospitals, police, fire service, ambulance service (or paramedic team), armed services and coastguards. Although the initial response is predetermined the particular type of disaster will often result in unforeseen actions having to be undertaken. The sequence of events that would normally follow a major disaster can be simplified.

Sequence of events and arrangements

1. The occurrence of the incident is followed by the alerting of the emergency services. A senior police officer or senior ambulance officer (or paramedic) makes the decision that a major incident has in fact occurred.

2. Local hospital switchboards are then notified by the police or ambulance (or paramedic) service. Hospitals may be designated first or second line. Each telephone switchboard then follows a pre-arranged plan of alerting key personnel, by role and priority. Preparation is made to receive and treat the number of casualties expected, by clearing reception areas, wards and operating theatres. Action cards, held in the accident and emergency (A and E) department, give written instruction to each key member of staff as they report for duty. A secondary call-up of further staff can commence.

3. The command structure within the hospital consists of a senior medical officer, a senior nursing officer and a hospital administrator. The senior medical officer appoints from available staff, a triage officer, a doctor in charge of each: A and E department, operating theatre and reception wards.

4. A site medical officer is conveyed to the scene of the incident. His task is to act as a professional medical adviser to the other emergency services, to liase between the emergency services and the hospitals, to act as site triage officer and to assess the need for further medical assistance. He must not get involved in medical treatment.

5. Should further medical assistance be deemed necessary a Mobile Medical Team is despatched from a local hospital. (The ambulance service usually provide the transport.) An anaesthetist will generally be a key member of this team. A primary aid kit will be carried by the team. The type and quantity of each item will have been decided previously and then packed into portable containers. Each kit will consist of intravenous fluids, cannulas and infusion sets; airways and endotracheal tubes; self-inflating bags; chest drainage cannulas and flutter valves; tracheostomy or cricothyroidotomy sets; suction apparatus; laryngoscopes; portable oxygen cylinders; limb splints; dressings and drugs. Team members, who include doctors and nurses, will wear fluorescent and protective clothing marked noticeably with an individual's role.

6. The Mobile Medical Team provide initial and lifesaving medical care when evacuation to hospital is delayed due to large numbers of casualties or trapped persons. General

anaesthetics are administered only in exceptional circumstances, such as limb amputation of a trapped person where no other course of action is possible.

7. Casualties will be transported to hospital at the earliest opportunity; the most seriously injured, hopefully, taking priority. The receiving hospital will have been advised by radiocommunication link or telephone as to the number and type of casualties that it is likely to receive.

8. On receiving casualties the hospital will triage them and start documentation. Triage would normally result in three groups of patients.

   - Those requiring immediate medical attention.
   - Those requiring admission, but not immediate medical attention.
   - Those who can probably be allowed home after treatment.

9. A nurse is allocated to each patient to be admitted. She remains with that patient as he or she passes from the A and E department to the ward. The seriously injured receive initial treatment in the A and E department. This treatment should be only relatively lifesaving with the institution of stabilizing measures, such as airway control and control of haemorrhage, but to include analgesia. Further treatment and radiography can take place once casualties have left the A and E department. Current patients will be discharged from their beds or moved to other wards, so that a ward area becomes available to the disaster casualties. Triage and assessment will continue for priority for radiographs and surgery.

10. Clinical treatment will depend on the types of injury, whether traumatic, burns, inhalational, near-drowning, radiation, etc.

11. Other aspects of the hospital care have to be considered.

    Documentation: prepared multiple copy admission forms should be used; casualties are each allocated a number, which is marked on a record card, a wrist bracelet and all radiology and pathology forms.

    Communications: a radio link will be established at the hospital by the ambulance service. Ex-directory telephones will speed the initial alerting of the hospital.

    Mortuary arrangements: an emergency mortuary may have to be set up in an appropriate nearby building.

    Relatives' enquiries: the Police will arrange for a casualty bureau to be set up, and for its telephone numbers to be advertised. Relatives will be notified, and the dead identified.

The Press and crowds: one hospital spokesman will communicate with the Press. Hospital security staff will control movement of people and vehicles within the hospital boundaries.

Role of the anaesthetist

On site

As a member of the Mobile Medical Team, an experienced anaesthetist will supervize and perform resuscitation and the administration of analgesia. In exceptional circumstances he may undertake general anaesthesia for the releasing of casualties. Analgesia will usually be undertaken with one of the following:

- IV opiates,
- Entonox (50 per cent oxygen and nitrous oxide mixture: pre-filled cylinder),
- ketamine 0.5 mg/kg IV or 1 mg/kg IM.

General anaesthesia may be conducted as follows.

- Ketamine 2 mg/kg IV or 8 mg/kg IM with oxygen added to the spontaneously inspired air.
- Pre-oxygenation, cricoid pressure, ketamine IV, suxamethonium (succinylcholine), endotracheal intubation, IPPV, air plus added oxygen via a self-inflating bag, intermittent bolus doses of ketamine, intermittent suxamethonium plus atropine, or vecuronium. Ketamine could be replaced by etomidate, especially in the head-injured casualty.

In the accident and emergency department

The anaesthetist will be involved in:

- resuscitation, including securing airways, IV infusion, insertion of chest drains and commencement of IPPV
- analgesia

In the intensive care unit (ICU)

The anaesthetist will be involved in:

- resuscitation
- commencement or continuation of IPPV
- postoperative care

In the operating theatre

- a senior anaesthetist coordinates the compiling of theatre lists,
- he delegates the administration of anaesthetics to the available anaesthetists.

Further reading

Kirby NG, Blackburn G, (eds). *Field Surgery Pocket Book*. London: Her Majesty's Stationery Office, 1981.

Moles TP. Planning for major disasters. *Br.J. Anaesth.* 1977; **49**: 643-9.

Richardson JW, (ed). *Disaster Planning*. Bristol: Wright, 1975.

Rutherford WH. Planning for major disasters. In: Odling-Smee W, Crockard A (eds). *Trauma Care*. London: Academic Press, 1981: 117-26.

Stoddart JC. *Trauma and the Anaesthetist*. London: Baillière Tindall, 1984.

Williams DJ. Disaster planning in hospitals. *Br. J. Hosp. Med.* 1979; **22**: 308-22.

20

Anaesthesia in Developing Countries

Raymond M Towey and Frank N Prior

General considerations
Premedication
Anaesthetic equipment
Anaesthetic techniques
    Local blocks
    Intravenous anaesthetic agents
    Inhalational agents
Specific problems for the anaesthetist
    Hydatid disease
    Tetanus
    Gas gangrene
    Ruptured uterus
    Camel bites and bear mauling
    Snake bites
Training

General considerations

Anaesthesia in developing countries raises special problems because of the severe financial restraints which are imposed, the small numbers of trained medical and paramedical support staff, and the often physical isolation and consequent difficulty in obtaining necessary supplies and servicing. In the urban capitals these problems may not be so much in evidence. In rural areas where most of the population live, the challenge is most pressing and this chapter is more appropriate for the rural hospital.

Emergency anaesthesia in the developing world has also to take into account the physical conditions under which it must be practised in terms of heat and cold. Extremes of heat and cold may be encountered in developed areas but their effects are largely mitigated by ensuring stable and acceptable temperature conditions in all parts of a hospital. Elsewhere, this may not be so. Even if the operating theatre has some form of air-conditioning, the wards seldom have and this is where patients spend most of their time.

Again, abnormalities of fluid balance, chronic anaemia and nutrition have to be taken into account. These factors form a background to the discussion of all conditions peculiar to the developing world and so will be considered first.

Ambient temperatures up to 44°C are often encountered and operating theatres, in spite of fans and air-conditioning, even if these are available, are likely to be 32–35°C. Higher temperatures are found in conditions of dry heat and, although obvious sweating is much less than where there is high humidity, fluid loss is greater and will be the more dangerous in pathological conditions where intake is restricted. Patients are liable to develop hyperpyrexia on the operating table with the added hazards of towels and operating lights. Simple measures to combat this include draping towels over a Mayo table instead of directly on the patient and repeatedly applying wet towels wherever possible, between the thighs being the most effective. Small table fans playing in the wet areas help further as does crushed ice in plastic bags, though these must be kept moving for fear of ice 'burns'.

Patients lose heat very rapidly during operations when the ambient temperatures are 4–15°C. Hot water bottles will help as long as they are not applied directly to the skin. Rapid surgery is most important, especially with babies.

Dehydration is very quickly produced in hot weather if fluid intake is restricted because of disease. Even those who are able to drink normally will often have a much reduced urine output. Principally water is lost, but also salt. So replacement must exceed measured loss in emergency situations. If the venous pressure is measured and 500 ml fluid administered rapidly (5–10 min) raises it by 2–3 cm, falling again rapidly, more fluid is needed. Only if the central venous pressure (CVP) is raised by 5–10 cm and is maintained, should caution be observed in giving more. It is useful to measure the urine output which can be kept up to about 0.5–1.0 ml/kg/hr and to do this as much as 4 litres of fluid may be needed in a 2–3 hr operation, in addition to blood replacement.

Anaemia is often associated with poor nutrition from many causes, especially intestinal infestations, but can present an acute problem when at 3–4 g/dl. The patient is in, or on the verge of, cardiac failure but has a near normal blood volume. Therefore, any infusion must be given with extreme caution. Also, such a patient will need very small amounts of anaesthetic drugs, e.g. 50 mg thiopentone (thiopental) may be quite adequate for induction. A central venous line is very helpful in monitoring such patients (*see* p. 65). The heart is unable to cope with an increased load and will easily fail.

Premedication

Sedative or narcotic drugs must be used with due regard to conditions such as those mentioned above. This will often mean very small doses or none at all.

Caution is also needed in giving belladonna derivatives. Their anticholinergic activity will mean impairment of the sweat glands and hence the danger of hyperpyrexia in hot weather. The danger is greatest in babies and children up to 5–6 yr and, to a lesser extent, up to 15 yr. Above this age there is little danger but there is also little need so the best advice is to omit these drugs altogether. Hyperpyrexia will be most likely as the ambient temperature reaches 28–30°C.

Anaesthetic equipment

From the point of view of capital investment and running costs, a draw-over air and oxygen apparatus is the most logical choice[1] (Table 20.1). The Epstein, Macintosh, Oxford Vaporizer (EMO), is a calibrated temperature compensated accurate diethyl ether vaporizer with a low internal resistance designed for draw-over use.

Table 20.1   Cost of equipment (in UK, in 1986)

Equipment	Cost (£)
EMO with bellows and connections	711
OMV vaporizer alone	225
Boyle's anaesthetic machine without accessories	3775

Together with the Oxford Miniature Vaporizer, (OMV), in which halothane and trichloroethylene, and also most other volatile inhalational agents may be used, the EMO system[2] provides the most appropriate choice of anaesthetic apparatus for virtually every emergency in the adult (Fig. 20.1). The Oxford Inflating Bellows (OIB) provides a means of hand ventilation.

It is best to replace the distal Heidbrink expiratory valve with an Ambu E dual purpose one-way valve, in which case the distal valve on the OIB must be immobilized with the special magnet provided to prevent the Ambu E value from sticking (Fig. 20.1). The OIB may alternatively be replaced by a Penlon bellows with a distal

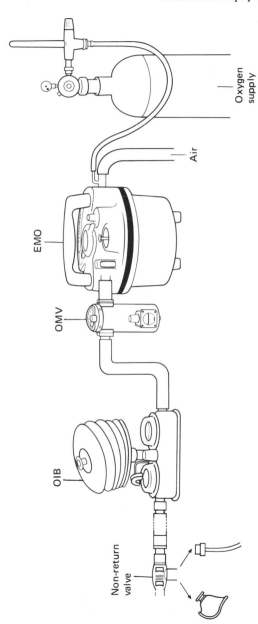

Fig. 20.1 The OIB, OMV and EMO draw-over apparatus (*see text*).

Ambu E valve in position. Supplementary oxygen is recommended. With a 2 litre/min oxygen flow rate, 25–40 per cent concentration is obtained depending on the minute volume. It is safe to use industrial oxygen cylinders if only these are available. They usually contain about 95 per cent oxygen, the rest being made up of nitrogen, carbon dioxide, rare gases and, in a large industrial area, acetylene; all in small and harmless concentrations.

For children under 15 kg draw-over techniques are not feasible. A standard paediatric T-piece may be attached to the outlet of the OIB and the bellows used to provide a continuous gas supply by slow expansion and compression (8–10 cycles/min). This is somewhat cumbersome and a paediatric entrainer has been designed which requires 2 litres/min of oxygen to generate a 10 litre flow of 35 per cent oxygen in air. The vaporizers function then as continuous-flow machines, and the T-piece is attached as before to the OIB. Alternatively the OMV with a continous flow of oxygen and T-piece provides satisfactory oxygen and halothane anaesthesia (Fig. 20.2). The flow of oxygen required will depend on the weight of the child and the physical characteristics of the OMV under continuous flow conditions.

A simply constructed foot-operated suction apparatus is an essential requirement.

Anaesthetic techniques

Local blocks (*see also* Chapter 21).

For the single-handed surgeon working with limited trained staff, local analgesic techniques are often the safest and most satisfactory and have the added advantage of being inexpensive. Spinal block using, e.g., heavy nupercaine (dibucaine) 0.5 per cent in 6 per cent glucose or lignocaine (lidocaine) 5 per cent with glucose, is satisfactory for a number of surgical emergencies. Careful monitoring of blood pressure and access to an intravenous route is recommended. The volume of local analgesic to be injected depends on the height of block required; 2 ml is usually a maximum dose. Other blocks, e.g. epidural, brachial plexus and Bier's, may also be used with success by anaesthetists or the single-handed surgeon trained in these techniques.

Intravenous anaesthetic agents

- Intermittent thiopentone (thiopental) for short surgical procedures is often satisfactory if limited to 10–15 min.
- Intravenous agents together with local anaesthetic infiltration

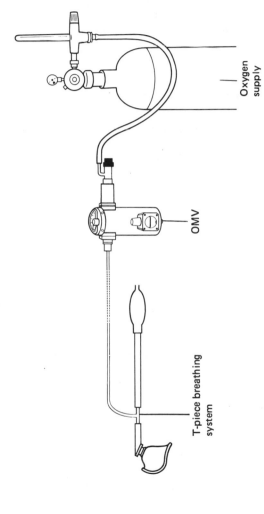

Fig. 20.2   Halothane and oxygen using the OMV and T-piece breathing system for children.

often prove successful in experienced hands. Pethidine (demerol) 50 mg, promethazine 25 mg, diazepam 10 mg given IV may prolong the action of local techniques, e.g. after delivery of the child in Caesarean section having previously infiltrated the wound site with lignocaine (lidocaine).

- Ketamine anaesthesia has been a major advance in anaesthesia in developing countries both for the trained anaesthetist and the single-handed surgeon. For surgical procedures in children which do not require muscle relaxation 4–10 mg/kg IM provides good surgical conditions for 10–15 min. Pre-operative atropine is recommended unless the ambient temperature is high as excessive salivation can cause severe laryngospasm. Patients often maintain a good airway.

Intravenous induction with ketamine can be produced by a dose of 2 mg/kg and supplementary doses or a continuous IV infusion containing 1 mg/ml can maintain anaesthesia for many prolonged surgical procedures not requiring muscle relaxation. The possibility, during recovery, of unpleasant dreams and hallucinations are best managed by prophylactic diazepam. A technique involving continuous IV ketamine, muscle relaxation and IPPV using air and supplementary oxygen after endotracheal intubation, has been described which could be used for any surgical emergency.[3] At the present time ketamine is an expensive agent.

Inhalational anaesthesia

Inhalational anaesthesia with or without muscle relaxation is the main anaesthetic technique for general anaesthesia in the developing world. Diethyl ether is the most appropriate agent and one of the cheapest, and halothane is also very suitable (Table 20.2). Ether in air is inflammable although not explosive but with oxygen it is explosive; however, many hospitals in remote areas do not have diathermy machines so ether may be used more safely. For a spontaneous respiration technique a thiopentone (thiopental), air, oxygen, halothane technique is appropriate using

Table 20.2 Cost of anaesthetic drugs

Agent	Ventilating concentrations		Approx cost/hr (UK pence in 1986)	Comments
	Controlled	Spontaneous		
Diethyl ether	2–3%	6–8%	12–50	
Trichloroethylene	0.3–0.5%	Unsuitable	3	
Halothane	0.5%	1–2.5%	30–70	
Nitrous oxide	5 litres/min		80	Transport problems

the OMV. If muscle relaxation is required a technique of pre-oxygenation, thiopentone (thiopental), suxamethonium (succinyl-choline) endotracheal intubation and IPPV using ether 2–4 per cent and air, oxygen and a relaxant such as tubocurarine provides excellent surgical conditions. In the presence of ether only about half the normal dose of nondepolarizing muscle relaxant is required. Powdered suxamethonium bromide can be made up in solution immediately before use to avoid its breakdown in the heat.

Specific problems for the anaesthetist

Hydatid disease

This may occur almost anywhere in the body, even including the retina, but hazards due to hydatid are greatest if the parasite is in the liver or lungs, or indeed both, for a cyst in the liver can extend into the lungs. During an operation for the removal of hydatid cysts, rupture may occur and lead to an acute anaphylactic reaction: corticosteroids and adrenaline (epinephrine) must be ready for immediate use, the steroids in large doses. Formalin or hypertonic saline may be used for injection into the cyst to kill the daughter cysts, but if spilt into the abdominal cavity it may cause problems. The former may be quickly mopped up as the smell reveals it but saline may be absorbed and lead to extreme hypernatraemia and death.

Some liver cysts grow to such huge proportions that the peritoneal cavity is obliterated and removal can be performed with a simple local anaesthetic infiltration and a small incision into the cyst. Such cysts may contain as much as 6 litres, and are often infected but infection does at least kill the scolices. Any spill is onto skin and is therefore harmless.

If in a lung, hydatid presents two hazards for anaesthetists. One is spill into the airways, this is best minimized by using a double-lumen tube. If communication with a bronchus has already occurred, it is safest to induce in a steep head-up tilt until the tube is in place. When only an ordinary endotracheal tube is available induction is safest, though messy, with the patient in a left lateral head-down tilt and subsequent operation in a head-down, Parry Brown (prone) position. The other hazard is, as above, anaphylaxis.

Tetanus

It is not proposed to deal with the overall treatment of tetanus but it should be emphasized that thorough debridement of any known portal of entry is needed as an emergency; this includes the uterus if a procured abortion is the cause. These cases are usually very severe and, of course, uterine dilatation and curettage may make things worse so that the patient must be fully relaxed with neuro-muscular blocking drugs as well as deep sedation using endo-tracheal intubation.

Gas gangrene

There is no reason why these patients, often suffering from septic shock and requiring urgent surgery, should not have the benefit of a main operating theatre with all its facilities for resuscitation and anaesthesia. The usual organism, *Clostridium welchii*, is in a site where it can threaten the patient's life but is the same organism as may contaminate any bowel (especially emergency) operation.

Ruptured uterus

This is unfortunately common in developing areas often due to the activities of untrained practitioners who use oxytocin inadvisedly. It can also be caused by grossly neglected labour in remote areas. The problem for an anaesthetist is to judge when to allow opera-tion, where blood may be lost more rapidly than supplies can be found to replace it. Generally, having secured good IV infusion (in a collapsed patient the internal jugular can be very useful) it is best to operate straightaway to control the bleeding. A very light anaes-thetic will be required with, preferably, muscle relaxants.

Camel bites and bear mauling

These are often severe, involve the face and, hence, raise airway problems. It may be possible to clean, suck out and find a way to the trachea with an endotracheal tube but it is probably best to make an early decision to make a tracheostomy. These wounds are also heavily infected.

Snake bites

Neurotoxins or haemolytic toxins may be involved, or both. The former can be dealt with by tracheal intubation and ventilation with support of the cardiovascular system as needed. The latter may be helped by corticosteroids and often lung ventilation as well. In all cases, antivenene is important if available.

Training

Medical and paramedical personnel are desperately needed in the rural areas of virtually all developing countries. In the urban capitals anaesthetic practice is often similar to Europe and North America and special training hospitals for draw-over techniques and local blocks are necessary. If the surgical need in the rural areas is to be met then paramedics and nonspecialist physicians will need to be trained in appropriate techniques. A detailed teaching manual called 'Primary Anaesthesia' published recently by the Oxford University Press is designed to help meet this need.

References

1. Prior FN. Appropriate technology: anaesthetics. *Br. Med. J.* 1984; **288**: 1750–3.
2. Boulton TB, Cole PV. Anaesthesia in difficult situations. *Anaesthesia* 1966; **21**: 268, 379, 513 and 1967; **22**: 101, 435.
3. Kamm GDR, Bewes PC. Ketamine anaesthesia by continuous intravenous drip. *Tropical Doctor* 1978; **8**(2), 68–72.

Further reading

Atkinson RS, Rushman GB, Lee JA. *Synopsis of Anaesthesia, 9ᵗʰ ed.* Bristol: Wright, 1982.

Eriksson E. *Illustrated Handbook of Local Anaesthesia.* Denmark: Munksgaard, 1979.

Farman J. *Anaesthesia and the EMO System.* London: English Universities Press, 1973.

King M. *Primary Anaesthesia.* Oxford: Oxford University Press, 1986.

Lee JA, Atkinson RS. *Lumbar Puncture and Spinal Analgesia.* London: Longman, 1978.

Lee JA, Bryce-Smith R. *Practical Regional Analgesia.* Amsterdam: Excerpta Medica, Elsevier, 1976.

Macintosh RR, Bryce-Smith R. *Local Analgesia – Abdominal surgery.* Edinburgh: Churchill-Livingstone, 1953.

Macintosh RR, Ostlere M. *Local Analgesia – Head and Neck.* Edinburgh: Churchill-Livingstone, 1955.

Prior FN. *A Manual of Anaesthesia for the Small Hospital, 2nd ed.* New Delhi: Voluntary Health Association of India, 1977.

21

Regional Anaesthesia

Gordon M C Paterson

Drugs
Toxicity
Methods of local and regional anaesthesia
    Surface analgesia
    Local infiltration
    Field block
    Peripheral nerve block
    Central neural blockade
    Intravenous regional analgesia (IVRA)
Equipment
Application of local anaesthesia for emergencies
    'In the field'
    In the casualty department
    In the ward and operating department
What blocks can be useful in emergencies?
    Head and neck
    Upper limb
    Lower limb
    Trunk and perineum
General considerations
    Pre-operative management
    Intra-operative management
    Failed blocks
    Postoperative management

Regional or local anaesthesia is the abolition of pain from a part of the body by the temporary interruption of conduction in associated sensory nerves. Motor function may also be affected, and autonomic blockade will occur, which if extensive can have marked effects on the cardiovascular system.

In clinical practice, the aim is to control pain with minimal danger or discomfort for the patient by the use of appropriate volumes and concentrations from the wide range of local anaesthetic drugs now available.

Methods used range from simple techniques requiring little experience to those requiring a sound knowledge of anatomy and physiology, and of technical skills best gained during the practice of local techniques for elective surgery under the supervision of experienced anaesthetists.

Compared with modern general anaesthesia, only simple equipment and monitoring are required and the methods are generally economical of staff and resources.

Local anaesthesia may be used alone, or combined with pre-, intra- and postoperative sedation or systemic analgesia; or to provide analgesia, muscular relaxation and autonomic blockade in a balanced general anaesthetic technique.

Local anaesthetics are toxic drugs that must be used with care and attention. As with general anaesthesia, no technique should be used without checking the availability of equipment and drugs for dealing with toxic effects that are potentially lethal. The quantity to be administered must be within the maximum permitted dosage assessed in relation to the patient's size, age and general condition. This applies equally to the vasoconstrictors often added to increase the efficiency and reduce the toxicity of local anaesthetic drugs.

The efficacy and safety of local compared with general anaesthesia and systemic analgesia should always be considered for pain relief in surgery and trauma, but efficacy and safety depend always on the knowledge and experience of the practitioner.

Drugs

Drugs used specifically to produce local anaesthesia are either esters of benzoic or para-aminobenzoic acids, such as cocaine, procaine, and amethocaine, or are amides, such as lignocaine (lidocaine), prilocaine, mepivacaine, bupivacaine, etidocaine and cinchocaine (dibucaine) (Table 21.1).

They are dispensed as water-soluble hydrochlorides in ampoules, or in multidose containers with added preservatives. Vasoconstrictors such as adrenaline (epinephrine) may also be included, except with cocaine which itself has a powerful vasoconstrictor action. Amides are generally more stable than esters and can be sterilized in solution. Lipid-soluble bases are released on contact with the relatively alkaline tissues and can then act upon nerve fibres. Local tissue acidosis, as in inflammation or ischaemia, is therefore likely to impair the efficiency of local anaesthesia. Moreover, systemic acidosis may enhance uptake of the water-

Table 21.1 Some local anaesthetic agents

Agents	Average duration (hr)	Range of concentrations used (%)	Maximum single dosage (mg/kg) Plain	Maximum single dosage (mg/kg) with adrenaline (epinephrine)* 1:200 000 (5 micrograms/ml)	Main uses
Cocaine HCl (EP & USP)	1–2	4–25	2.5	—	Vasoconstrictor. Topical use only. Controlled drug.
Procaine HCl (BP & USP)	0.5–1	1–2	7	8.5	Infiltration, nerve block. Now little used.
Amethocaine HCl (BP) (Tetracaine HCl (USP))	3–4	0.1–1	1.5	—	Spinal. Little used in United Kingdom.
Lignocaine HCl (BP) (Lidocaine HCl (USP))	1–2	0.5–5	3	7	Topical. Infiltration, nerve block, extradural, spinal.
Prilocaine HCl (BP & USNF)	1–2	0.5–3	5.5	8.5	Topical. Infiltration, nerve block, extradural, spinal. 0.5% recommended for IVRA.
Mepivacaine HCl (USP)	1.5–2	1–2	3	7	Similar to lignocaine. No longer marketed in United Kingdom.

Bupivacaine HCl (BP & USAN)	4–8	0.25–0.75	2	3.5	Infiltration, nerve block, extradural, spinal. Long duration, not significantly increased by addition of adrenaline. Relatively poor motor block.
Etidocaine HCl (USP)	4–8	0.5–1.5	3	5.5	Infiltration, nerve block, extradural. Long duration. Relatively profound motor block. Not marketed in the United Kingdom.
Cinchocaine HCl (BP) (Dibucaine HCl (USP))	3–4	0.5	0.7	—	Spinal anaesthesia

* A concentration of more than 1:200 000 (5 micrograms/ml) adrenaline (epinephrine) is unnecessary.
The maximum dose is 7 micrograms/kg — 0.5 mg or 100 ml in a fit adult.

soluble hydrochlorides by the central nervous system (CNS) and so aggravate toxicity following inadvertent intravascular injection.

The addition of vasoconstrictors such as adrenaline (epinephrine) or felypressin is intended to reduce bleeding after local infiltration, or to intensify the local block and limit systemic absorption from the site of injection, especially when lignocaine (lidocaine) or prilocaine is used.

Adrenaline (epinephrine) itself can be dangerous to the myocardium and vascular system, especially in the presence of halogenated general anaesthetics, and tricyclic and other anti-depressants, or in hypertensive and degenerative vascular disease. Its use is also contra-indicated in the digits and the penis, where the resulting constriction of end arteries can lead to necrosis.

The amount of drug in a given volume and concentration of solution should always be known for both local anaesthetic and vasoconstrictor. Large volumes from multidose containers should not be used for techniques such as epidural or intravenous regional analgesia because of the possibility of local tissue damage, or of systemic toxicity from added preservatives.

There is nowadays a wide choice of drugs of differing durations and capabilities. In general, the intensity of blockade is related to the concentration used and can range from autonomic to complete blockade involving even the largest motor fibres. Anomalous responses may, however, occur as in the case of amethocaine and etidocaine, which readily produce relatively profound motor blockade, or with bupivacaine, following which motor blockade is poor, but these differences can be exploited in clinical practice.

Results may benefit from using mixtures of drugs. For example, the rapid onset but short duration of lignocaine (lidocaine) can be combined with the slower onset but much longer duration of bupi-vacaine analgesia, provided that the final concentrations in the mixture are adequate. If adrenaline (epinephrine) is used to limit systemic absorption of lignocaine (lidocaine), then it should be added immediately before use, or the acid stabilizer it contains can impair the efficiency of the lignocaine. In practice, it may there-fore be simpler to inject the two agents sequentially.

Other agents such as cold, or tissue poisons such as alcohols and phenols, may also block conduction, as in refrigeration analgesia, or more permanently as in neurolytic blockade for intractable pain.

The extension of the principles of local anaesthesia to include the use of opioids has now opened up a whole new approach to the control of pain with conventional narcotic analgesics, particularly in the field of pain relief following surgery and trauma.

Toxicity

This may be due to allergy or sensitivity to the agent used, although such is rare with the now commonly used amide-linked drugs. Toxicity is more likely to result from drug overdosage or inadvertent intravascular injection. An overdose can most readily occur when the site of administration is highly vascular, as from mucous membranes in surface analgesia, and following intercostal nerve block and sacral epidural anaesthesia.

Toxicity following an overdose is commonly manifest as CNS excitation that may culminate in generalized convulsions followed by unconsciousness. Simultaneous cardiovascular and respiratory stimulation may likewise be followed by depression and the combined effects are potentially lethal.

Measures must always be available to combat convulsions, hypotension, bradycardia and arrhythmias, and apnoea. By far the most important are ventilation of the lungs with oxygen and the IV administration of anticonvulsant and vasopressor drugs. Such will offset the respiratory and metabolic acidoses that can enhance further uptake by the CNS of the water-soluble hydrochloride from the site of injection and aggravate brain toxicity.

Toxicity is not likely to occur when the right drug is given in the right dose by the right technique, with injections made slowly and carefully to avoid high blood levels, especially from inadvertent intravascular injection. Toxicity is not likely to have serious consequences if it is always anticipated so it can then be treated promptly and efficiently (Table 21.2).

Table 21.2 Management of local anaesthetic toxicity

1. Airway
2. Ventilate lungs with oxygen
3. CNS Excitation
   a. Benzodiazepines
   b. Barbiturates
   c. Neuromuscular blockade (with intubation + IPPV)
4. Vasodilatation
   a. Raise cardiac filling pressure: Elevate limbs, IV fluids.
   b. Vasopressors
5. Myocardial depression
   a. Bradycardia – atropine, etc
   b. Hypotension – inotropes
   c. External cardiac massage
6. Vasoconstriction – β-adrenergic blockade
7. Allergy – Antihistamines
8. Anaphylaxis

Methods of local and regional analgesia

These include surface analgesia, local infiltration, field block, nerve block: peripheral and central, and IVRA; and they are well described in the many detailed and fully illustrated texts and articles that are readily available.

All have their uses, either alone or in combination, and their particular advantages and limitations must be appreciated. Topical, local infiltration and field block, together with IVRA, whilst technically easy, reliable and requiring of minimal equipment, are especially prone to toxicity if simple precautions are not taken. Peripheral and central nerve blocks, however, whilst providing pain relief over wide areas using small amounts of drug and a minimum number of injections, require much more skill and knowledge and are therefore more prone to failure than to toxicity in inexperienced hands.

Central blockade in the form of spinal intradural or epidural anaesthesia inevitably involves segmental autonomic sympathetic and sacral parasympathetic preganglionic fibres. This can lead to systemic hypotension for which appropriate treatment must be available. Visceral structures innervated by afferents in cranial parasympathetic pathways will not be completely affected by spinal anaesthesia and allowance for this must be made if the technique is used for upper abdominal surgery by providing specific visceral nerve blockade or, more conveniently, light general endotracheal anaesthesia.

For many other procedures also it may be preferable, in practice to combine more than one method of local anaesthesia or to provide sedation or general anaesthesia to complete pain relief, especially during surgery. This may be essential if the block has been incomplete and cannot be improved upon, or because the surgery has proved more extensive or prolonged than was expected, or because the patient has proved unable to tolerate the procedure from anxiety or physical discomfort.

Surface analgesia

Cocaine, lignocaine (lidocaine), prilocaine and other agents are applied directly to mucous membranes, or even to wounds and abrasions, and overdosage is always a risk. Minor surgery of the eye, nose, eardrum, or instrumentation of the upper respiratory tract or the urethra are all amenable to this form of anaesthesia, using sprays, lotions, gels, ointments, etc.

Local infiltration

Lignocaine (lidocaine), prilocaine and other agents may be injected in the vicinity of the affected site if no inflammation is present. Adrenaline (epinephrine) is usually added to reduce bleeding during surgery. Administration can be painful and the number of injections should be limited, but even so patient co-operation may be inadequate, especially with children.

Inadvertent IV injection is possible if the needle is not kept moving and the volume injected at any point should not exceed 2 ml. This is the normal method of analgesia for extraction of teeth, other than the lower molars for which a nerve block is usually necessary. It has many other applications such as wound suturing and as a convenient way of using adrenaline (epinephrine) to reduce bleeding during plastic and other delicate surgical procedures especially around the face and neck.

Field block

Lignocaine (lidocaine), prilocaine and other agents are injected so as to lay a barrage across the pathway of nerves from an operation site such as the scalp, the inguinal, or the paracervical uterine region. Though large volumes may be necessary, the concentration used may be low and intravascular injection is easily avoided.

Peripheral nerve blocks

Lignocaine (lidocaine), prilocaine, bupivacaine and other agents must be injected with accuracy so as to make contact with nerves in the trunk or extremities. Skill and a sound knowledge of anatomy are necessary to gain a high success rate and to avoid complications such as pneumothorax, damage to structures such as blood vessels and tendon sheaths, or inadvertent spinal blockade.

Commonly used nerve blocks include inferior dental, lingual and mental for procedures on the lower teeth; brachial plexus and wrist block in the upper limb; femoral, lateral femoral cutaneous, obturator and sciatic nerve blocks, and ankle blocks in the lower limb. Maxillary, mandibular, intercostal and digital nerve blocks are further examples of this approach.

When anatomical landmarks are poor, such as for the brachial plexus in the neck, or the sciatic nerve from the front of the thigh and in obese patients, some practitioners routinely employ a peripheral nerve stimulator to locate the nerves more accurately.

Central neural blockade

Most agents are, or have been, used in the vicinity of the spinal cord and emerging spinal nerve roots to produce spinal anaesthesia. This may be intradural (subarachnoid or intrathecal) when the drug is injected into the spinal fluid at lumbar puncture; or epidural (extradural, peridural). Unqualified, the term 'spinal anaesthesia' commonly refers to intradural block whilst extradural block is commonly termed epidural. Epidural anaesthesia may be administered at the thoracic, lumbar or sacral level of the vertebral column. Compared with epidural anaesthesia, the intradural approach is technically easy, is more rapid and reliable in onset, requires smaller amounts of drug and can be confined to one side of the body. Epidural analgesia is, however, amenable to replenishment if a catheter is used. All spinal anaesthesia is followed by blockade of sympathetic and sacral parasympathetic preganglionic fibres and by hypotension, for which suitable measures must be available.

Intravenous regional analgesia (IVRA)

An agent is injected into a vein in a limb that has been exsanguinated and isolated from the general circulation by an arterial tourniquet. Provided the volume and concentration injected are adequate, analgesia and muscular relaxation develop rapidly and completely and persist until the circulation is restored. The method is easy and reliable and generally safe, and its duration can be controlled and even extended for long periods if necessary by repeating the process. The extent of the block can also be controlled and when the circulation is restored recovery is rapid and usually complete so that full use of the limb is then possible.

The main disadvantages are that a tourniquet is always required, the exsanguination process may be painful or even impractical in an injured limb and further measures are required for postoperative pain.

- Toxicity may occur when the tourniquet is released or if it fails during the procedure, and it is therefore important to limit the amount of drug used.
- Prilocaine is preferred to lignocaine (lidocaine) because of its greater therapeutic ratio and a concentration of 0.5 per cent is adequate.
- Adrenaline (epinephrine) must *not* be used and tourniquet release should not occur within 30 min of the original administration to avoid high systemic blood levels.
- Forty ml of solution should be adequate for a forearm or

hand procedure with the tourniquet on the upper arm, but the volumes required for lower limbs can be followed by toxicity unless the concentration is reduced or the procedure is confined to the ankle or foot with the tourniquet on the calf.
- The technique should be avoided in the presence of sickle cell disease, in which the use of tourniquets and also of general anaesthesia may be contra-indicated.
- Peripheral vascular disease and systemic hypertension may also raise practical difficulties and the method should also be avoided in epileptics, whose seizure threshhold could be reached when blood levels rise in the phase immediately following tourniquet release.

The method has its main use in procedures on the forearm and hand where postoperative pain can if necessary be controlled by other means.

Equipment

Equipment required for local anaesthesia is minimal compared with general anaesthesia. Trays should be available with a selection of basic requirements for producing a sterile field and injecting local anaesthetics free from contamination by antiseptic lotions or other drugs. Needles should have short bevels to minimize trauma to nerve fibres and 'security beads' to prevent insertion to the junction of shaft and hub where breakage may occur. There are many forms of disposable tray available commercially, but reusable equipment is more economical if the items to be included can be agreed upon.

- *Resuscitation* if necessary may involve positive pressure endotracheal ventilation with oxygen, and the administration of IV infusions and drugs to combat convulsions, bradycardia, hypotension and metabolic acidosis. Patients should always be on tipping trolleys when local anaesthesia is performed and efficient suction equipment must be available.
- *Monitoring* should always include heart rate and blood pressure, and patients must always be accompanied by personnel who can make these observations. It is important to decide in advance what changes in blood pressure are acceptable.

The administrator must always check all drugs and equipment personally, just as for general anaesthesia, deciding in advance the amounts of local anaesthetic drugs that the patient may safely receive so that the volumes and concentrations of agents then used do not lead to overdosage.

- Antiseptics should always be kept away from needles and syringes, and local anaesthetic drugs should always be kept away from drugs for resuscitation or general anaesthesia.

Application of local anaesthesia for emergencies

The relief of pain, muscular relaxation and autonomic blockade with local anaesthesia are advantages that can be applied to patients following trauma or during and after emergency or elective surgery and obstetrical procedures.

'In the field'

Local anaesthesia has possible uses even in the immediate care of civilian and military casualties (*see* p. 228). The main requirement is for analgesia, for which narcotics and ketamine are generally used, but they may be unreliable and of short or uncertain duration, and are often cumulative. Narcotics are particularly unreliable when injured patients must be moved and they are contra-indicated in suspected head injury, chest injuries, and in facial injuries when the stomach may contain much swallowed blood.

Local anaesthesia of a limb or limbs can be accomplished with minimal systemic upset to permit initial wound cleansing, splinting, reduction of fractures or dislocations, and removal of foreign bodies, while awaiting or during transport to the military or civilian hospital. Assessment, radiology and further treatment may then follow whilst the analgesia is still effective, or has been reinforced. Problems of minimal equipment, head injury and full stomach are kept in perspective if general anaesthesia is avoided and patients can be left in the care of relatively unskilled personnel, leaving anaesthetists free to deal with more complex problems.

There are obvious disadvantages that will apply in many cases. Local anaesthesia can be slow and unreliable when undertaken by unskilled anaesthetists or surgeons. Multiple injuries requiring several blocks and large doses of drugs would not seem amenable, but even one block can be better than none if it can deal with a particularly painful injury; e.g. femoral nerve block in cases of fractured shaft of femur. Trauma may distort anatomy or preclude correct positioning for performing blocks, and working conditions may make the risk of infection or other complications of these procedures too high.

In the casualty department

Local anaesthesia can permit completion of treatment and early discharge of the patient, which is always an advantage, especially if it involves the simplest block possible. Wound suture, reduction of fractures and dislocations, removal of foreign bodies and minor surgery of the face, lips, tongue, teeth, eardrum, eye, etc., and drainage of distally located abcesses, can be accomplished if patients, doctors and nurses are all in favour and adequate time is allowed for blocks to be administered gently and safely and to take full effect. The possibility of treatment without delay and early return home will often tempt the relatively reluctant patient to accept local anaesthesia.

A local anaesthetic technique that provides prolonged analgesia can be of further advantage, but patients must then be made aware of their vulnerability from any residual anaesthesia or paralysis once they leave the hospital.

In the ward and operating department

Here especially, local anaesthesia can be as safe as, if not safer than, general anaesthesia, especially if treatment can then begin without delay when, for example, head injury, full stomach, diabetes, sickle cell disease, etc. complicate acute surgical and obstetrical emergencies. In the management of chest injuries with fractured ribs, intercostal nerve blocks or segmental thoracic epidural analgesia can render endotracheal positive pressure ventilation unnecessary. Within the hospital, blocks of all types become feasible for almost all sites, even for emergencies, and again the need is for skill and experience and a commitment to make the most possible use of the features of local anaesthesia.

Whilst surface infiltration and IV regional anaesthesia can be accomplished quickly and reliably by relatively inexperienced personnel, many apparently difficult and unusual nerve, plexus or intradural blocks become equally feasible using combinations of drugs and methods once experience has been gained with elective cases, so that the anaesthetist's own confidence in a high success rate can be communicated and then put to effect in the patient. Even epidural blockade, though of relatively slow onset, can have applications in emergencies such as severe renal colic, or the hypertensive crises of eclampsia (*see* p. 275) when other measures may be unavailable or less safe.

Whilst local anaesthesia alone may seem appropriate for short operations on the extremities, the addition of sedation or light general anaesthesia will usually be necessary when the patient is a child, of low intelligence, confused or otherwise unco-operative, or when there is a language barrier.

When surgery is liable to become prolonged or extensive, or when some discomfort is inevitable as with abdominal surgery under field block or even under central neural blockade, local anaesthesia alone cannot be expected to suffice, either for patient or operators.

A carefully chosen combination of techniques can provide the best and safest anaesthesia for many emergencies, even when time is short; the advantages of rapid recovery and postoperative analgesia without respiratory depression, and even early ambulation and discharge can amply justify the initial effort.

What blocks can be useful in emergencies?

Head and neck

Scalp	– Field block
Eardrum	– Surface analgesia
Eyelids	– Local infiltration. Periorbital nerve blocks.
Conjunctiva	– Surface
Eye	– Retro-ocular. Facial (at orbital margin or in parotid gland).
Nasal cavity	– Surface
Oral cavity	– Surface. Local infiltration.
Upper respiratory tract	– Surface
Teeth	– Local infiltration. Inferior dental, lingual and mental nerve blocks.
Face	– Local infiltration. Maxillary, mandibular nerve blocks (trunks or terminal branches).
Neck ⎫ Tracheostomy ⎬	– Superficial cervical plexus Local infiltration

Upper limb

	– Local infiltration, or
Shoulder and upper arm	– Interscalene ⎫ Brachial plexus Supraclavicular ⎬ blocks
	(The possibility of pneumothorax and of phrenic nerve blocks precludes the use of supraclavicular or interscalene brachial plexus blocks in out-patients or bilaterally in any patient!)

Elbow and forearm	– Axillary brachial plexus and intercostal nerve blocks. IV regional.
Wrist and hand	– Brachial plexus blocks, wrist block. Digital nerve blocks. IV regional. (Solutions containing vasoconstrictors must *not* be used for digital nerves or IV regional blocks.)

Lower limb

	– Local infiltration or central neural blockade (intra- or epidural),
Hip	– Sciatic, obturator nerve blocks
Groin	– Field block
Thigh	– Femoral, lateral femoral cutaneous nerve blocks
Knee	– Femoral, lateral femoral cutaneous, obturator, sciatic nerve blocks
Foot	– Ankle block. Digital nerve blocks. IV regional. (Solutions containing vasoconstrictors should not be used for digital nerve or IV regional blocks.)
Calf and ankle	– Sciatic. Femoral nerve blocks. IV regional.

Trunk and perineum

	– Local infiltration, or
Chest wall	– Intercostal nerve blocks. Segmental thoracic epidural blockade.
Abdominal wall	– Intercostal nerve blocks and field blocks.
Abdominal cavity	– Field block. Central neural blockade. (The abdominal viscera are sensitive to handling in the presence of inflammation and general anaesthesia may then be necessary in addition.)
Renal colic	– Lumbar epidural blockade

Obstetrics   – Lumbar ⎫
                            Sacral ⎬ epidural blockade
                            Low or mid-intradural blockade.
                            Pudendal, paracervical nerve blocks.
Eclampsia   – Lumbar epidural blockade
Urethra   – Surface, sacral epidural blockade
Penis   – Field block, sacral epidural
                            blockade. (Solutions containing
                            vasconstrictors must not be injected
                            into the penis.)

In general, a combination of techniques such as nerve block, local infiltration and surface analgesia, supplementary distal blocks to cover inadequacies, or light general anaesthesia with field block or central neural blockade can provide a high overall success rate.

General considerations

Pre-operative management

A history of local anaesthesia should be sought, together with its outcome and any suggestion of drug allergy. The attitude of the patient to local anaesthesia and the choice between local and general anaesthesia should be assessed both for the patient and the procedure concerned.

The general physical status of the patient should be noted. Extremes of age, obesity, and arthritic and other deformities may render both local and general anaesthesia difficult.

As with general anaesthesia, intercurrent illness, particularly hypertensive and ischaemic heart disease, respiratory disease, epilepsy, alcoholism and coagulopathy can be of crucial importance. Also medication with tricyclic and other anti-depressants renders vasoconstrictors particularly dangerous.

In the fit patient, general anaesthesia is usually very safe and local anaesthesia often has dubious advantages unless the patient requests it. The unfit reluctant patient needs persuading that local anaesthesia is safe and effective, that recovery is quick, side effects and postoperative discomfort are minimal, that the operation cannot be seen, that the patient will not be left alone and that sedation or possibly unconsciousness can still be provided if necessary.

Discussion and explanation must be appropriate to the patient's age, intelligence and native language, but if local anaesthesia is not acceptable, undue persuasion should not be used.

Other contra-indications include lack of equipment and drugs, especially for resuscitation, and lack of experience with patients under local anaesthesia on the part of anaesthetists, surgeons and nursing staff. Infection at the site of injection and deformities that render correct positioning for the block too difficult are equally as important as when the patient is found to have neurological or peripheral vascular disease or injuries that could be aggravated by the local anaesthetic technique.

The decision to embark on local anaesthesia and the choice of agents to be used leads to consideration of the need for additional medication to relieve anxiety, residual pain and restlessness that can mar success.

The choice begins with premedication, for which many drugs have been used. Benzodiazepines have now proved superior to phenothiazines and butyrophenones for sedation, whilst narcotic analgesics are rarely indicated, especially as they may negate the advantages of a local technique in an unfit patient. Narcotics may also lead to nausea and vomiting, but if pain is too severe for the patient to co-operate until the block is accomplished, small IV doses of opiates or of ketamine may be necessary. However, these can further delay gastric emptying and render an eventual general anaesthetic induction more hazardous.

Intra-operative management

Even with a successful local block, it remains necessary to attend to details for the patient's comfort and general condition.

- As with general anaesthesia, the procedure begins with the provision of reliable venous access for additional medication and the safe management of toxicity, the appearance of which can be delayed, particularly if IVRA is used.

Additional medication may be required for anxiety, restlessness, or because the environment is unsuitable. Pain may exist in another part of the body or may arise at the operation site because the block is incomplete or is waning during a prolonged operation. A decision to provide sedation or general anaesthesia may have been made in advance and the choice may be related to the premedication already provided. General anaesthesia may be intravenous, using chlormethiazole, etomidate or propofol; or inhalational, using nitrous oxide and a volatile agent, but tracheal intubation may then be necessary, particularly during upper abdominal surgery.

Cyanosis due to methaemoglobinaemia may occasionally develop after the use of large doses of amide drugs, usually prilocaine. It can be counteracted with IV 1 per cent methylene blue, 1–2 mg/kg if necessary because of anaemia or during obstetrical procedures.

Failed blocks

If failure is total it must be accepted that the technique was at fault, unless an unstable agent was used that had deteriorated during storage. More often the failure is only partial and may not show until the operation has progressed. Clinical signs of successful blockade can be misleading and good surface analgesia may not be reflected in the deeper tissues of the surgical field or underlying a tourniquet.

- The right choice of agent or combination of agents, the addition of a vasoconstrictor and the injection of an adequate volume and concentration of agent well in advance of the surgery are essential for success.

Pain can be controlled by the use of more local anaesthesia, either before surgery by reinforcing the original block, by blocking specific nerves more distally as required, or by local infiltration by the surgeon during the operation. In such cases, the possibility of toxicity must be anticipated as an overdose can occur.

If additional local anaesthesia is impracticable or unsafe, the wishes of the patient and the needs of the surgeon will usually require the provision of intravenous analgesia or general anaesthesia unless the operation is almost complete.

Postoperative management

Local anaesthesia with minimal sedation should present few postoperative management problems, and nor should a successful block covered by light general anaesthesia, from which recovery should be rapid and complete. Postoperative pain when the block wanes may be slight if injuries are splinted and elevated and only simple analgesics may be needed. If long acting agents have been used, the dangers of tight splints and tissue swelling may not be appreciated; patients and nursing staff must be warned.

Patients hoping to return home must be accompanied during and after the journey until the possible dangers of residual anaesthesia are passed. Written instructions must be given regarding possible complications and simple analgesics prescribed with a warning that severe pain should be reported without delay.

- Brachial plexus blocks in the neck may be followed by pneumothorax and phrenic nerve paralysis, and should never be performed bilaterally.

The effects of pneumothorax, which may also follow intercostal blocks for fractured ribs and postoperative pain, may be delayed and patients must remain in the hospital after such procedures.

- Discharge home must likewise be delayed after nerve blocks in the lower limb, until motor power is fully recovered and ambulation is safe.
- Central neural blockade may be followed by hypotension and urinary retention in addition to motor paralysis for which the patient must be kept under observation, often for more than 24 hr if spinal opiates have been used. Hypotension may be due to bleeding rather than residual blockade, and restlessness may be due to bladder distension rather than waning analgesia. The management of such complications requires the availability of trained nursing and medical staff, provision of which should have been arranged in advance. Such disadvantages must be borne in mind when these techniques are selected with the intention of avoiding general anaesthesia and conventional narcotic analgesia in the interests of patient safety.

Conclusion

The successful practice of local techniques in emergency anaesthesia depends ultimately on the ability of the anaesthetist to apply skills based on a sound knowledge of anatomy, physiology and pharmacology so that the patient can be relieved of pain with minimal danger and discomfort. Enthusiasm for and determination to make the best use of local anaesthesia must always be tempered by the wishes of the patient, the needs of the surgeon and the availability of skilled nursing support before, during and after the procedure.

Further reading

Atkinson RS, Rushman GB, Lee JA. *A Synopsis of Anaesthesia, 9th ed.* Bristol: Wright, 1982.

Bromage PR. *Epidural Anaesthesia.* London: Saunders, 1978.

Cousins MJ, Bridenbaugh PO. *Neural Blockade in Clinical Anesthesia and Management of Pain.* Philadelphia: Lippincott, 1980

Cousins MJ, Mather LE. Intrathecal and epidural administration of opioids. *Anesthesiology* 1984; **61**: 276–310.

Eriksson E. *Illustrated Handbook in Local Anaesthesia, 2nd ed.* London: Lloyd-Luke, 1979.

Henderson JJ and Nimmo WS. *Practical Regional Anaesthesia.* Oxford: Blackwell, 1983.

King M. *Primary Anaesthesia.* Oxford: Oxford University Press, 1986.

Lee JA, Atkinson RS. *Macintosh's Lumbar Puncture and Spinal Anaesthesia*. Edinburgh: Churchill-Livingstone, 1978.

Lee JA, Bryce-Smith R. *Practical Regional Anaesthesia*. Amsterdam: Excerpta Medica, 1976.

Macintosh RR, Bryce-Smith R. *Local Analgesia: Abdominal Surgery, 2nd ed*. Edinburgh: Churchill-Livingstone, 1962.

Macintosh RR, Ostlere M. *Local Analgesia: Head and Neck, 2nd ed*. Edinburgh: Churchill-Livingstone, 1967.

Williams PL, Warwick R. *Gray's Anatomy, 36th ed*. Edinburgh: Churchill-Livingstone, 1980.

Winnie AP. *Plexus Anaesthesia: Volume I*. Edinburgh: Churchill-Livingstone, 1984.

22

Obstetric Emergencies

W Robert Casson and Penelope B Hewitt

Physiological changes of pregnancy
Anaesthesia for the pregnant patient
Local analgesic techniques
    Lumbar epidural analgesia
    Caudal epidural analgesia
    Spinal analgesia
    Paracervical block
    Pudendal block
    Local infiltration
General anaesthesia
    Induction
    Failed intubation drill
    Maintenance of anaesthesia
    Post-partum procedures
Pregnancy related pathology
    Pre-eclampsia
    Amniotic fluid embolism
    Heart disease

The similarity between the blood-brain and placental barriers in terms of drug transmission implies that anything given to depress the mother's central nervous system will also have a depressant effect on the unborn child. Safe obstetric anaesthesia depends on a knowledge of this fact and of the physiological and pathological processes associated with pregnancy.

Physiological changes of pregnancy

Salt and water retention is an integral part of any normal pregnancy. Although interstitial fluid accumulates only in the third trimester, intravascular volume increases from the sixth week onwards; this reaches a level of about 50 per cent above normal by 30 weeks. Red cell volume also increases but less so, so that at term there is a relative anaemia (haemoglobin concentration of 12 g/dl and a haematocrit of 35 per cent).

Cardiac output rises markedly in the first trimester (30–34 per cent above pre-pregnancy values), associated with a rise in pulse rate of 15–20 beats/min. This is maintained until term. Systolic and diastolic blood pressures tend to fall up to the 28th week of pregnancy (diastolic more than systolic) and then recover to pre-pregnancy values by the 36th week.

Progesterone appears to stimulate the medullary respiratory centre so that hyperventilation occurs early in pregnancy and continues up to term. The increase in minute volume is achieved mainly by an increase in tidal volume although there is also a small increase in respiratory rate. The arterial carbon dioxide tension falls to about 30 mmHg (4 kPa) and this is accompanied by a mild compensatory metabolic acidosis (base deficit about 3 mmol/l). There is a reduction in functional residual capacity, particularly when the patient lies supine, as a consequence of splinting of the diaphragm by the expanding uterus. Closing capacity appears to remain at pre-pregnancy values, so that ventilation–perfusion mismatch could occur if dependent airways then closed during tidal respiration. However, studies of arterial oxygen tensions have only shown a larger variability of values around the pre-pregnancy norm. Oxygen consumption is increased by 15 per cent during pregnancy.

Smooth muscle relaxation, as a consequence of a rise in progesterone, is a concomitant of all normal pregnancies; this leads to constipation and ureteric dilatation, but the main potential problem of concern to the anaesthetist is the effect on gastric emptying. The most recent Report on Confidential Enquiries into Maternal Deaths in England and Wales (1979–81) has yet again emphasized the relatively high incidence of regurgitation and aspiration of gastric contents during anaesthesia for obstetric procedures. However, the generally accepted assumption of a delay in gastric emptying is not supported by the data presently available. Paracetamol absorption studies have shown only a small, and not statistically significant, delay in gastric emptying at term; similarly, during labour there appears to be no hold up until narcotics are administered for pain relief, retention of gastric contents then becoming a significant complication. What is clear, however, is that the competency of the gastro-oesophageal junction is suspect in the pregnant woman, particularly if she has suffered from heartburn.

There is an increase in both coagulation and fibrinolysis during pregnancy with the delicate balance being slightly in favour of the former. This explains the increased incidence of deep venous thrombosis during and immediately after pregnancy. Also, there is increased potential for this delicate balance to be upset (*see* below).

Anaesthesia for the pregnant patient

Operative intervention during pregnancy may be for obstetric or non-obstetric reasons. Caesarean section may be necessary because of fetal distress or failure to progress in labour; the incidence of major anaesthetic complications may be minimized by the use of local analgesic techniques such as epidural or subarachnoid block. The anaesthetic management of a patient presenting for a surgical procedure unconnected with the pregnancy should be aimed towards the avoidance of induction of premature labour. No technique has been convincingly shown to minimize this complication. β-2 receptor stimulants (e.g. salbutamol, terbutaline) are useful inhibitors of premature labour.

The presence of an experienced anaesthetist, with adequate assistance and equipment, is mandatory in any hospital where operative intervention might be necessary during pregnancy. The following equipment must be immediately available.

- An operating table which can be tilted head down rapidly if necessary.
- Powerful suction apparatus with pharyngeal sucker attached and tracheal catheters available.
- Some means of tilting the patient to her left side so that the inferior vena cava is not compressed by the gravid uterus; this is usually in the form of a 'Crawford wedge' positioned under the right buttock; various types of inflatable devices are also available.
- Two working laryngoscopes with adult standard and large Macintosh blades, and one with a Magill blade; a Macintosh polio blade may be useful if large breasts interfere with the introduction of a standard laryngoscope.
- A wide bore stomach tube.
- Endotracheal tubes with introducers and bougies to help in the manipulation of the tip.
- Magill intubating forceps.
- A standard anaesthetic machine with nitrous oxide, oxygen and vaporizers for halothane, enflurane and isoflurane.
- Intravenous infusion equipment designed for rapid blood transfusion.
- Two units cross-matched or (in an acute emergency) 2 units group O Rh negative blood.
- Standard anaesthetic drugs; drugs for resuscitation; an

antacid e.g. 0.3 M sodium citrate; oxytocin (superior to ergometrine which causes vomiting and hypertension).

An experienced assistant must be available at all times when an obstetric anaesthetic is to be undertaken. This will usually be a trained Operating Department Assistant or anaesthetic nurse; he or she should be able to apply cricoid pressure correctly and should know the location of all the anaesthetic equipment which may be needed in an emergency. If the anaesthetist has any doubt the assistant must be fully instructed in the use of Sellick's manoeuvre before anaesthesia is induced (*see* p. 7).

Local analgesic techniques

Lumbar epidural analgesia

The use of epidural block for pain relief during labour and to provide analgesia for Caesarean section is becoming more widespread. An anaesthetist who is skilled in endotracheal intubation and treatment of cardiovascular collapse must be available on site at all times when epidural blocks are in progress.

Epidural analgesia is contra-indicated in the presence of defective coagulation or sepsis (such as infected spots) on the back. Relative contra-indications include neurological disease (although it is an accepted technique for patients with multiple sclerosis) and a history of back pain, especially with nerve root compression.

It is customary to inject a 3 ml test dose of local analgesic before instituting the analgesia. Subarachnoid block may be detected at this point but intravascular placement may not. Thus, it is important that the full dose is given slowly so that early symptoms of toxicity (numb lips, tinnitus, etc.) may be detected before the development of later, and more dangerous, manifestations.

For the relief of pain in labour, bupivacaine is the drug of choice; it is a useful agent due to its high tissue binding and lack of tachyphylaxis. The ideal epidural block would provide analgesia without ablating the urge for the mother to push in the second stage. Lower concentrations of local anaesthetic are probably beneficial in this respect; 0.5, 0.375 and 0.25 per cent have been used successfully. The maximum dose recommended for bupivacaine is 2 mg/kg in any 4 hr period (about 30 ml of 0.5 per cent).

For forceps delivery, if an epidural is in progress, a further 'top up' may be needed. If an acute emergency Caesarean section is necessary it is unlikely that there will be time to institute an epidural. If there is a catheter *in situ* then great care is needed if it is necessary to increase the depth of analgesia. Grand mal convulsions, occurring 20 min after the final injection, have been reported after the supplementation of prolonged epidural blocks with large doses of bupivacaine (> 95 mg).[1] Bupivacaine and etidocaine are particularly hazardous, especially if they are injected intravascularly, since strong myocardial binding requires prolonged resuscitation. If Caesarean section become necessary after prolonged epidural anaesthesia a less toxic local analgesic, such as prilocaine, may be safer or it may even be less dangerous to proceed to general anaesthesia.

Complications

Hypotension may occur due to sympathetic blockade (which extends about two segments higher than the level of analgesia); this is usually corrected by turning the patient on her left side (to take pressure off the inferior vena cava), tilting the bed 'foot up' and rapidly administering IV fluids (including some colloid); oxygen should be given by face-mask. If the blood pressure does not rise it sometimes responds to turning the patient onto her right side. If the blood pressure still does not rise then IV ephedrine (5–10 mg) may be given. Rarely, high epidural block or inadvertent total spinal block occur; these must be treated with circulatory support and, if respiratory paralysis supervenes, with intubation and positive pressure ventilation.

The epidural catheter may be left *in situ* and used to administer postoperative pain relief.

Caudal epidural analgesia

Rarely used in modern obstetric practice because of the high volumes of local analgesic which must be injected. It may be a useful form of analgesia for forceps delivery and is a quick and relatively easy approach to the epidural space. Access is via the sacral hiatus and 20–30 ml of local analgesic (e.g. 0.25 per cent bupivacaine) is injected which should give a block to about the level of T10–T12.

Spinal analgesia

Appears to be regaining favour since the advent of small gauge needles. It is an easier, quicker and more reliable technique than lumbar epidural block. The incidence of post-spinal headaches, even in this young population, is very small if 25 G or smaller needles are used. It is not advisable to leave a catheter in the subarachnoid space and therefore further analgesic cannot be given if surgery is prolonged.

Lumbar puncture is performed, using a 25 G needle through a Size introducer. As with epidural blocks, a smaller volume of local analgesic is necessary in the pregnant, compared to the non-pregnant individual. When there is free flow of CSF 1.6–2.4 ml of 'heavy' bupivacaine (0.5 per cent) is injected; the patient is turned to the supine position, whilst the uterus is manually pushed to the left side by an assistant to avoid caval compression.

By tilting the patient 'head down' the desired level can be reached and if the hips and knees are flexed the block is unlikely to extend above T4 due to the curvature of the thoracic spine. When the local analgesic has 'fixed' the patient is tilted to the left side and surgery can begin. Hypotension is treated as with epidural block. Plain isobaric bupivacaine has also been used successfully by this route.

Paracervical block

This technique, where local analgesic solution is injected into both lateral vaginal fornices in order to block the sympathetic nerve plexus has been largely abandoned due to the high incidence of fetal bradycardia.

Pudendal block

This is a nerve block usually performed bilaterally by an obstetrician in order to provide analgesia for forceps delivery. The pudendal nerve (S_2, S_3, S_4) may be approached via a transvaginal or perineal route.

If the former route is used the needle (usually one with a guide such as a Kobak) is guided behind the ischial spine and through the sacrospinous ligament; a definite 'click' is usually felt as the ligament is penetrated; after negative aspiration 10 ml of either 1 per cent lignocaine (lidocaine) or 1 per cent prilocaine is injected.

The perineal route is an alternative approach to block the pudendal nerve. After skin infiltration, halfway between the dorsal commissure of the vagina and the ischial tuberosity, the needle is introduced and, using the other hand as a guide, 5–10 ml of 1 per cent lignocaine (lidocaine) or prilocaine is injected to block the nerve at the level of the ischial spine. Some solution should be placed posteriorly to the ischial tuberosity to block the perineal branch of the posterior cutaneous nerve of the thigh. Supplementary local analgesic may need to be injected into the perineum.

A lumbar or caudal epidural block, or a spinal block allows easier manipulation of the baby's head within the pelvis.

Local infiltration

Caesarean section may be carried out under local infiltration and this can be a useful technique in some patients. Up to 100 ml of 0.25 per cent lignocaine (lidocaine) with adrenaline (epinephrine) is used. Two skin wheals are raised about 3 cm lateral to the linea alba. Injection from the symphysis pubis to a point 5 cm above the umbilicus achieves the necessary block of the lower six intercostal and the lumbar nerves.

General anaesthesia

During the years 1979–81 there were 22 maternal deaths in England and Wales directly attributable to anaesthesia for obstetric patients,[2] eight of these being due to problems with endotracheal intubation and/or regurgitation of gastric contents with pulmonary aspiration (some of the latter leading to Mendelson's syndrome) (*see* page 12).

• Inexperience of the anaesthetist and inadequate assistance and/or equipment are repeatedly implicated in these disasters.

The likelihood of a patient presenting for an emergency obstetric procedure having retained gastric contents is high; antacids should be given to raise the pH of these contents and, if possible, their volume should be reduced. The passage of a large-bore stomach tube or apomorphine induced vomiting have been advocated prior to induction. However, most anaesthetists prefer to attempt to raise the pH of the gastric contents. In modern British practice most women will have received an H_2 receptor blocker, e.g. ranitidine,[1] or an antacid regularly throughout labour in the form of Magnesium Trisilicate Mixture (MTM), 15–20 ml 2-hourly. There is some evidence to suggest that the particulate antacids, such as MTM, may themselves cause pulmonary damage should aspiration occur. Also, mixing within the stomach may be incomplete and so a clear solution of 0.3 M sodium citrate is preferred as a single dose (30 ml) just prior to induction. Metoclopramide may improve gastric emptying but needs to be given at least 1 hr before induction of anaesthesia (*see* p. 105). H_2 receptor antagonists also have a place in reducing volume and increasing pH of gastric contents during labour (Fig. 22.1, and page 105).[3]

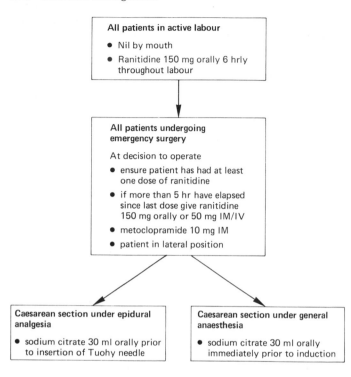

Fig. 22.1   Protocol for use of ranitidine and sodium citrate for prophylaxis against acid aspiration syndrome in obstetric patients.[1]

Induction

The patient is positioned supine with left lateral tilt and pre-oxygenated via a *well-fitting* face-mask (Fig. 22.2) for 3 min (there is some evidence to suggest that five large breaths may be adequate so long as there are no air leaks). Anaesthesia is induced with a predetermined dose of thiopentone (thiopental) or methohexitone (methohexital), whilst cricoid pressure[4] is applied by a trained assistant. The induction agent is immediately followed by suxamethonium (succinylcholine) and rapid orotracheal intubation after relaxation has occurred; suxamethonium (succinylcholine) is used because of its rapid onset of action and metabolism (allowing spontaneous respiration to return in the event of a failed intubation). In the event of failed intubation if the surgery is not urgent the patient can be awakened and a local analgesic technique used.

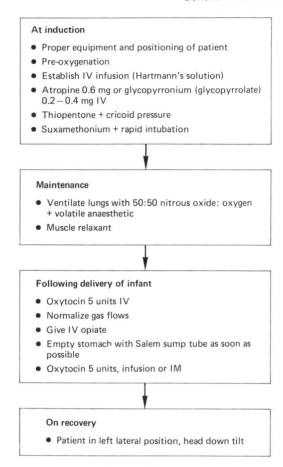

Fig. 22.2 General anaesthetic techniques.

Failed intubation drill

The initial management of a failed intubation should be along the lines of the 'drill' recommended by Tunstall.[5]

1. Maintain cricoid pressure.
2. Put patient head down and in complete left lateral position (request surgeon and scrub nurse to 'unscrub' and help).
3. Oxygenate by IPPV; it may be difficult; try different positions and sizes of Guedel airway; get someone else to squeeze the bag if necessary. *Aspirate the pharynx as required.*

4. If airway obstruction persists, try effect of releasing cricoid pressure.

5A. *If ventilation and oxygenation are easy*, ventilate with N_2O, O_2 and either diethyl ether or halothane. Establish surgical anaesthesia with spontaneous ventilation using the face mask.

6A. Pass a 33–36 French gauge stomach tube via the mouth; aspirate; instill 30 ml 0.3 M sodium citrate solution; withdraw tube and clear pharynx.

7A. Level table and place patient supine with left lateral tilt and right buttock wedge. Allow operation to proceed using inhalational anaesthesia with a face-mask. Ask for an experienced paediatrician to be present at delivery.

5B. *If oxygenation is difficult*, allow suxamethonium (succinylcholine) to wear off and let the patient wake up.

6B. Proceed as in 6A. If practicable ask the patient to roll over through 360 degrees so that the antacid is distributed throughout the stomach.

7B. Use local or regional analgesia. Alternatively, undertake an inhalational induction and continue as in 7A. Bear in mind that the airway may be difficult to maintain if 5B applies. *Get senior help*.

NB Initial posture as in (2) is critical. If aspiration occurs after posturing, only one lung is likely to be affected. Caval compression must be avoided at all times so as to prevent a reduction in cardiac output due to mechanical causes.

A fibreoptic laryngoscope may be a useful aid to intubation if the larynx cannot be visualized by conventional means. Other alternatives include a cricothyroidotomy (*see* p. 160) or the use of a 'Gordon and Don Michael Esophageal Gastric Tube Airway.'[6]

Maintenance of anaesthesia

The patient's lungs are ventilated, aiming to maintain the $PaCO_2$ at 30 mmHg (4 kPa). The incidence of awareness is low in emergency Caesarean sections. Patients are best maintained on the regimen recommended by Moir of 50/50 nitrous oxide and oxygen with a small concentration of volatile agent. Small supplements of volatile agent (e.g. 0.5 per cent halothane) are not associated with increased uterine bleeding. Most nondepolarizing relaxants are highly ionized at body pH and therefore do not readily cross the placenta; only gallamine and alcuronium have been found in cord blood in significant quantities. Muscle relaxation can be provided by an infusion of suxamethonium (succinylcholine) or alternatively pancuronium, tubocurarine, vecuronium or atracurium may be used. Once the baby is delivered, a dose of oxytocin (5–10 unit bolus followed by an infusion) is administered and an opiate supplement may be given.

Post-partum procedures

Induction risks, apart from caval compression, are just as high for post-partum procedures. Thorough preparation before anaesthetizing a patient with a retained placenta is vital. Halothane may be used to allow cervical dilatation and evacuation of retained products, although there is a risk of increased blood loss when high concentrations of any of the volatile agents are administered.

Pregnancy related pathology

Pre-eclampsia

This condition, of unknown aetiology, occurs after the 20th week of gestation. Symptoms include headache, abdominal pain, vomiting and visual disturbances.[2] Hypertension (systolic pressure greater than 140 mmHg and diastolic greater than 90 mmHg) and/or proteinuria are present but the presence of peripheral oedema is not essential for diagnosis. Disseminated intravascular coagulation (DIC) occurs in the microvascular beds of many organs, including the placenta, lungs, kidneys and liver resulting in fibrinolysis, an increase in fibrin degradation products (FDPs) and defective coagulation. Increased vascular permeability and reduced serum albumin leads to an increase in tissue fluid and hypovolaemia. If the condition progresses to eclampsia, with generalized grand mal convulsions, then this poses a threat to both mother and baby. It is associated with cerebral oedema and coagulation in the small cerebral vessels.

The successful management of this condition depends on controlling the blood pressure and avoiding an eclamptic fit, whilst minimizing central nervous depression of the already compromised fetus; the need to expedite delivery, as a consequence of deteriorating placental function, may well mean that labour is induced before term, with all the risks that this causes to a small and immature baby. If the patient's coagulation is normal, then epidural analgesia is indicated; as well as causing vasodilatation, the analgesia will avoid the pressor response to pain.

These patients are hypovolaemic and fluid therapy may be needed as the sympathetic block occurs (colloid being preferred). Anticonvulsant sedation with a chlormethiazole (0.8 per cent) infusion and diazepam is in common usage, although the baby will also be sedated by these agents.

Thus, the neonate may be underdeveloped, immature and sedated and an experienced paediatrician should be present at the delivery. If these measures fail to control the blood pressure then vasodilators are used. In the United Kingdom, hydralazine is preferred, although in the United States magnesium sulphate (1 g/hr) by IV infusion or 5 g 4-hrly IM is commonly employed. The latter agent will increase the effects of nondepolarizing neuromuscular blocking agents. It may be necessary to administer hydralazine prior to induction of anaesthesia to minimize the pressor response to laryngoscopy and intubation. Ergometrine should not be administered at any time.

Amniotic fluid embolism

This thankfully rare condition has a high mortality. It may occur during precipitous labour or during Caesarean section, especially if the placenta is incised. The main dangers are obstruction to the pulmonary circulation and consumptive coagulopathy. In the acute phase central venous pressure measurements are mandatory whilst administering intravenous fluids if right heart failure is not to occur. If the patient survives this the massive generalized activation of clotting factors and consequent severe haemorrhage is best managed by a specialist haematologist. Heparin, to minimize further activation, and transfusion of clotting factors and platelets may be indicated.

Heart disease

As long as preload is maintained, then epidural analgesia is indicated in most situations. However, it should not be used if a reduction in systemic vascular resistance may be detrimental (e.g. Eisenmenger's syndrome). If cardiac failure is a risk then ergometrine is contra-indicated.

References

1. Thorburn J, Moir DD. Bupivacaine toxicity in association with extradural analgesia for Caesarean section. *Br. J. Anaesth.* 1984; **56**: 551–3.
2. Turnbull AC, Tindall VR, Robson JG, Dawson IMP, Cloake EP, Ashley JSA. *Report on Confidential Enquiries into Maternal Deaths in England and Wales 1979–81.* London: HMSO, 1986.

3. Gillett GB, Watson JD, Langford RM. Ranitidine and single dose antacid therapy as prophylaxis against acid aspiration syndrome in obstetric practice. *Anaesthesia* 1984; **39:** 638–44.
4. Sellick BA. Cricoid pressure to control regurgitation of stomach contents. *Lancet* 1961; **ii:** 404– 6.
5. Tunstall ME. Failed intubation drill. *Anaesthesia* 1976; **31:** 850.
6. Tunstall ME, Geddes C. 'Failed intubation' in obstetric anaesthesia. An indication for the use of the 'Esophageal Gastric Tube Airway'. *Br. J. Anaesth.* 1984; **56:** 659–61.

Further reading

Bonica JJ. *Obstetric Analgesia and Anaesthesia.* Amsterdam: World Federation of Societies of Anaesthesiologists, 1980.

Bromage PR. *Epidural Analgesia.* Philadelphia: Saunders, 1978.

Crawford JS. *Principles and Practice of Obstetric Anaesthesia, 5th ed.* Oxford: Blackwell; 1984.

Eriksson E. *Illustrated Handbook in Local Anaesthesia, 2nd ed.* London: Lloyd-Luke; 1979.

Hunt CO, Rubin AP. Spinal Anaesthesia for Obstetrics. In: Ostheimer GW (ed). *Clinics in Anaesthesiology.* 1986; **4:** 135–43.

Mendelson CL. The aspiration of stomach contents into the lungs during obstetric anaesthesia. *Amer. J. Obstet. Gynecol.* 1946; **52:** 191–205.

Moir DD. *Obstetric Anaesthesia and Analgesia, 3rd ed.* London: Baillière Tindall; 1986.

Tunstall ME. Anaesthesia for obstetric operations. *Clin. Obstet. Gynecol.* 1980; **7:** 665–94.

23

Paediatric Anaesthesia

Charles L Schleien

Pre-operative assessment
Transport to the operating theatre
Preparation for anaesthesia
Fluid balance
Anaesthesia
Specific surgical conditions
   Pyloric stenosis
    Tracheo-oesophageal fistula
    Diaphragmatic hernia
    Gastroschisis/omphalocele
    Bronchoscopy
Postoperative care

Emergency paediatric anaesthesia of the newborn, infant and older child is a discipline tied into the general concepts of anaesthetic care and the particular needs of the paediatric patient. Since the older child is similar to the adult in physiological make-up, emphasis is given in this chapter to the emergency anaesthetic for the newborn infant with reference to the older child where material differences arise.

Pre-operative assessment

The pre-operative assessment begins with rapid history taking from the chart, medical personnel, and parents. In older children the usual information is obtained with special regard to the presence of allergies, drug therapy, bleeding diatheses and personal and family history of general anaesthesia especially with regard to the malignant hyperthermic syndrome. Information concerning the circumstances at birth should be obtained, e.g. birth asphyxia, maternal drug abuse. Nursing staff responsible for the present care of the baby provide important information about haemodynamic and respiratory liability.

All organ systems need to be reviewed as the premature or new-born infant requiring surgery often has multisystem disease. Respiratory distress is common in preterm infants: hyaline membrane disease is frequently present in infants born before 31–32 weeks of gestation.[1]

Further information is required about:

- The presence of respiratory distress syndrome or bronchopulmonary dysplasia.
- The presence of pneumonia as ascertained from physical examination, white blood cell count and a smear of the tracheal aspirate.
- Periodic breathing or apnoea (common in preterm infants); infants with a history of apnoea will not breathe during anaesthesia and usually are worse after operation than before in this respect.
- Inspired oxygen concentration (F_{IO_2}).
- Ventilator settings (including peak inspiratory and end-expiratory pressures, inspiratory and expiratory times (I:E ratio, rate).
- Recent arterial pH and blood gas status.
- Infant's lability during movement and suctioning.

Physical signs in the respiratory system include râles, wheezes, and intercostal muscle retraction. Chest wall retraction is commonly due to the highly compliant chest wall of the infant; severe retraction is a sign of pulmonary disease with decreased lung compliance or increased airway resistance. Atelectasis with a resultant decrease in lung compliance is common due to the decreased alveolar size: airway closing volume tends to approximate to normal tidal volume. Once the infant lung has become atelectatic, expansion becomes more difficult because the highly compliant chest wall does not allow for significant increase in the subatmospheric pressure generated during spontaneous breathing.

Dead space ventilation is 50 per cent in the preterm infant, 40 per cent in the term infant and reduces to the adult value of 30 per cent at one month of age.[2] The functional residual capacity (FRC) is 30 ml/kg, the same as for adults, but because of the small lung capacity of the infant the closing volume is reached at a higher lung volume, so predisposing to atelectasis. Normal tidal volume in the infant is 7 ml/kg, with a respiratory rate of 30–60 breaths/min. Oxygen consumption is 6 ml/kg compared to 3–4 ml/kg in adults.

Examination of the cardiovascular system is directed to the detection of murmurs, cyanosis, or congestive heart failure. The presence of congenital heart disease in the newborn is usually obvious from the history (lethargy, decreased feeding, failure to thrive, diaphoresis), physical examination (cyanosis, pulses, heart murmur, signs of congestive heart failure): echocardiography and cardiac catheterization confirm the exact nature of the lesion(s).

In the preterm infant, failure of the ductus arteriosus to close is common with resultant left-to-right shunting of blood. The signs consist of increased pulmonary blood flow, pulmonary oedema, bounding pulses, heart murmur, and signs of congestive heart failure.

The normal heart rate in preterm infants is 130–170 beats/min. The 1 kg infant has a systolic blood pressure of about 40–50 mmHg, the 2 kg infant 50–60 mmHg, and the term infant 60–65 mmHg. By one year of age the blood pressure is about 100/65 mmHg.[3] The ECG shows right ventricular hypertrophy and right axis deviation up to six months of age. The cardiac index of infants is 30–50 per cent greater than that of adults with an increase in metabolic demand due to rapid growth and the decrease in the release of oxygen to tissues by fetal haemoglobin.[4]

The P_{50} value (i.e. oxygen tension value at which haemoglobin is 50 per cent saturated) is only 2.53 kPa (19 mmHg), compared to 3.73 kPa (28 mmHg) in the adult situation. The blood volume of infants is higher than in adults with a value of 85 ml/kg during the first month of life, decreasing to 80 ml/kg by one year of age and reaching the adult value of 70 ml/kg in adolescence.[5] The haemoglobin concentration in newborns is elevated at about 19 g/dl, decreasing to 16.5 g/dl by one week of age, and reducing to its lowest levels of 11 g/dl in term infants and 8.5 g/dl in preterm infants at six weeks of age.

The rest of the clinical examination consists of palpation of the abdomen for masses – when present they are usually of renal origin – and observation of the onset and quantity of urine. Ninety-five per cent of infants have passed urine by 24 hr of life.[6] The liver is usually palpable 1–2 cm below the costal margin and frequently a spleen tip can be palpated.

Central nervous system damage increases with degrees of prematurity. Note the Apgar score at birth, the presence of seizures and the presence of signs of flaccidity or hypertonia. Head sonography or CT scan should be reviewed (for the presence of intraventricular haemorrhage).

Laboratory studies should be obtained prior to surgery if the emergency situation permits. Optimum haemoglobin concentration > 14 g/dl in the newborn or > 10 g/dl for older infants subjected to emergency surgery.

Serum electrolyte concentrations should be closely monitored in the preterm or sick newborn before surgery as derangements are common. Serum Na^+ and K^+ concentrations change frequently, especially in the preterm infant with respiratory distress syndrome or a patent ductus arteriosus; care must be taken to evaluate:

- state of hydration
- the possibility of excessive Na^+ or water administration
- the response to therapy with diuretics.

Serum concentrations of calcium and glucose are frequently lower than acceptable in preterm infants.

Coagulation factors V, VII and VIII are reduced in infants asphyxiated at birth; thrombocytopenia may also be present. Platelet transfusion should be given if the platelet count is below 20 000/mm³ or bleeding is manifest to raise the count to 50 000/mm³. More platelets may be given during surgery of long duration. If vitamin K therapy has been inadvertently omitted during the resuscitation of the sick newborn or preterm infant – as may often occur – pre-operative administration is helpful in postoperative management. Many newborn surgical patients have disseminated intravascular coagulopathy and rapid treatment with fresh frozen plasma before surgery is necessary (*see* p. 49).

Transport to the operating theatre

Transporting sick infants anywhere is a hazardous venture. An anaesthetist should always accompany the infant during the journey from the intensive care unit (ICU) to the operating room so that continuous observation and monitoring may be carried out; i.e. ECG, direct arterial pressure (if a catheter is in place) and a precordial stethoscope to listen to breath sounds and heart tones.

Intravenous lines are kept patent and infusion pumps are continued at their current settings. Ventilation is supported during transport at similar settings to those obtaining in the ICU wherever possible; a manometer is attached so that the correct inspiratory pressures may be achieved during manual ventilation. The inspired O_2 concentration should be kept at the same value as was previously found suitable: an air/O_2 blender facility on the transporting system is most valuable; if this is not available 100 per cent inspired O_2 should be administered until the infant reaches the operating theatre. Heat conservation during transportation is essential in maintaining normal homeostatic function of the infant. Extreme heat loss to the environment occurs in infants for several reasons:

- increased skin blood flow
- the presence of only a thin layer of subcutaneous fat
- the large surface-to-volume ratio of the infant (especially preterm).

Oxygen consumption and use of energy for heat conservation are increased when the patient is outside the neutral environment.[7] Heat production in infants is achieved by nonshivering thermogenesis through an increase in O_2 consumption by brown fat metabolism. Heat losses from the infant by way of radiation, convection and conduction are reduced by wrapping the infant in a 'space-blanket' foil wrap, especially covering the head and extremities; a cap over the head and warm swaddling blankets. The design of modern incubators has overcome most of the problems (e.g. in-built ventilators, blender, heat and humidity controls). Operational policies should expedite transport to the operating theatre (e.g. the elevator waiting for the patient, etc.).

Preparation for anaesthesia

The operating theatre must be warmed to a high temperature prior to the arrival of the patient and all necessary equipment should be assembled and tested. A heating pad or mattress is placed under the infant and all exposed parts of the body are kept wrapped up as far as possible consistent with surgical access. A neonatal operating table incorporating a radiant heater is useful.

Anaesthesia equipment should include all the routine equipment appropriate for paediatric anaesthesia. A variety of sizes of endotracheal tubes, airways, face-masks, laryngoscopes (with straight blades for neonates and small children), appropriate sized suction catheters, etc. are needed. All routine drugs and other drugs for cardiovascular support should be made up in appropriate dilutions in syringes ready for use, e.g. atropine, induction agent, e.g. thiopentone (thiopental) or methohexitone (methohexital), suxamethonium (succinylcholine), narcotic, nondepolarizing muscle relaxant, etc. Details appear in standard textbooks of paediatric anaesthesia.

In the older child for emergency surgery monitoring is similar to that for adults (*see* Chapter 7). Temperature monitoring and ECG monitoring are essential in all children; a precordial stethoscope permits monitoring of heart sounds and breathing whilst some designs of oesophageal probe permit all these parameters to be obtained. Arterial pressure may be obtained directly if necessary by invasive monitoring using a 22 G catheter (24 G in the preterm infant) inserted into the radial or the posterior tibial artery or noninvasively by use of the 'Infrasonde' device or blood pressure cuff with a Doppler sensor placed over a radial artery. Invasive monitoring is preferred if large blood or fluid losses are anticipated, the child is pre-term (less than 35 weeks gestation) or has multi-system disease, e.g. respiratory distress syndrome. A pulse oximeter (e.g. Nellcor) is valuable as arterial oxygen saturation and heart rate are continuously displayed and the sensor can be positioned over extremities such as the finger, nose or across the heel.

Fluid balance

Evaporative water losses are large especially in preterm infants because of their large surface-to-volume ratio, thin skin, rapid respiratory rate and relatively large minute volume. Intravenous access in the sick child is usually established some time pre-operatively but care should be taken to ensure that this is adequate; if large losses of blood are anticipated two IV lines should be established. Use of a central vein is convenient. All fluids should be administered through a microdrip infusion set or syringe pump so as to avoid accidental overload.

The volume of fluid required depends on a number of factors. Normal maintenance fluids are administered as 5 per cent dextrose and 0.2 per cent isotonic saline solution at a rate of 4 ml/kg/hr for the first 10 kg body weight. This regimen delivers 3.5 mg dextrose/kg/min which is approximately 50 per cent of the 3-5 mg/kg/min glucose requirements of the newborn. The blood glucose level should be closely monitored (blood glucose photometry, Dextrostix, Chemstix). Blood glucose concentrations should be maintained in the range 4.5-5.0 mmol/l (45-90 mg/dl). Third space losses and blood are replaced with Ringer's lactate administered through a separate IV line whenever possible.

Abdominal and thoracic surgical procedures cause large third space losses and administration of 7-10 ml/kg/hr for this need may be expected. Blood should be warmed to body temperature and administered to maintain the haematocrit at 30 per cent or above 40-45 per cent in the newborn. Since the blood volume of a 1 kg infant is only 85 ml, meticulous care should be taken to follow blood losses closely by weighing sponges and watching the operative area; an 8-10 ml loss equals 10 per cent of the blood volume of the infant.

Anaesthesia

An adult anaesthesia breathing system can be used for children over 10 kg body weight. The Mapleson E-system (i.e. Ayre's

T-piece) is recommended for smaller children; for manual ventilation the Jackson Rees modification by the addition of a double ended 500 ml reservoir bag is simple and efficient. The inspired gases should be warmed and all other heat conservation procedures should be maintained. Measurement of body temperature is important in all children. The very ill child, especially the newborn, should also be closely monitored (e.g. arterial pressure, CVP, urine output, pH and blood-gases, other clinical chemistry e.g. Na^+, K^+, Ca^{2+}, glucose and haematology, etc.).

A supply of medical air on the anaesthesia machine is valuable as a carrier gas; this enables oxygen enriched air to be given if necessary and provides a means of controlling inspired O_2 concentrations and hence PaO_2 at normal values in newborns (50–80 mmHg). High oxygen concentrations may produce toxic effects in the eyes of premature infants; retrolental fibroplasia producing blindness is a condition seen in 10–17 per cent of preterm infants produced by PaO_2 concentrations over 100 mmHg for a period of perhaps minutes to hours, depending on the infant's gestational age. It usually occurs in infants less than 35 weeks of gestational age and weighing less than 2 kg.[8] The condition can also occur in more mature infants.

Automatic ventilators for anaesthesia should be as simple as possible; dead space and resistance should be very low and there should be facilities for humidification and the provision of PEEP.

In the older child a rapid sequence induction after pre-oxygenation using thiopentone (thiopental), suxamethonium (succinylcholine) and cricoid pressure is suitable provided that the patient is normotensive and adequately hydrated. Ketamine is advocated in patients who are less fit. In the newborn infant less than 1 month of age an awake intubation is preferred after pretreatment with atropine. The endotracheal tube must be securely fixed in place and care taken to avoid the all too frequent problem of kinking.

Any kind of anaesthetic may be given, e.g. halothane. The least amount of anaesthetic consistent with preventing increases in blood pressure should be administered to the newborn as deep anaesthesia causes more circulatory depression in these patients than in older children. Because of a lack of baroceptor responses, reductions in blood pressure are not usually accompanied by increases in heart rate in preterm and newborn infants. Since the newborn depends primarily on increases in heart rate to maintain cardiac output, loss of baroceptor response makes it difficult to respond to hypotension. Nitrous oxide reduces the baroceptor response to the same extent as 0.5 MAC halothane and decreases in blood pressure can cause cardiac arrest in pre–term infants. The MAC for halothane in neonates is 0.87 per cent, i.e. lower than in infants (1.20 per cent).[9] Fentanyl (10–30 micrograms/kg IV) is sometimes preferred for the maintenance of anaesthesia to attenuate increases in heart rate or blood pressure when the skin is incised. Muscle relaxants are used to prevent movement and help reduce the amounts of anaesthetics required; pancuronium is useful although atracurium or vecuronium may prove to be the drugs of choice. Neonates require much lower doses of the non-depolarizing muscle relaxants than older children and adults;[10] it is best to err on the side of low dosage as more drug can be given if necessary.

Specific surgical conditions

Pyloric stenosis

Infantile pyloric stenosis is the most common cause of obstruction of the gastrointestinal tract in paediatric patients. Patients with this disorder present with regurgitation and vomiting, frequently projectile in nature. These infants may be hypovolaemic with hypochloraemic alkalosis. These abnormalities should be strictly corrected before surgery by administration of IV isotonic saline, potassium and chloride.

A rapid-sequence induction is required because of the obstruction at the pyloric outlet. An endotracheal tube is passed and lung ventilation controlled with anaesthesia maintained by inhalational agents. The patient should be extubated when awake at the conclusion of surgery.

Tracheo-oesophageal fistula

The most common type of tracheo-oesophageal fistula is oesophageal atresia and distal tracheo-oesophageal fistula (80–90 per cent). Other congenital abnormalities should be sought, including the common association with Vater syndrome (vertebral anomalies, anal atresia, tracheo-oesophageal fistula, and renal and radial anomalies). Cardiac malformations, especially ventricular septal defect, are also commonly associated with tracheo-oesophageal fistula. Patients with tracheo-oesophageal fistula may have respiratory problems due to respiratory distress syndrome or aspiration. If respiratory distress is moderate or severe, surgery should be delayed until the condition clears.

Induction is performed following the placement of an endotracheal tube with the patient awake. Anaesthesia is induced with either volatile or IV agents. Every effort should be made to maintain spontaneous ventilation so that air is not forced into the stomach. Placement of the endotracheal tube should be very precise so as to occlude the opening to the fistula in the distal trachea. Once the surgeon has performed the preliminary gastrostomy, the endotracheal tube is pulled back to the mid-trachea position and the infant is paralysed. The fistula is then surgically ligated and repair of the oesophagus is undertaken if possible. The ligation of the tracheo-oesophageal fistula makes ventilation easier. Intra-operative monitoring is performed with a radial arterial line and a central venous line because of the additional possibility of extracellular fluid losses. At the end of the procedure, the endotracheal tube is left in place and the lungs mechanically ventilated in the postoperative period.

Diaphragmatic hernia

Patients with congenital diaphragmatic hernia have a mortality rate of approximately 50 per cent. The usual cause of death in these patients is hypoxia and acidosis due to lung hypoplasia, atelectasis, and persistent fetal circulation. Persistent fetal circulation is associated with right-to-left shunting of blood through the foramen ovale and ductus arteriosus, and pulmonary hypertension. Most patients arriving in the operating theatre will already be intubated. Ventilation is performed so that the chest is moved slightly with inspiration. High airway pressures are associated with a high incidence of pneumothorax. Anaesthesia is maintained with inhalational anaesthetic or IV agent, e.g. fentanyl. The patient should be maintained on 100 per cent oxygen due to the lability of blood-gas status, and hyperventilated to a pH >7.5 in order to reduce pulmonary artery pressures and improve oxygenation. As usual, body temperature, and the plasma concentrations of glucose and calcium should be closely monitored. Sometimes these patients may do well during surgery but develop severe pulmonary hypertension within hours to a few days later. If the pulmonary artery pressure increases and hypoxia ensues, vasodilators such as tolazoline may be administered although systemic artery pressure is usually also decreased; inotropes may be needed in those instances.

Gastroschisis/omphalocele

Gastroschisis is a defect in the abdominal wall not associated with either the midline or the umbilical cord. An omphalocele is a midline defect in the abdominal wall related to the umbilical cord. Both lesions are associated with malrotation of the gut, bowel atresia and other congenital anomalies. Pre-operative assessment of these patients should include strict attention to the state of hydration and electrolyte status (calcium, glucose) and body temperature. The patient should be intubated awake. Monitoring includes the insertion of arterial and central venous catheters. Fluid losses are very large during surgery and hypothermia is a common problem both during and after operation. At abdominal closure, serious decreases in heart rate, blood pressure or oxygen saturation may prompt the surgeon to suspend the gut in a silo with deferment of formal closure of the abdomen for a few days.

Bronchoscopy

The pre-operative evaluation of paediatric patients for emergency bronchoscopy and oesophagoscopy should highlight the status of oxygenation and degree of stridor or wheezing. These procedures are usually performed on an emergent anaesthetic basis in order to remove a foreign body. Maintenance anaesthesia should be performed using an inhalational anaesthetic so that close to 100 per cent oxygen can be administered. The cough reflex should be suppressed (by muscle paralysis) during insertion of the bronchoscope. Care should be taken to ensure adequate ventilation through the bronchoscope and not to obstruct or dislodge an endotracheal tube. Jet ventilation may force an inhaled foreign body more distally and is not advised.

Postoperative care

After emergency anaesthesia very small children are usually maintained with an endotracheal tube *in situ* in the intensive care unit. Care during transport is necessary as already described.

References

1. Usher RH, Allen AC, McLean FH. Risk of respiratory distress syndrome related to gestational age, route of delivery, and maternal diabetes. *Am. J. Obstet. Gyn.* 1971; **111**: 826.
2. Gregory GA. Pediatric anesthesia. In: Miller RD (ed). *Anesthesia*. New York. Churchill-Livingstone, 1981, 1200.
3. Kitterman JA, Phibbs RH, Tooley WH. Aortic blood pressure in normal infants during the first 12 hours of life. *Pediatrics* 1969; **44**: 959.
4. Daily WR, Klaus M, Meyer HB. Apnea in premature infants: monitoring incidence, heart rate changes and an effect of environmental temperature. *Pediatrics* 1969; **43**: 510.
5. Linderkamp O, Versmold HT, Reigel KP, Betke K. Estima-

tion and prediction of blood volume in infants and children. *Eur. J. Paed.* 1977; **125**: 227–34.

6. Clark D. Times of first void and first stool in 500 newborns. *Pediatrics* 1977; **60**: 457.

7. Hey EN. The relation between environmental temperature and oxygen consumption in the newborn baby. *J. Physiol.* 1969; **200**: 589.

8. Daum JD. Retrolental fibroplasia. *Dev. Med. Child Neurol.* 1979; **21**: 385.

9. Lerman J, Robinson S, Willis MM, Gregory GA. Anesthetic requirements for halothane in young children 0–1 month and 1–6 months of age. *Anesthesiology* 1983; **59**: 421.

10. Fisher D, O'Keefe C, Stanski RD, Connelly R, Miller RD, Gregory GA. Pharmacokinetics and pharmacodynamics of d-tubocurarine in infants, children, and adults. *Anesthesiology* 1982; **57**: 203–8.

Further reading

Beasley JM, Jones SEF. *A Guide to Paediatric Anaesthesia.* Oxford: Blackwell, 1980.

Brown TCK, Fisk GC. *Anaesthesia for Children.* Oxford: Blackwell, 1979.

Hatch DJ. Acute upper airway obstruction in children. In: Atkinson RS, Adams AP (eds). *Recent Advances in Anaesthesia, 15th ed.* London: Churchill-Livingstone 1985.

Hatch DJ, Sumner E. *Neonatal Anaesthesia and Perioperative Care, 2nd ed.* Current topics in anaesthesia – 5. London: Edward Arnold, 1986.

Rees GJ, Gray TC. *Paediatric Anaesthesia. Trends in current practice.* London: Butterworths, 1981.

Smith RM. *Anesthesia for Infants and Children, 4th ed.* St Louis: C.V. Mosby, 1980.

Steward DJ. *Manual of Pediatric Anesthesia, 2nd ed.* London: Churchill-Livingstone, 1985.

24

Emergency Anaesthesia in the Elderly

Elizabeth L Rogers

Physiological alterations with ageing
    Cardiovascular function
    Pulmonary function
    Renal function
    Neurological changes
    Nutritional status
Pharmacological alterations with ageing
    Pharmacokinetics
Pre-operative assessment
Intra-operative management
Postoperative care

Anaesthesia cannot be contra-indicated simply because the patient is elderly.[1,2] However, caring for the elderly requires knowledge of how the ageing process makes them physiologically and pharmacologically different from healthy young adults and how these factors may affect anaesthetic, surgical, and peri-operative planning.

The elderly are not just older healthy adults. They differ in definable physiological ways which are heightened by the increased probability of concomitant chronic disease processes in the elderly. Knowledge of the physiology, biochemistry, and pharmacokinetics of ageing has grown at a geometric rate over the last decade. As our basic understanding of ageing physiology increases, our ability to refine our approach to the elderly will further improve. Already, information is available on how the elderly differ from the young adult in the areas of cardiac, respiratory, renal, and neuro-physiology. This information is reviewed to plan for appropriate emergency anaesthetic care of the elderly.

Physiological alterations with ageing

The literature in the area of cardiac physiology in the elderly has many inconsistencies because many of the studies have traditionally observed the sick elderly in acute care facilities and assumed that they represented normal elderly people.

Cardiovascular function

One of the best studies on healthy, ambulatory adults has been the Baltimore Longitudinal Study on Ageing.[1] By following a large cohort of healthy adults over many years, it has been possible to clarify which physiological changes occur simply because of ageing versus those which occur because of disease processes. For example, it has been shown in this study that although the elderly are prone to atherosclerotic cardiovascular disease with concomitant impairment of cardiovascular function, ageing alone leads to no obligatory decline in cardiovascular function.

If atherosclerosis or aortic valvular sclerosis does not occur, the elderly do not suffer decrease in cardiac output (CO) or cardiac index (CI) at rest. Cardiac output response to exercise is likewise similar to that of the younger adult. However, the increase of CO with stress in the elderly is accomplished by an increased stroke volume rather than the tachycardic response seen in young adults.[1]

Ageing is associated with changes in aortic compliance and cardiovascular response to stress which importantly change the elderly person's response to surgery. With age, the aorta develops increased stiffness, less elasticity, and less diastolic recoil. The resulting increase of systolic blood pressure with ageing is associated with increased after-load on the heart and left ventricular hypertrophy as an adaptive mechanism. The increased ventricular wall stiffness seen in early diastole may lead to incomplete filling and cardiac compromise in the elderly when tachycardia occurs due to fever or drugs.

The elderly patient who has experienced atherosclerotic disease may well have hypokinesia of the ventricular wall and therefore have decreased CO and decreased ability to respond to stress. In these patients, there is a delicate balance between the work necessary to maintain CO, myocardial oxygen demand, and coronary blood flow. In the elderly with coronary artery disease, myocardial ischaemia can develop with modest decreases in oxygenation or mild increases in cardiac work.

Pulmonary function

The cardiac/thoracic ratio on chest radiography increases in the elderly due mainly to a decreased thoracic diameter due to stiffness of the chest wall.[1, 3] In addition to increased chest wall rigidity, mild kyphosis of the spine, lowered diaphragm during tidal breathing, and loss of internal alveolar surface area, all contribute to the loss of pulmonary function seen with ageing. Because there is less ascent of the diaphragm, the residual volume is increased while vital capacity decreases with age.

Airways become more narrow with loss of strength of the elastic recoil fibres so that there is high flow resistance at low lung volumes, with greater difficulty in keeping the airways open. Therefore, a greater airway volume is needed to keep the small airways from collapsing in the elderly. This is known as the closing volume.

The forced expiratory volume at one second (FEV_1) also decreases with age by 2 per cent per year after age 20, further leading to progressive ventilatory insufficiency with age. With ageing there is progressive decrease in arterial oxygen tension (PaO_2). Further decrease in PaO_2 of 6–10 mmHg (0.8–1.3 kPa) occurs with the supine position because of the effect of the supine position on closing volume, the decrease in functional residual capacity (FRC) as the abdominal contents push upon the diaphragm, and the increased shunting seen with a low ventilation to perfusion ratio. An 85-year-old nonsmoker with normal ageing lungs may therefore have a resting PaO_2 of 75 mmHg (10 kPa) which is adequate for sedentary living, but leaves little reserve for stress. The expected hypoxaemia will be worsened if there is anaemia or decreased CO from heart disease.

The incidence of pneumonia in the critically ill elderly is high due to a number of factors. The high closing volume may lead to airway closure with each breath, especially in the supine position, predisposing the elderly to atelectasis. Increased secretions in the elderly further potentiate the possibility that the closed airways will not get enough air flow with the next breath to re-open.

- A decreased cough reflex in the elderly also increases the chance of aspiration with ensuing pneumonia if not reflex respiratory arrest.

Pulmonary function may be further compromised by the occurrence of pulmonary emboli from which the elderly are at increased risk. The reason for the increased incidence of pulmonary emboli in the elderly is probably multifactorial, including decreased ambulation, an increased tendency to calf vein thrombosis, and decreased cardiac return with failure.

Renal function

Renal function is also impaired in the elderly. This is due both to loss of nephrons as well as decrease of renal plasma flow with age. Loss of renal function appears to be a process that is demonstrably progressive beginning in young adulthood. This results in a glomerular filtration rate (GFR) that falls by 50 per cent over the years from age 20 to 90.[1]

Along with decreased ability to clear creatinine is a decreased capacity to conserve water and a blunted response to sodium shifts.

- The elderly are at greater risk from volume depletion, hyponatraemia from diuretics, and hypernatraemia or fluid overload from iatrogenic sodium administration.[3]
- Decreased urinary excretion of drugs also make the elderly at risk for drug toxicity.

Neurological changes

Perhaps most frustrating to the patient and family of the elderly are the neurological changes that occur with ageing. In general, many of the changes which are seen are due to autonomic nervous system dysfunction. This may result in orthostatic hypotension, decreased sexual function, impaired body temperature regulation, altered gut motility, impaired bladder emptying, and decreased heart rate response to stress.

- Maintenance of cerebral blood flow (CBF) requires a higher perfusion pressure in the elderly. In a sense, the traditional autoregulatory curve of cerebral blood flow is shifted to the right.[4]
- Cerebral blood flow becomes more dependent on mean arterial pressure, and avoidance of iatrogenic hypotension becomes even more important.

The elderly experience clinical, biochemical, and histological deterioration of the nervous system, resulting in impaired glucose utilization by the brain[4] as well as altered mental state, muscular performance, peripheral sensation, and tendon reflexes in addition to the autonomic changes described above. These changes are all enhanced by the disease processes of the elderly such as cerebrovascular accidents due to atherosclerosis, presenile dementia in Alzheimer's Disease, and Parkinson's disease.

Nutritional status

Integral to understanding the physiological and biochemical changes in the elderly is an awareness of the altered nutritional state of many elderly. This altered nutritional state may result in

- obesity
- deficiencies of isolated nutrients
- generalized nutritional depletion.

Obesity is frequent in the 50–70-year-old patient and should not be equated with a 'well nourished' condition, for obesity is frequently associated with excess carbohydrate but inadequate protein ingestion, and subsequent protein malnutrition.

- The obese elderly is more susceptible to hepatotoxins, to prolonged effects from lipid-soluble agents such as anaesthetics, and to infection.

Isolation, idiosyncracy, poor dentition, financial considerations, lack of mobility, or lack of cooking utensils make the elderly prone to dietary deficiencies. This can result in either unbalanced diets with isolated nutrient deficiencies, or else severe protein, calorie, and nutrient deficiencies. Malnutrition *per se* will increase the morbidity and mortality from hospitalization and surgery.

- The chance of developing significant infection, delayed wound healing, and other complications is higher in the malnourished patient.

Pharmacological alterations with ageing

Pharmacokinetics

The elderly are frequently the repository of polypharmacy and are the ones most sensitive to the adverse effects of drugs. They are therefore at increased risk from the individual drugs as well as from drug–drug or anaesthetic–drug interactions.

- The elderly have altered pharmacokinetics for they frequently have decreased absorption, decreased excretion and decreased metabolism of drugs. Because there are so many factors involved, not all drugs have their pharmacokinetics altered in the same way.

Oral drugs may be less effectively absorbed in the elderly due to decreased gastrointestinal motility, decreased enzyme activity at the brush border, decreased gastric acid and peptide production, and decreased pancreatic enzyme release.

- Absorption of IM and SC administered drugs may also be delayed, resulting in delayed effects or needless repetition of administration to achieve an effect.
- Drugs which require urinary excretion can be expected to accumulate due to decreased renal clearance if their dose or frequency is not decreased.
- Drugs which require activation by the liver may require larger amounts because the P450 system is less active in the elderly, while drugs which are deactivated by the liver will be toxic unless reduced in amount.

With malnutrition, the serum albumin is frequently lowered in the elderly, leading to less protein binding of drugs, thus increasing the amount free in the serum.

Examples of altered pharmacokinetics in the elderly include:

- Increased toxicity seen with digoxin which can lead to an increased plasma level for a longer half-life unless the dose is reduced.
- Nephrotoxicity from aminoglycosides increases to 10 per cent if the serum creatinine is greater than 1.0.
- Susceptibility to the toxic effects of cimetidine and haloperidol.
- Increased sensitivity to effects of sedatives, hypnotics and analgesics compared with young adults.[5]

Narcotic-induced depression of the CNS is thought to occur with smaller doses than in younger adults and the dose of thiopentone (thiopental) required to achieve early burst suppression of the EEG decreases linearly with age.[6] It is important to stress, however, that these are complicated problems and that, for example, brain sensitivity to thiopentone dose not change with age and is not responsible for the observed dose changes in burst suppression seen in the elderly. It appears that a smaller initial distribution volume in the elderly is responsible in that it results in higher serum levels after a given dose of thiopentone.

The minimum alveolar concentration (MAC) of inhalation anaesthetics consistently decreases with age although the exact reasons for it are not entirely understood.[7,8]

Pre-operative assessment

The elderly patient can expect to be at higher risk of having a fatal complication from surgery than a younger adult. Mortality is highest in those over the age of 95.[2]

Communication between physician, surgeon, and anaesthetist is necessary to optimize care of the elderly patient. A history of exercise intolerance, cardiovascular or pulmonary disease, previous anaesthetic difficulties, polypharmacy, and drug allergies may place the patient at greater risk. The elderly are, likewise, more likely to have problems of hearing, vision, and orientation which may make their peri-operative experience frightening or confusing (*see* p. 354). Unfortunately, with emergencies, the elderly are often confused and unable to give a coherent history and the anaesthetist must rely on a physical examination and laboratory data.

The American Society of Anesthesiologists' (ASA, *see* p. 4) classification system for risk evaluation is quite good at predicting mortality, even in the elderly. A review of the results of 500 patients, over the age of 80 years, found that mortality for healthy octogenarians would be similar to that expected for young adults. Mortality would rise slightly above young adults for ASA class 3 patients, and would rise dramatically if the patient was ASA class 4.[9] Mohr demonstrated a similar stepwise pattern, but with somewhat higher percentages.[2] In that series, patients were at increased cardiac risk if they were greater than 70 years of age or if they had underlying heart disease (17 per cent). Mohr also described increased mortality if diabetes (26 per cent) or dementia (45 per cent) were present.[2]

All elderly patients should have screening laboratory studies performed. This should include:

- complete blood count
- blood urea nitrogen
- serum creatinine
- liver function tests.

Also recommended (particularly in confused or debilitated patients) are measurements of:

- pH and arterial blood gases
- pulmonary function tests
- creatinine clearance.

Fowler has reviewed the procedure for approaching noncardiac surgery in the elderly patient with severe heart disease.[10] He recommended pre-operative assessment including pulmonary wedge pressure and mixed venous oxygen saturation for ASA class 3 and 4 patients. Surgery should perhaps be delayed in elderly patients in order to stabilize their cardiovascular system and reduce their mortality risk, since elderly patients who cannot have their underlying pulmonary and cardiovascular problems corrected prior to surgery may face a very high mortality rate.[8]

• Since emergency surgery carries higher mortality rates than does elective surgery for patients over the age of 65 years, whatever time is available should be spent optimizing the patient's clinical status.

Pre-operative care, time permitting, should focus on control of blood pressure; therapy of congestive heart failure with diuretics, pre-load and after-load reduction; control of serum glucose; correction of fluid and electrolyte abnormalities; correction of anaemia preferably to a haematocrit > 30 per cent and treatment of infections with initiation of antibiotics.

Intra-operative management

There is no 'golden rule' for choice of anaesthetic technique or agents but a sophisticated analysis of the medical condition of the patient, surgery to be performed, and anticipated complications is necessary.

It is common to consider that some operations in the elderly such as repair of a fractured hip are best performed under regional techniques;[11,12] this has been assumed to be safer than general anaesthesia, but the data for it are not entirely convincing.

• Elderly patients are somewhat confused and may require much more sedation than is anticipated, even if the successful regional anaesthetic technique is performed.
• Regional anaesthesia of any sort may be difficult in elderly patients because of abnormalities of body habitus, spinal deformities, nonco-operation in position, etc.
• The sensitivity of the elderly to spinal and epidural anaesthetics requires much more attention to dosage. For example, the dose of local anaesthetic required for epidural anaesthesia decreases with age until, about 60-years-of-age, it is only one-third the normal dose.[13,14]
• There is no impetus to perform regional anaesthesia rather than general anaesthesia.

Describing complications of regional anaesthesia does not mean that general anaesthesia is any safer.[14,15] In patients with chronic debilitation, demineralization of bone, and abnormalities of the spinal column, it is easy to have complications of endotracheal intubation secondary to arthritis of the mandible, twisting of the neck, or other musculoskeletal problems. Great care should be exercised in these procedures and the same attention should be directed at an elderly patient with multiple medical conditions as is generally directed at a critically ill emergency neonate – and for the same reasons. The latitude of safety afforded the anaesthetist before serious patient complications develop is very narrow. This applies not only to techniques such as intubation but to anaesthetic and associated drug use as well. The decreasing MAC of inhalation anaesthetics with age and the increased sensitivity of the elderly to hypnotics and sedatives such as narcotics and barbiturates has already been mentioned. It also applies to muscle relaxants. Because hepatic and renal function decrease with age, plasma clearance of muscle relaxants may be delayed and neuromuscular blockade prolonged in elderly patients.

- Chronically administered diuretics, digitalis, anti-hypertensive medicines, and a host of other drugs to interfere with the anaesthetic plan must always be considered.
- Prescribed dosage and administration of drugs such as digitalis cannot always be assumed to actually be followed by the elderly, confused patient. Attention to digitalis dose, e.g., compared to evidence of bradycardia or tachycardia may reveal that the prescription with which the patient arrives for pre-operative evaluation is not the medical regimen which is actually being followed.

The net result of all of these considerations is that the anaesthetist must translate pre-operative concern about hypotension and tachycardia into an appropriate anaesthetic plan which may be general anaesthesia with or without endotracheal intubation; or regional anaesthesia, as the case requires.

Postoperative care

There is very little difference about the postoperative care of the elderly to distinguish their care from other patients other than the increased susceptibility to complications. Confusion, drug induced respiratory depression, and need for longer periods of postoperative ventilation are all to be anticipated. Depending on associated medical problems, cardiac, neurological, respiratory, or an organ system compromise can occur but are not age specific. Perhaps the most important point for the anaesthetist to remember in caring for the elderly is a need for increased vigilance (*see* p. 354).

Summary

The explosion of interest in the process of ageing has resulted in attention to the unique medical, including anaesthetic, problems in the elderly. As the speciality of geriatrics develops, it can be anticipated that specific knowledge in geriatric anaesthesia will follow and that this will result in this field becoming a specialty in its own right.

References

1. Andres, R, Bierman EL, Hazzard WR. *Principles of Geriatric Medicine.* New York : McGraw Hill Book Co., 1985.
2. Mohr DN. Estimation of surgical risk in the elderly, a correlative review. *J. Am. Ger. Soc.* 1983; **31**: 99–102.
3. Rosberg B, Wulff K. Haemodynamics following normovolaemic haemodilution in elderly patients. *Acta Anaesth. Scand.* 1981; **25**: 402–6.
4. Kuhl DE, Metter EJ, Riege WH, Phelps ME. Effects of human ageing on patterns of local cerebral glucose utilization determined by the (18F) fluorodeoxyglucose method. *J. Cerebral Bl. Flow Metab.* 1982; **2**: 163–71.
5. Saunders RJ. Anesthesia and the geriatric patient. *Otolaryn. Clin. N. Am.* 1982; **15**: 395–403.
6. Homer TD, Stanski DR. The effect of increasing age on thiopental disposition and anesthetic requirement. *Anesthesiology* 1985; **62**: 714–24.
7. Gregory GA, Eger EI II, Munson ES. The relationship between age and halothane requirement in man. *Anesthesiology* 1969; **30**: 488–91.
8. Stefansson T, Wickstrom I, Haljamae H. Cardiovascular and metabolic effects of halothane and enflurane anaesthesia in the geriatric patient. *Acta Anaesth. Scand.* 1982; **26**: 378–85.
9. Djokovic JL, Hedley-White J. Prediction of outcome of surgery and anesthesia in patients over 80. *JAMA* 1979; **242**: 2301–6.
10. Fowler NO. Noncardiac surgery in the elderly patient with heart disease. *Cardiovasc. Clin.* 1981; **12**: 211–20.
11. Duncalf D, Kepes ER. In: Rossmon I (ed). *Geriatric Anesthesia in Clinical Geriatrics.* Philadelphia: JB Lippincott, 1971; 421–37.
12. Davis FM, Laurenson VG. Spinal anaesthesia or general anaesthesia for emergency hip surgery in elderly patients. *Anaesth. Intens. Care* 1981; **9**: 352–8.
13. Miller RW, Coulthard SW. Anesthesia for the elderly and debilitated patient. *Otolaryn. Clin. N. Am.* 1981; **14**: 715–22.
14. Carli F, Clark MM, Wollen JW. Investigations of the relationships between heat loss and nitrogen excretion in elderly patients undergoing major abdominal surgery under general anaesthesia. *Br. J. Anaesth.* 1982; **54**: 1023–9.

15. Freund PR, Ward RJ. Anesthesia for geriatric patients. In: Andres R (ed). *Principles of Geriatric Medicine*. New York: McGraw Hill, 1985; 933–8.

Further reading

Chapple WA, White IWC, Burman AL. Anaesthesia and the elderly. *South African Med. J.* 1982; **62**: 399–402.

Del Guerico LRM, Cohn JD. Monitoring operative risk in the elderly. *JAMA* 1980; **243**:1350.

Sidi A, Pollack D, Floman Y, Davidson JT. Hypobaric spinal anesthesia in the operative management of orthopedic emergencies in geriatric patients. *Israel J. Med. Sci.* 1984; **20**: 589–92.

Spreadbury TH. Anaesthetic techniques for surgical correction of fractured neck of femur. A comparative study of ketamine and relaxant anaesthesia in elderly women. *Anaesthesia* 1980; **35**: 208–14.

Wickstrom I, Holmberg I, Stefansson T. Survival of female geriatric patients after hip fracture surgery. A comparison of five anaesthetic methods. *Acta Anaesth. Scand.* 1982; **26**: 607–14.

25

Renal Disease

W Robert Casson and Ronald M Jones

Chronic renal failure
Anaesthesia for the patient with chronic renal failure
Acute renal failure
Nephrotic syndrome

Advances in the medical treatment of patients with renal disease, and the more widespread availability of dialysis facilities, means that they have a longer life expectancy. A corollary of this is that patients are increasingly presenting for surgery which, because of the nature of the underlying medical problem, is often urgent in nature. This may be directly related to their underlying disease, such as a renal transplant or a vascular access procedure, or it may not, for example emergency appendicectomy. Patients with chronic renal failure, who are undergoing haemodialysis or continuous ambulatory peritoneal dialysis (CAPD), are the most commonly encountered but other conditions with anaesthetic significance include acute renal failure and the nephrotic syndrome.

Chronic renal failure

This is said to be present when chronic renal impairment, from whatever cause, results in abnormalities of plasma biochemistry. This usually occurs when the glomerular filtration rate (GFR) falls to below 30 ml/min and may be subdivided into early (GFR 10–30 ml/min), late (GFR 5–10 ml/min) and terminal (GFR < 5 ml/min) renal failure.

The anaesthetic considerations include abnormalities in fluid and electrolyte balance and in drug handling as well as various complications which may not be reversed by dialysis. These include:

- anaemia
- hypertension
- pericarditis
- cardiomyopathy
- lung complications
- retention of gastric contents
- peripheral neuropathy
- skeletal abnormalities
- blood coagulation disorders
- psychological problems.

Anaemia

The secretion of erythropoietin from the kidney appears to bear an inverse relationship with the blood urea concentration; reduced secretion of this hormone leads to bone marrow suppression. Gastrointestinal bleeding is also common and this will contribute to the anaemia, as will the reduced red cell survival time due to intrarenal damage.

Thus, anaemia is often associated with chronic renal failure and haemoglobin concentrations of 4–5 g/dl are not uncommon. Oxygen carriage is dependent on cardiac output, as well as the concentration and oxygen saturation of haemoglobin. Therefore, if anything untoward should occur during anaesthesia leading to a decrease in cardiac output and/or arterial oxygen tension then, in the presence of anaemia, a critically low level of oxygen delivery may occur. However, the presence of renal failure leads to a shift of the oxyhaemoglobin dissociation curve to the right due to increased red cell 2,3-diphosphoglycerate activity and the metabolic acidosis; this shift causes a reduction in the affinity of haemoglobin for oxygen – tending to optimize oxygen delivery to the tissues.

Until recently it was common practice to avoid pre-operative blood transfusion in these patients if they were undergoing renal transplantation, lest the immune system should be sensitized leading to rejection of the transplanted tissue. However, recent work has demonstrated an increase (about 20 per cent) in graft survival after pre-operative blood transfusion. For this reason many centres now transfuse with fresh blood (low in potassium) prior to renal transplantation. However, transfusion should be avoided in patients known to have (or who develop) cytotoxic antibodies; if transfusion is strongly indicated, on general medical grounds, these patients should receive leucocyte depleted blood.

Hypertension

Elevated blood pressure and ischaemic heart disease are common in these patients. The hypertension is often a concomitant of salt and water retention and may respond to dialysis. However, a minority of patients have severe hypertension as a result of increased renin output and this group does not respond well to antihypertensive drug therapy.

- These patients are at an increased risk during induction of anaesthesia due to the pressor response to laryngoscopy and tracheal intubation. Intracerebral bleeding or left ventricular failure may occur. The pressor response may be attenuated by the prior administration of droperidol (alpha blocking effect) or a 'loading dose' of a narcotic analgesic such as fentanyl or alfentanil. Vasodilators such as hydralazine may also be useful in this respect as may β-adrenergic antagonists. The latter are administered intravenously, titrating the dose against the pulse rate. The individual response to β-adrenergic antagonists is variable so they should be administered in small divided doses. The authors' usual practice is to give 0.5 mg aliquots of propranolol at 3 min intervals in order to reduce the resting heart rate by 10 bpm. Intravenous β-adrenergic antagonists should not be administered to patients who are receiving other agents which influence atrioventricular nodal conduction, for example verapamil.
- It is mandatory to give patients treated in this way an anti-cholinergic (glycopyrronium [glycopyrrolate] or atropine) prior to the administration of suxamethonium (succinylcholine) or a profound bradycardia may occur.
- Large fluctuations in blood pressure may occur intra-operatively and these will require appropriate fluid and drug therapy.

Pericarditis

The painless pericarditis associated with chronic renal failure is not such a problem since the demise of systemic heparinization for haemodialysis. The use of 'regional heparinization' seems to have lessened the risk of intrapericardial bleeding and subsequent tamponade. However, there is a tendency for chronic pericardial effusions to develop in patients with renal failure. If this interferes with venous return, cardiovascular function may be compromised and an anaesthetic technique with minimal effects on the heart and peripheral vasculature should be employed. This may be particularly important during induction of anaesthesia.

Cardiomyopathy

This occurs only after several years but may have a profound effect on myocardial contractility and may contribute to the cardio-vascular instability.

Lung complications

So called 'uraemic lung' is an ill defined radiographic appearance of consolidation within the pulmonary hila ('butterfly wing'); it may well be due to a degree of left ventricular failure.

Also of relevance to the anaesthetist is the high incidence of chest infections occurring in this type of patient, particularly if they are being treated with immunosuppressant drugs. Aggressive pre-operative treatment of such complications should be undertaken.

Retention of gastric contents

Renal failure patients have prolonged gastric emptying times (especially when on dialysis), hyperacidity and increased gastric volume; they are therefore at risk of regurgitation and aspiration of stomach contents. Pre-oxygenation and a rapid sequence induction of anaesthesia are therefore indicated.

Peripheral neuropathy

This occurs commonly in patients in renal failure and it is probably wise to avoid regional analgesia if it is clinically evident. Autonomic neuropathy may also occur with a loss of cardio-vascular compensation for blood loss or positive pressure ventilation. Muscle denervation may lead to a hyperkalaemic response to suxamethonium (succinylcholine) administration.

Skeletal abnormalities

Osteomalacia often results from chronic renal failure and extra care should be taken when moving these patients. Secondary hyperparathyroidism, due to reduced phosphate excretion and calcium absorption, results in metastatic calcification and osteitis fibrosis cystica, with a tendency to spontaneous fractures.

Blood coagulation disorders

A bleeding tendency is common in these patients and pre-operative tests of coagulation are mandatory. However, this appears to be mainly related to toxic inhibition of platelet function by agents which are removed by haemodialysis.

Psychological problems

These patients are often introspective and distrustful of medical staff they do not know. Despite (or because of) the numerous skin punctures they have been subjected to they are often more frightened than average of needles. This may be because of previous problems with venous cannulation, involving numerous attempts, since they tend to have 'difficult' veins. A pre-operative visit will help if the anaesthetist can build up a rapport with the patient.

Anaesthesia for the patient with chronic renal failure

Pre-operative assessment

The patient may be receiving a large number of drugs. These often include antihypertensive and anti-anginal drugs which have significant interactions with anaesthetic agents. It is important that these drugs should be continued up to the time of surgery. A careful history and physical examination is important, paying particular attention to the assessment of extracellular fluid volume. Haemodialysis has usually taken place prior to the patient presenting for anaesthesia and surgery and they may therefore be relatively hypovolaemic. However, emergency surgery occurring a prolonged period of time after dialysis will mean that the patient may be relatively hypervolaemic. Pre-operative control of blood pressure is necessary and signs of long standing elevations in systemic pressure, such as evidence of left ventricular hypertrophy, may be detected.

Investigations should include:

- urea and electrolytes
- creatinine
- acid base status
- haemoglobin and platelets
- coagulation screen
- ECG
- chest radiograph.

There will usually be a mild metabolic acidosis and slight hyponatraemia (due to water retention), but the most significant potential electrolyte abnormality is hyperkalaemia. If possible, surgery should be delayed if the serum potassium level is greater than 5.5 mmol/litre; if dialysis is impossible the potassium may be reduced with dextrose/insulin (e.g. 50 ml of 50 per cent dextrose and 10 i.u. of soluble insulin) or ion exchange resins. In extremely urgent situations calcium may be administered (10 ml of 10 per cent calcium chloride, or gluconate, given slowly).

Premedication

Despite their familiarity with hospitals these patients are often unusually nervous prior to surgery. The wish to reduce this pharmacologically should be balanced against the increased sensitivity of patients with terminal renal failure to depressant drugs. Conservative doses of standard premedicant drugs are usually suitable.

Anaesthetic induction

Maintenance of a gas tight seal around a face-mask may be difficult in children who have been on steroids and this factor, along with the anaemia, makes pre-oxygenation necessary. Any of the standard IV agents may be used to induce anaesthesia with the usual care necessary for any patient with hypertension and/or ischaemic heart disease. The measures which can be taken to avoid the exaggerated pressor response to laryngoscopy have already been mentioned.

Suxamethonium (succinylcholine) may be used safely if the serum potassium level is normal and may be indicated if rapid sequence induction is deemed necessary. The nondepolarizing relaxant of choice is atracurium since it does not rely on intact renal or hepatic function for its metabolism; significant histamine release may be avoided if the intubating dose (0.5 mg/kg) is administered slowly. Other relaxants such as tubocurarine and pancuronium have longer durations of action, not only because of decreased elimination, but also because the relatively small volume of distribution for these highly ionized drugs means that blood levels are closely related to the rate of excretion. Conservative doses of vecuronium may also be used safely in these patients because it relies mainly on the liver for its excretion and because its volume of distribution is relatively larger (due to its increased lipid solubility compared to agents such as pancuronium).

An aseptic technique must be followed at all times in an attempt to minimize the risk of infection.

Maintenance of anaesthesia

The patient's lungs should be ventilated to maintain a slight respiratory alkalosis (to compensate for the metabolic acidosis and to reduce serum potassium). Anaesthesia may be maintained, and muscle relaxation supplemented, with a volatile anaesthetic agent. Enflurane administration is associated with a greater level of inorganic fluoride production (compared with halothane or isoflurane) although the values reached are not, in themselves, nephrotoxic. As there are few clinical situations where enflurane has clearly superior properties to alternative agents, many anaesthetists would consider it an unwise choice in patients with a pre-existing renal abnormality.

The remarkably low metabolism of isoflurane (about 0.2 per cent) does suggest that the potential for organ toxicity of the agent will be small – it may therefore be regarded as the agent of choice. In addition, certain procedures such as renal transplantation are known to be associated with an increased likelihood of a disturbance in cardiac rhythm (probably due to a release of vasoactive hormones); the greater stability of cardiac rhythm which is associated with isoflurane anaesthesia again suggests this agent as the volatile anaesthetic of choice.

- Intra-operatively, particularly if the patient is undergoing renal transplantation, it is vital to maintain intravascular volume; CVP monitoring (*see* p. 82) may be helpful in assessing this compartment and the administration of colloid (plasma or whole blood) should keep it well filled.
- Blood loss may occur rapidly and a large bore IV cannula is necessary.
- Forearm veins should be avoided as they may be needed for future arterio-venous fistulae or shunts; the dorsum of the hand is probably the most suitable site for the cannula.
- Blood pressure and ECG monitoring are mandatory but intra-vascular systemic, pulmonary artery and pulmonary capillary wedge pressure measurements are probably only indicated in the patient with associated ischaemic heart disease.

Although the duration of action of atracurium is unaffected by the absence of renal function its rapidity of offset may lead to intra-operative problems. For this reason, we would recommend routine monitoring of neuromuscular blockade. This may also be reassuring when the time comes to reverse the relaxant.

The advent of immunosuppression with cyclosporin A means that the need to give drugs such as azathioprine or methyl prednisolone intra-operatively is reduced. Azathioprine may potentiate the depolarizing neuromuscular blockade produced by suxamethonium (succinylcholine); it also has the potential to antagonize the nondepolarizing neuromuscular blocking drugs. Methyl prednisolone may cause hypotension if it is given too rapidly.

During a renal transplant a small dose of dopamine (<2.5 micrograms/kg/min) may be necessary to improve renal blood flow.

Postoperative care

Analgesia may be provided intra- and postoperatively with narcotic analgesics or, in the case of a transplant, with lumbar epidural analgesia. Intravenous analgesic infusions or patient controlled analgesia (PCA) devices may be useful. Postoperative fluid balance is best managed by specialists in renal medicine.

Regional analgesia

As previously mentioned a lumbar epidural block may be useful intra- and postoperatively in patients undergoing renal transplantation. The normal stress response to surgery may be inhibited to some extent by epidural analgesia. This will minimize the salt and water retention which normally accompanies surgery and in this way may improve urine flow.

A brachial plexus nerve block (using the axillary, supraclavicular or interscalene approaches) is a useful technique for a patient who requires an arterio-venous shunt or fistula to be formed prior to haemodialysis. The accompanying sympathetic block will cause arterio- and venodilation which will improve surgical access. Axillary block may not reach the musculocutaneous nerve, the sensory component of which (lateral cutaneous nerve of forearm) supplies the radial aspect of the forearm which is often the site of surgery, and supplementation with local infiltration may be necessary (great care being taken not to exceed the recommended dose of local analgesic; *see* p. 248). If vascular access proves impossible in the blocked limb and the surgeon wishes to continue on another limb then general anaesthesia should be used. Local analgesic nerve blocks are contra-indicated in the presence of a bleeding diathesis.

Acute renal failure

This is due to a sudden decrease in GFR to less than 2 per cent of normal. Oliguria (< 0.5 ml/kg/min) ensues and biochemical abnormalities such as a rise in blood urea and serum creatinine, metabolic acidosis, hyperkalaemia, hypocalcaemia and hyperphosphataemia occur.

From the anaesthetist's standpoint the main priority in the management of the acutely oliguric patient is to differentiate outflow obstruction (postrenal) from prerenal and renal causes. Having ruled out postrenal causes it is essential to determine whether there is a reduced effective extracellular fluid volume or a low perfusion pressure, both of which will cause a fall in GFR. The response of the kidney to decreased perfusion is to retain sodium and water and so a highly concentrated urine is produced ($>$ 500 mOsm/litre). The urinary sodium will be less than 20 mmol/litre whilst the potassium will be in excess of 1.2 mmol/litre. This is in contrast to those patients with parenchymal disease where the urine will be dilute ($<$ 350 mOsm/litre) with a high sodium ($>$ 40 mmol/litre) and low potassium ($<$ 1.2 mmol/litre). The method for maintaining optimum blood flow will depend on the underlying cause and fluid and inotropic therapy will depend on measurements of pre-load, after-load and heart rate.

- It is pointless (and may be harmful) administering diuretics to hypovolaemic patients.

Acute tubular necrosis (ATN) has a significant mortality and should be prevented if at all possible. It may follow hypovolaemia or sepsis and may be caused by drugs such as aminoglycoside antibiotics (thus it is important to monitor trough and peak levels).

- Patients with obstructive jaundice are also at risk of developing ATN if their urine flow is poor.
- Careful intra-operative monitoring of urine volume is mandatory for those at risk with particular attention to fluid replacement; administration of mannitol (as an osmotic diuretic) or frusemide (furosemide) may be necessary if urine flow is reduced.

Acute renal failure may occur in Goodpasture's syndrome, an auto-immune condition affecting basement membranes in the renal glomeruli and alveolar/capillary septa. Anaesthetists may be particularly involved in the management of these patients if respiratory failure also supervenes.

If, despite the preventative measures, a patient presents for anaesthesia and surgery with ATN then the management is similar to that of a patient with chronic renal failure.

Nephrotic syndrome

This refers to the clinical association of heavy proteinuria, hypoalbuminaemia (due to the former) and generalized oedema.

There are numerous underlying causes including:

- congenital
- connective tissue diseases (e.g. systemic lupus erythematosus)
- renal vein thrombosis
- toxins
- idiopathic (e.g. minimal change nephritis).

Pre-operatively the plasma albumin and electrolytes must be estimated and corrected as indicated. An albumin infusion (up to 50 g) will restore blood volume and may initiate a diuresis. In an emergency situation blood volume may be rapidly restored with human albumin solution (HAS). The low plasma protein levels may cause alterations in the effect of drugs which are significantly protein bound. Thus, the doses of muscle relaxants and barbiturates should be conservative and the degrees of neuro-muscular blockade must be monitored. Central venous cannulation is advisable in all but the most minor surgery.

Further reading

Black, D, Jones NF (eds). *Renal Disease, 4th ed*. Blackwell : Oxford, 1979.

Strunin L, Pettingale KW. Renal disease. In: Vickers, MD (ed). *Medicine for Anaesthetists, 2nd edn.*, Blackwell : Oxford, 1982.

Weir, HC, Chung FF. Anaesthesia for patients with chronic renal disease. *Canad. Anaesth. Soc. J.* 1984; **31**: 468–80.

26

Liver Disease

Elizabeth L Rogers

Acute liver dysfunction
Chronic liver dysfunction
Pre-operative interventions
    Clinical examination and investigations
Stabilization of patients and timing of surgery
Anaesthetic and surgical factors which affect liver function after operation
Interactions of liver disease and anaesthetic agents
Approaches to minor and major emergency procedures
Intra-operative monitoring
Protection of the anaesthesia team from liver disease

The patient with liver disease is at increased risk of developing postoperative complications. The decisions of when to time surgery and even whether to undergo surgery should be based on the consequences of delaying or avoiding the procedure versus the acuteness and reversibility of the liver and liver-related systemic processes.

Acute liver dysfunction

The patient with acute liver dysfunction may be best served by delaying surgery when urgent but non-life threatening conditions are being contemplated; e.g. a patient undergoing repair of a hip fracture who has acute liver disease due to viral or drug hepatitis may have an increased mortality of 10–80 per cent based on the severity of the liver disease and associated complications. While urgent, even a short delay of a few days or a week may be in the best interest of the patient. Likewise, patients with alcoholic hepatitis undergoing surgery experience an increased mortality by 10 per cent simply based on the existence of Mallory Bodies and inflammatory changes on biopsy. As a result, while patients with viral or alcoholic hepatitis may require up to a year to maximize hepatic enzymatic function and hepatic reserve, their ability to tolerate surgery and anaesthesia will be dramatically improved by at least waiting until evidence of acute liver cell necrosis has disappeared.

Chronic liver dysfunction

Patients with advanced chronic liver disease (such as cirrhosis, regardless of aetiology) or neoplastic disease, have an increased surgical mortality related to the severity of the liver failure.[1] With poorly compensated liver disease, the surgical mortality from even simple major procedures may reach 90 per cent. Patients with chronic liver disease will have improved outcomes if their metabolic, nutritional, and haematological parameters are improved as much as possible prior to surgery. Other than the time necessary to improve any correctable factors expeditiously, mortality is not improved by further delay of surgery.

When emergency surgery for life threatening problems must be performed in patients with liver disease, best care of the patient involves:

- recognition of liver disease
- pre-operative interventions to decrease surgical morbidity
- understanding of the factors predisposing to intra-operative and postoperative morbidity
- effect of anesthetic agents on the liver.

Pre-operative interventions

Successful management requires knowledge and skill to

- recognize liver disease
- assess the clinical risk of anaesthesia due to the presence of liver disease.

Even in emergency situations, the timing of surgery and stabilization of the patient prior to surgery then become important issues.

One-half of all patients with even mild pre-operative abnormalities of liver function have loss of liver function post-operatively as demonstrated by an up to 30 per cent retention of bromosulphthalein dye.[3] Liver disease should be suspected in a patient with previous history of jaundice or with symptoms of malaise, fatigue, anorexia, and/or pruritus. Drug induced liver disease frequently leads to symptoms first then jaundice later.

Commonly used drugs associated with liver disease

Patients with the above symptoms and who are taking the following drugs shall definitely be suspected of having liver disease until proven otherwise.

- alcohol (> 4 drinks/day)
- isoniazid
- α-methyl dopa
- chlorpromazine
- acetaminophen
- monoamine oxidase inhibitors
- sulphonamides.

Clinical examination and investigations

Physical examination is useful in differentiating acute from chronic liver disease. Acute liver disease such as that seen with drug or acute viral hepatitis is usually associated with hepatomegaly but without the stigmata of chronic liver disease such as gynaecomastia, ascites, splenomegaly, spider telangiectasias, or Dupuytren's contractures.

Prolonged protein calorie malnutrition in patients with chronic liver disease or alcoholism is associated with:

- limb muscle atrophy
- loss of subcutaneous fat
- the presence of asterixis (liver flap)
- slurred speech
- confusion
- easy bruising
- bleeding gums
- scleral icterus.

These are all signs of decompensated liver disease whether acute or chronic in nature.

The degree of hepatic encephalopathy may indicate the degree of liver dysfunction and the amount of stress being applied to the patient and his liver at the time.

Encephalopathy can be classified on a scale of 1–4.

- *Grade 1*: altered sleep habits, altered affect, and loss of spatial orientation.
- *Grade 2*: Slurred speech, drowsiness and the presence of asterixis.

- *Grade 3*: The stuporous patient arousable only with noxious stimuli.
- *Grade 4*: the unresponsive patient.

Patients with liver disease will frequently vacillate from one grade level of encephalopathy to the next based on the presence or absence of infection, bleeding, medication, protein intake, and electrolyte balance.[2]

Evidence of liver disease may be uncovered in patients with previously unsuspected liver disease (due to chronic active hepatitis or cryptogenic cirrhosis) by laboratory studies demonstrating decreased hepatic synthesis or function. Useful tests in adults include:

- serum bilirubin
- serum albumin
- prothrombin time.

Elevation of the hepatic enzymes in serum, such as transaminases and alkaline phosphatase, indicate the presence of an active process and are therefore useful from that point of view, but they do not represent hepatic reserves or function. Understanding that even asymptomatic patients have underlying liver disease is important, for they are at risk of 'activation' of liver disease. Altered hepatic architecture places them at increased risk of hepatic damage from even mild ischaemic insults during anaesthesia.

Patients with severe liver failure have more than an 80 per cent risk of mortality. With only minimal liver failure, this mortality reduces to less than 30 per cent. Table 26.1 summarizes a modification of Child's classification scheme for liver failure, and thus the risk of surgery, by evaluating the degree of pre-operative liver function.[3]

Table 26.1 Child's assessment of clinical risk, modified

Factors	Minimal	Moderate	Severe
Encephalopathy	none	provoked	Grade 2–4
Ascites	none	controlled	uncontrolled
Nutrition	good	good	poor
Bilirubin (mg/dl)	2	2–3	3
Bilirubin (μmol/litre)	34	34–50	50
Prothrombin time prolongation (sec)	2	2–3	3
Albumin (mg/dl)	3.5	3–3.5	3
Albumin (g/litre)	35	30–35	30

In addition to giving the anaesthetist information on risk, physical examination can also suggest specific complications that the patient with liver disease may expect. For example, patients with encephalopathy may need reduced amounts of inhalational anaesthetics and less IV sedation with hypnotics and narcotics. Avoidance of inhalation anaesthetic overdose in patients with encephalopathy therefore requires individual titration of anaesthesia.[4] Ascites may act as a reservoir for drugs given during anaesthesia; this may both delay onset of action, by dilutional effects, and prolong the duration of action of IV administered medications.[4] Because of the increased abdominal wall tension in patients with ascites, intragastric pressure may be elevated, thus further predisposing the patient to gastro-oesophageal reflux and aspiration.

Some patients with liver disease have diffuse intravascular coagulopathy as well as deficient synthesis of clotting factors. This coagulopathy may be activated by:

- bleeding
- infection
- stress of surgery.

Spinal and epidural blocks, and regional anaesthetics carry increased risks if such a coagulopathy exists due to local bleeding. Problems of hypovolaemic hypotension due to bleeding may be accentuated in these patients. Peripheral vasodilatation may precipitate profound hypotension.

- Spinal and epidural anaesthesia may be poorly tolerated in the liver patient with active bleeding.

In addition to the obvious risk due to hepatic failure, patients with liver disease have additional medical problems which increase operative risk. These are:

- respiratory alkalosis
- hypoglycaemia
- electrolyte imbalance
- decreased renal function
- susceptibility to infection
- poor temperature control.

Respiratory insufficiency and respiratory alkalosis are associated with intrapulmonary and systemic arterio-venous shunts, displacement of the oxygen affinity curve to the right, and respiratory changes secondary to disturbances in the CNS.

Mild hypoxaemia is frequent in patients with liver disease,

associated with the development of anatomically verified intra-pulmonary shunts.

Ventilation–perfusion inequality is responsible for hypoxaemia. This frequently results in a hypoxaemia driven tachypnoea with resulting respiratory alkalosis. A reduced affinity of haemoglobin for oxygen, moreover, is seen as decreased oxygen saturation. Pulmonary oedema and hyperventilation related to CNS changes are also reported.

The hyperkinetic vascular system also demonstrates shunting around the liver when portal hypertension is present.[6]

Hypoglycaemia due to decreased hepatic stores of glycogen can be a severe problem, requiring continuous infusion of IV glucose.

Dilutional hyponatraemia is also frequently found due to secondary hyperaldosteronism and may be aggravated by administration of IV fluids to a critically ill patient.

Functional renal failure is seen in patients with liver disease and mostly appears to be due to perception of inadequate intravascular volume by the kidney; part of the problem may be due to bile acids interfering with renal medullary function. Although the patient may have a greatly expanded intravascular and extravascular volume, much of this fluid is sequestered in third spaces and intra-vascularly behind the liver because of portal hypertension. The kidney therefore responds as though there is a decreased intra-vascular flow (prerenal failure); this leads to further sodium and water retention and eventually urinary insufficiency.

Stabilization of patients and timing of surgery

Patients with acute liver problems should have elective surgery delayed, if possible, until the liver disease has improved or resolved. Patients with acute or chronic liver disease who need emergency surgery should have this timed so correction of anaemia, hypoxia, and serum electrolyte concentrations can at least be started.

- Except for the patient who is exsanguinating from varices despite medical therapy, most can have surgery delayed sufficiently long to allow transfusion with packed red blood cells to raise the haematocrit to 30 per cent.
- When tracheal intubation is required for control of hypoxia use of the nasal route may be associated with an increased risk of bleeding.
- Serum glucose, potassium, and sodium levels can be brought towards normal levels.

- Severe coagulopathy may be corrected by administration of fresh frozen plasma and platelets.
- Vitamin K rarely helps patients with severe liver failure and coagulopathy.

If time permits, improvement in nutrition, control of ascites and encephalopathy will all improve the prospects of survival; also hepatic enzymes have a chance to return to normal values.

Anaesthetic and surgical factors which affect liver function after operation

Postoperative hepatic dysfunction is determined by the degree of existing dysfunction, the length of surgery, the complications presenting during surgery, the degree of hypoxaemia, changes in hepatic blood flow, and exposure to hepatotoxins.

- The most important factor is shown consistently to be the degree of previous liver damage. This will affect the ability of the liver to tolerate damage during anaesthesia.
- The most important task of the anaesthetist is to prevent or minimize hypotension and hypoxia during surgery so that damage to the liver may be minimized.

The greatest danger from anaesthesia is hepatic hypoxia. The liver receives most of its oxygen supply through the portal venous system; oxygen extraction continues until the blood leaves the liver through the central veins leading towards the inferior vena cava. The centrilobular hepatocyte is thus the part of the liver that is most sensitive to a reduced oxygen delivery. Distortion of hepatic architecture by previous necrosis or cirrhosis makes the centrilobular area even more vulnerable to changes in oxygen delivery. Portal hypertension secondary to cirrhosis or severe acute hepatic disease will also leave the liver with a reduced portal flow.

The three factors most important in decreasing oxygen delivery are:

- reduced portal blood flow
- increased CVP
- reduced oxygen content of blood.

Portal venous flow to the liver is related to splanchnic arterial flow in normal circumstances.

The major factors which acutely decrease portal venous flow to the liver are:

- systemic hypotension

- decreased cardiac output
- splanchnic vasoconstriction
- increased CVP
- reflexes secondary to surgical manipulation of the abdominal cavity.

Hypoxia also reflexly increases splanchnic vascular resistance so that blood flow through the splanchnic circulation is decreased and in turn decreases portal venous return to the liver. This decrease of hepatic blood flow in its turn enhances ischaemic tissue necrosis.

Hypovolaemic hypotension is the most serious problem affecting hepatic blood flow that is faced by a patient with liver disease. Hepatic blood flow is drastically reduced because of two interrelated factors: the reduction in portal blood flow due to splanchnic vasoconstriction, and the reduction in hepatic artery flow due to systemic hypotension.

- Hypovolaemic hypotension must be avoided at all costs.

Spinal and CNS reflexes induced by laparotomy alone can lead to acute decrease of hepatic blood flow.[6] This is due to decreased portal blood flow which cannot be compensated by mild increases in hepatic arterial flow.

Hypothermia leads to a decrease in mean arterial pressure and decreased hepatic blood flow, but also decreases hepatic metabolism and oxygen requirements. The hypothesis that these two activities are parallel and equal has been argued without good resolution. Although hypothermia alone may not harm the liver, hypothermia associated with hypoxia and the stress of surgery may be dangerous. Control of patient's body temperature during surgery is therefore recommended.

A precipitous decrease in hepatic blood flow may be associated with the induction of anaesthesia using a wide variety of agents; this effect tends to recover with time.[7,8] Although inhalation agents were believed to be worse than epidural or high spinal anaesthetics, the 25 per cent decrease in estimated hepatic blood flow during spinal anaesthesia is similar to values reported for volatile anaesthetics such an halothane.[9] In general, the deeper the anaesthesia, the greater the decrease in hepatic blood flow. Halothane results in decreased perfusion pressure due to decreased cardiac output; however, the liver can usually tolerate this if it is the only variable causing liver damage. Methoxyflurane is associated with a greater decrease of hepatic blood flow than halothane due to decrease in mean arterial pressure as well as increased splanchnic resistance.

Drugs with high hepatic extraction ratios such as lignocaine (lidocaine) and propranolol are very sensitive to alterations in hepatic blood flow. Metabolism of these drugs is therefore influenced by the decrease of hepatic blood flow caused by anaesthetic agents in patients with liver disease.

Interactions of liver disease and anaesthetic agents

Patients with liver disease, in general, present difficulties during anaesthetic induction and emergence as well as being more susceptible to anaesthetic toxicity. The liver is necessary to convert polar, fat-soluble drugs to active forms and to the water-soluble forms necessary for excretion. When determining drug usage and drug dose, it is necessary to evaluate the degree of altered hepatic metabolism.

In liver disease there is altered biotransformation, decreased excretion, and altered protein binding of drugs. Increased microsomal enzyme induction, especially in alcoholics and in patients on phenobarbitone (phenobarbital), may be seen despite liver disease. This will result in increased metabolism and activation of drugs requiring the microsomal cytochrome P450 enzyme system for metabolism. Cytochrome P450 is a haemoprotein found in the endoplasmic reticulum of hepatocytes which plays the role of an electron transferring agent, encouraging oxidative and reductive processes to occur.

This induction of cytochrome P450 acounts for the relative resistance of chronic, nonintoxicated alcoholics to diazepam, where they may appear to inactivate the drug almost as quickly as it can be administered.

Chronic ethanol consumption also leads to tolerance to the anaesthetic effects of some volatile anaesthetics which may be related to increased defluorination of inhalational anaesthetics. Acute, recent ethanol ingestion, on the other hand, inhibits hepatic metabolism of drugs and decreases the amount of anaesthetic required to produce general anaesthesia.

Although metabolism is not required for most inhalational anaesthetics to produce their effects, all the volatile anaesthetics currently in use undergo metabolism to some degree. Biotransformation, or metabolism of drugs, plays a role in the patient's handling of most IV and inhalational anaesthetics. Decreased biotransformation in liver disease will result in altered drug metabolism and increased excretion of a host of anaesthetic drugs including barbiturates, opioids, and muscle relaxants. Volatile anaesthetics may persist in liver and fat stores for weeks or months after a single exposure because of high lipid solubility. Enflurane and halothane are enzyme-inducing agents, resulting in increased cytochrome P450 activity. This may explain the finding of greater biotransformation activity occurring during anaesthetics which are repeated over a short time interval.

Altered binding of drugs to protein also occurs with liver disease. The effects will vary depending upon whether the drug binds to albumin or to globulins, the serum concentrations of which are respectively reduced and increased in liver disease. For example, the active portion of non-depolarizing muscle relaxants is the amount of the drug which remains in the blood stream unbound to protein. A decreased serum concentration of the particular protein necessary for binding results in an increase in pharmacological action at the myoneural junction due to increase of free drug. As the binding protein is not the same for all muscle relaxants, these drugs need to be carefully titrated to prevent overdosage. Atracurium is the most useful muscle relaxant in patients with liver disease because of its unique mode of destruction by the Hofmann elimination; vecuronium is excreted in bile and should probably be avoided.[10]

The simple presence of liver disease, therefore, does not mean that all drugs will present metabolic problems because of the potentially conflicting possible changes in metabolism. Only mild changes in overall metabolism are found in patients given thiopentone (thiopental) because three factors are operating simultaneously.[11] Decreased hepatic blood flow and decreased activity of drug metabolizing enzymes by the liver result in decreased hepatic intrinsic clearance. This is counteracted by decreased plasma binding, resulting in increased clearance related to the greater fraction which is unbound. Patients with liver disease are therefore probably only at small risk from the prolonged effects of thiopentone (thiopental), but may be more susceptible to hypotension from a single dose being toxic.[11]

Similarly, it is suggested that the amount of suxamethonium (succinylcholine), given as a single injection, required to produce paralysis need be no different in a patient with chronic liver disease and low plasma cholinesterase concentration because the clinical consequences of prolonged apnoea are relatively unimportant.[4] The potential for prolongation of action during continuous IV infusion, or after repeated injections makes this method of administration less wise.

Surgery itself results in mild abnormality of liver function, regardless of whether general or spinal anaesthesia is used.[1] Most of the original anaesthetic agents with direct hepatotoxic reactions (e.g. chloroform, trichloroethylene) have been discontinued. Most of the anaesthetic hepatotoxicity that is seen nowadays is thought to be due to an idiosyncratic or hypersensitivity type of reaction. These reactions to anaesthetic agents are unpredictable, occur infrequently, but seem to occur in patients with repeated exposures over a short period of time.

Halothane

Halothane hepatitis has been vigorously studied over the past two decades. Mild abnormality of serum transaminases may occur in as many as 20 per cent of patients exposed to halothane.[12] While some controversy continues, it appears that true halothane hepatitis is a rare but real phenomenon, occuring once every 10 000–30 000 anaesthetic exposures. It occurs most often in women, with obesity, and with short intervals between administration of the agent.[13] Most patients who develop halothane hepatitis have a history of fever, leukocytosis, and elevated transaminase levels after their previous halothane exposure. The course of halothane hepatitis is that of post-operative malaise, followed by fever, nausea and vomiting over the following 3–6 days, with jaundice appearing between the sixth and tenth day. In 70 per cent of jaundiced patients, massive hepatic necrosis will occur with rapidly worsening hepatic encephalopathy and death. Chronic active hepatitis has also been described in an occasional patient repeatedly exposed to halothane, as well as to several anaesthesia personnel with chronic exposure to halothane.[14]

It would seem wise to avoid unnecessary repeated administration of halothane, and before use to question the patient carefully on prior exposure. Development of unexplained fever or jaundice after prior halothane would seem to contra-indicate repeated exposure. Nevertheless, many patients, particularly young burn patients, have had repetitive exposure to halothane, some for over a hundred such episodes, without complications.

Halothane, however, is better than many anaesthetics in optimizing hepatic blood flow, hepatic tissue oxygenation, and stability of the patient. For these reasons, and because of the low incidence of halothane hepatitis in patients with liver disease, the overall mortality with halothane in these patients may be less than with other agents. For this reason, halothane may not be an inappropriate choice in patients with liver disease who have not demonstrated a previous sensitivity to halothane.

- Avoidance of hypoxia to reduce the chance of inducing anoxic biotransformation of toxic metabolites, however, is crucial.

Methoxyflurane

Methoxyflurane hepatitis also occurs, with even less frequency than halothane hepatitis, but similarly occurs most frequently in women with a prior exposure history. A similar course of fever followed by jaundice from day 6–10 is also seen. Rash and eosinophilia occur in less than 20 per cent, however. Renal failure occurs in 17 per cent of patients with methoxyflurane hepatitis, a finding not seen with halothane hepatitis. Mortality with methoxyflurane hepatitis seems slightly less (58 per cent) than after halothane hepatitis. There is a risk of cross-reactivity and cross-sensitivity between halothane and methoxyflurane, so it is better, when possible, not to use one when there is a history of sensitivity to the other.

Enflurane

Enflurane hepatitis is exceptionally rare (1:200 000 exposures).[15] The same centrizonal necrosis characteristic of halothane and methoxyflurane hepatitis is seen; however, the mortality is just 20 per cent; renal failure can occur.

Isoflurane

Isoflurane appears to be one of the safer inhalation anaesthetics to use in patients with liver disease.[16,17] It does not appear to produce liver injury even when given for long periods or during conditions of mild hypoxia. In normal volunteers not undergoing surgery, isoflurane (and enflurane) does not affect BSP retention.

Approaches to minor and major emergency procedures

If a given emergency procedure appears to be best handled with local, spinal or epidural anaesthesia, there are still important considerations in patients with liver disease. Amide local anaesthetics can quickly produce toxicity if given as continuous infusions because of metabolism. For this reason it has been recommended to give them only as a single dose.

Barbiturates, opiates, and phenothiazines should be used in small quantities if used at all, as there is increased sensitivity, increased duration, and enhancement of encephalopathy with these agents in patients with liver disease.

For major emergency procedures, light levels of anaesthesia plus full muscular paralysis have been recommended in an attempt to avoid the reduction in hepatic blood flow seen with deeper levels. Conduction of major emergency cases with only N_2O/O_2 and a muscle relaxant has been recommended. However, there is frequently increasing desaturation of oxyhaemoglobin with time, despite adequate ventilation, because of the ventilation–perfusion imbalance due to pulmonary shunting. This reduces the usefulness of N_2O.

As control of blood pressure, cardiac output, and artrial oxygen saturation is more important than the effect of any particular agent on liver function, the anaesthetic which is chosen should be that which best serves the patient in the experience of the anaesthetist. Because of their known qualities, halothane, enflurane or isoflurane are usually chosen.

As already mentioned, patients with encephalopathy may need reduced concentrations of inhalation anaesthetics and less hypnotics and narcotics.

Intra-operative monitoring

Minute-to-minute monitoring is required to prevent hypoxaemia and hypovolaemia.

- A radial artery catheter to allow observation and recording of blood pressure as well as the collection of frequent samples for pH, P_{CO_2} and P_{O_2} measurements is usually necessary.
- A pulmonary artery flotation catheter to monitor left and right sided pressures for minute-to-minute fluid control should be used in all major cases. The aim is to keep left atrial pressure appropriate for adequate cardiac filling while maintaining right atrial pressure between 3–8 mmHg to prevent the elevated central pressures that result in decreased portal flow. The central catheter also enhances venous access to obtain samples for analysis of electrolytes and glucose concentrations in prolonged cases.
- A urinary catheter to measure urinary output, an ECG to detect arrhythmias, and a rectal thermistor plus a temperature control blanket are usually necessary.

Because these patients are more unstable than may appear and because mortality and morbidity is high, meticulous care must be taken to maintain adequate anaesthesia records.

Protection of the anaesthesia team from liver disease

Anaesthesia teams are definitely at risk of developing liver disease. This risk comes from exposure to anaesthetic agents and from exposure to hepatitis viruses. Good ventilation, recognition of symptoms of liver disease, and perhaps even monitoring of liver enzymes and liver function may well prevent the development of serious liver problems.

Anaesthetists are at high risk for exposure to hepatitis B and hepatitis non A–non B viruses. Twenty to 30 per cent of anaesthesia personnel have demonstrated immunological evidence of exposure to hepatitis B. Avoidance of hepatitis contact requires that one should suspect everyone, be careful, and be prophylactically vaccinated with hepatitis B vaccine.

Rule 1: Suspect everyone. The carrier rate for hepatitis B virus varies from 0.1–20 per cent depending on the population being served. Anaesthesia teams are in intimate contact with large numbers of patients a day, therefore their chance of being exposed to asymptomatic carriers of hepatitis is high. The index of suspicion should be raised when there is a history of previous unexplained jaundice, when the patient comes from a geographic area where hepatitis is endemic, when there is a history of drug addiction, multiple sexual partners, or institutionalization in a penal or mental institution. Patients with a history of large volume transfusion, such as open heart patients or patients with sickle cell disease as well as haemodialysis patients are also at risk.

Rule 2: Be careful. Careful personal hygiene is essential. This includes washing hands frequently and adequately and wearing gloves when handling oral, urinary or other secretions. Sterilization of equipment is obviously essential. Learn and practise techniques to avoid accidental self innoculation with needles and report such accidents immediately to receive appropriate therapy. Hepatitis B immune globulin is far superior to regular immune serum globulin in preventing type B hepatitis.

Rule 3: obtain appropriate vaccination against hepatitis B virus. It is now well shown that personnel at risk from 'needle-sticks', and personnel exposed to blood products of potentially infected patients, will have less hepatitis (and less virulent hepatitis) if appropriately vaccinated against hepatitis B. There is no evidence of significant side effects from vaccination. There is very reasonable evidence that the system for inactivating the hepatitis B virus also kills similar viruses, such as those responsible for Acquired Immune Deficiency Syndrome (AIDS). Although expensive, the cost of vaccination is far less than the livelihood lost when hepatitis occurs.

Conclusion

Anaesthetic considerations in the patient with liver disease undergoing emergency surgery include recognizing the severity of the liver disease, assessing the clinical risk of the surgery, and stabilizing the patient as much as possible prior to surgery. The aim of anaesthesia during surgery is to maintain a stable haemodynamic condition with optimal tissue oxygenation. Under these conditions, the patient will have the best chance of avoiding progressive postoperative liver failure and mortality. Avoidance of liver disease on the part of the anaesthesia team requires vigilance, attention to aseptic techniques, and immunization.

References

1. Fairlie CW, Barss TP, French AB, Jones CM, Beecher HK. Metabolic effects of anesthesia in man. IV. A comparison of the effects of certain anesthetic agents on the normal liver. *New Eng. J. Med.* 1951; **244**: 615–22.
2. Rogers EL, Rogers MC. Fulminant hepatic failure and encephalopathy. *Ped. Clin. N. Amer.* 1980; **27**: 701–13.
3. Child CG. *The Hepatic Circulation and Portal Hypertension.* Philadelphia: Saunders, 1954.
4. Greene NM. Anesthesia risk factors in patients with liver disease. *Comtemp. Anesth. Pract.* 1981; **4**: 87–109.
5. del Guercio LRM, et al. Pulmonary arteriovenous admixture and the hyperdynamic cardiovascular state in surgery for portal hypertension. *Surgery* 1964; **56**: 57–74.
6. Bohrer SL, Rogers EL, Kohler RC, Traystman RJ. Effect of hypovolemic hypotension and laparotomy on the splanchnic and hepatic arterial blood flow in dogs. *Curr. Surg.* 1981; **38**: 325–8.
7. Thorshauge C. Hepatic blood flow during anaesthesia. *Acta Anaesth. Scand.* 1970; **37**: 205.
8. Cowan RE, Jackson BT, Thompson RPH. The effects of various anaesthetics and abdominal surgery on liver blood flow in man. *Gut* 1975; **16**: 839.
9. Kennedy WF. Simultaneous systemic and hepatic hemodynamic measurements during high spinal anesthesia in normal man. *Anesth. Analg.* 1976; **49**: 1016–24.
10. Adams AP, Hewitt PB. The new muscle relaxants: atracurium and vecuronium. In: Atkinson RS, Adams AP (eds). *Recent Advances in Anaesthesia–15.* London: Churchill-Livingstone 1985, 13–25.
11. Pandele G. Thiopental pharmacokinetics in patients with cirrhosis. *Anesthesiology* 1983; **59**: 123–6.
12. Wright R. Controlled prospective study of the effect on liver function of multiple exposures to halothane. *Lancet* 1975; **i**: 817–20.

13. Dundee JW, Prospective study of liver function following repeat halothane and enflurane. *J. Roy. Soc. Med.* 1981; **74**: 286-90.
14. Thomas FB. Chronic aggressive hepatitis induced by halothane. *Ann. Int. Med.* 1974; **81**: 487-9.
15. Lewis JH. Enflurane hepatotoxicity. *Ann. Int. Med.* 1983; **98**: 984-92.
16. Steven WC. Comparative toxicity of isoflurane, halothane, fluroxene, and diethyl ether in human volunteers. *Can. Anaesth. Soc. J.* 1973; **20**: 357-68.
17. Eger EI, Calverley RK, Smith NT. Changes in blood chemistries following prolonged enflurane anesthesia. *Anesth. Analg.* 1976; **55**: 547-9.

Further reading

Howell CW. Anaesthetic problems in the liver. In: Kaufman L. (ed). *Anaesthesia Review 3*. London: Churchill-Livingstone; 1985, 29.
Strunin L. *Liver and Anaesthesia. Major Problems in Anaesthesia 3*. London: W. B. Saunders, 1977.

27

Respiratory Insufficiency

A Terry Walman

Definitions
Causes of respiratory insufficiency
  Airway disease
  Alveolar (parenchymal) disease
  Extrapulmonary ventilatory failure
Basic measures in treatment
  Supplementary oxygen therapy
  Controlling the airway
  Laryngoscopy and intubation of the trachea
Management of acute (upper) airway obstruction
Causes of difficult intubation
Other therapeutic measures
Care of patients during surgery
  Premedication
General or regional anaesthesia

The anaesthetist is a key member of the emergency medical team in the situation of respiratory insufficiency. The diagnosis of inadequate oxygenation and/or ventilation demands immediate and aggressive intervention – including knowledge of airway management, muscle relaxation, tracheal intubation, and mechanical ventilation – and the anaesthetist is usually the most skilled practitioner in acute diagnostic and therapeutic manoeuvres for this emergency.

Strictly speaking, respiration is a cellular phenomenon. The actual site of aerobic metabolism occurs in the mitochondria of cells, producing carbon dioxide and water as by-products in the process. When we speak of 'respiratory insufficiency' we are really referring to inadequate oxygen delivery and carbon dioxide elimination. Interference with this process can occur at any point in the respiratory system – from the uppermost portions of the patient's airway to the lowermost functional unit of the lungs – the alveolus.

Definitions

While respiratory insufficiency is a concept, the anaesthetist is practically faced with problems of *oxygenation* – the ability to maintain an adequate arterial blood oxygen content, and *ventilation* – the capacity to remove carbon dioxide from the venous blood. Arterial oxygen tension (Pa_{O_2}) represents the driving pressure of oxygen in arterial blood available to the tissues. Arterial oxygen content (Ca_{O_2}) represents the amount of oxygen (in ml or mol) contained in unit volume of arterial blood. Arterial oxygen saturation (Sa_{O_2}) represents the percentage saturation of haemoglobin in the blood. Ca_{O_2} is difficult and tedious to measure but a most valuable concept. For convenience and speed Pa_{O_2} (and to a lesser extent Sa_{O_2}) are most used.

Although there are many signs and symptoms of *hypoxia* (oxygen deficiency in the tissues) with varying degrees of specificity and accuracy, all except for frank apnoea are ultimately clinical impressions that must be confirmed by arterial blood analysis. *Hypoxaemia*, or decreased oxygen tension in the blood, is generally defined in the adult as a Pa_{O_2} of less than 60 mmHg; this value represents oxygen tension at the threshold of near saturation of haemoglobin.[1] Normal Pa_{O_2} ranges between 80 and 110 mmHg when an individual is breathing room air. Hypoxaemia is a significant medical emergency that demands prompt institution of therapy as well as diagnostic measures to determine aetiology and pathophysiology. *Cyanosis* describes a dark blue or purplish colour of the skin and mucous membranes due to deficient oxygenation of blood suggestive of hypoxaemia, but it is not specifically an accurate measure of Pa_{O_2}; rather it is a finding that occurs when the level of reduced haemoglobin (deoxyhaemoglobin) in the blood exceeds 5 g/dl. The appearance of cyanosis can be affected by anaemia, colours of the environmental background, lighting, and observer variation.

Carbon dioxide is a normal end-product of aerobic metabolism and the amount of CO_2 circulating in the body is a function of both its production and elimination. Carbon dioxide production parallels O_2 consumption (the respiratory quotient R), and lacking an increase in O_2 consumption (and therefore CO_2 production) or a significant change in pulmonary blood flow, the Pa_{CO_2} is an accurate reflection of alveolar ventilation. Inadequate alveolar ventilation will lead to a concomitant increase in Pa_{CO_2}.

Hypercapnia is generally defined in the adult as a $Pa_{CO_2} >$ 50 mmHg and, although the condition may be suspected clinically from signs and/or symptoms, direct measurement on an arterial blood sample is the accurate method of diagnosis. Hypercapnia may become severe with subsequent haemodynamic and metabolic derangements that could lead to organ dysfunction and morbidity; except in the setting of acute CNS injury, severe hypercapnia can be tolerated by the body for moderate periods of time without the irreversible cellular damage that occurs with relatively brief periods of hypoxaemia.

In summary, Pa_{O_2} is a direct measure of the adequacy of oxygenation and Pa_{CO_2} is usually a direct measure of ventilation, and the compromise of either oxygenation or ventilation is what is meant by the term 'respiratory insufficiency'.

Causes of respiratory insufficiency

Respiratory insufficiency can result from a large variety of causes, but three major subdivisions help to categorize the various presentations.

Airway disease

Upper/lower airway obstruction

- foreign body
- bronchospasm
- tracheal stenosis
- tumour
- aspiration (acute)
- bronchopleural fistula.

Usually obstructive lesions involving either the larger upper air conduits such as foreign bodies or tracheal stenosis, or, disease processes affecting the smaller, more distal generations of bronchial airways such as bronchospasm. Airway obstruction increases resistance to air flow, leading to air trapping and collapse of unstable airways, thus hampering gas exchange. Therapy is directed at relieving or bypassing the obstruction.

The principles of airway management using artificial airways, tracheal intubation, and sometimes emergency tracheostomy come into use with these lesions. Supplemental oxygen may improve oxygenation in upper airway obstruction and positive pressure ventilation will overcome the increased resistance to airflow and improve gas exchange. For distal airway pathology such as bronchospasm, specific pharmacological therapy (bronchodilators) is indicated to relieve the obstruction to air flow.

Alveolar (parenchymal) disease

- necrotizing viral or bacterial pneumonia
- aspiration pneumonitis
- toxic vapours/smoke inhalation
- O_2 toxicity
- Adult Respiratory Distress Syndrome (ARDS)
- Hyaline Membrane Disease (newborn)
- pulmonary emboli
- congestive heart failure
- near drowning
- atelectasis.

Widespread disruption of a large enough area of pulmonary parenchymal tissue leads to inadequate gas exchange at the alveolar capillary membrane interface with resultant hypoxaemia and hypercapnia. Treatment involves supportive care with supplementary oxygen and, if necessary, mechanical ventilation while diagnosis of the underlying disease process and specific therapy are instituted.

Extrapulmonary ventilatory failure

Respiratory drive

- brain (medullary) injury
- sepsis
- drug overdose.

Bellows function

- muscle weakness
- quadriplegia
- obesity
- severe pain ('splinting')
- thoracic trauma (pneumothorax).

Primary ventilatory failure from disease or drug effects on the neurological system, or at the systemic level, that either inhibit respiratory drive or interfere with the bellows function of the chest cavity. In this type of respiratory failure the airway and parenchymal functions are virtually intact. Oxygen and CO_2 exchange are impaired only because ventilatory drive mechanics are inadequate. Therapy consists of improving pulmonary mechanics or, failing that, instituting mechanical ventilation.

Basic measures in treatment

In emergencies involving respiratory insufficiency, the underlying cause may not be readily discernable, but the institution of therapy cannot be delayed until a specific aetiology is identified. Fortunately, what may be specific treatment for one cause, such as intubation of the trachea to bypass an obstructing body, is also the indicated general supportive measure for securing the airway in any situation of respiratory failure. Likewise, mechanical ventilation may be specifically indicated for extrapulmonary causes of ventilatory failure, but it is also the appropriate therapy for severe alveolar disease that has progressed to a condition of hypercarbia. Essentially, there are a number of basic therapeutic modalities which may be used individually, in combination, or in series to treat the important end-results of respiratory insufficiency, namely hypoxaemia and/or hypercapnia.

Supplementary oxygen therapy

Administration of oxygen is indicated in virtually all circumstances for the treatment or prevention of hypoxia. An increase in the inspired fraction of oxygen with resultant increase in $Pa O_2$ will minimize the peripheral sympathetic discharge, hyperventilation, and increased cardiac output evoked by hypoxaemia. In patients with underlying severe chronic obstructive pulmonary pathology, supplemental oxygen must be used with great caution, as such patients often have attenuated responses to $Pa CO_2$ and their ventilation depends on hypoxic drive. In these individuals, a $Pa O_2$ much higher than their norm would no longer promote adequate ventilation, therefore oxygen administration is begun at very low concentrations, with close attention paid to arterial blood gas analysis for adequate improvement in $Pa O_2$ without unacceptable increases in $Pa CO_2$.

An additional complication of the use of supplemental oxygen is the possibility of alveolar damage from continual exposure to high concentrations of inspired oxygen. This is known as O_2 toxicity, and is not proven actually to occur with $FI O_2 < 0.6$. However, if a patient required $FI O_2 > 0.6$ to prevent hypoxia, then such therapy is the lesser of evils. As always, the only precise measure of response to oxygen therapy is repeated arterial blood–gas analysis, and the least $FI O_2$ necessary to restore normal oxygenation needs to be continually determined and administered.

In order for oxygen to be delivered in concentrations higher than 60 per cent, it is necessary to use a system which involves the addition of a reservoir bag to the face-mask or breathing circuit, so that room air is not entrained during inspiration thus diluting the inspired oxygen concentration. With the use of such a reservoir, an $F\text{IO}_2$ approaching 1.0 can be attained.

Controlling the airway

The concept of the airway in man includes the nasal passages, oral cavity, naso- and oropharynxes, larynx, and trachea. These are all rather large conduits for air movement that consist of muscular soft tissue covered by mucous membranes on a cartilaginous and bony framework. Endotracheal intubation is not always necessary to maintain airway patency, even in emergency situations.[2] The most common cause of compromised airway (soft tissue obstruction) is usually relieved by simple manoeuvres such as adjustment of head position, opening the mouth, and/or elevation of the temporal area of the mandible (so called 'jaw-thrust'). If these manipulations, along with removing any foreign substances present in the oral cavity or pharynx are not successful, then the placement of a nasopharyngeal or oropharyngeal airway may help.

Nasopharyngeal airways are easier to insert, as they do not require patient co-operation for mouth opening. However, the nasal passages are highly vascularized, fragile, and therefore easily damaged. Nasopharyngeal airways must be narrow and soft enough to pass through the inferior turbinates without causing bleeding or mucous membrane damage, but long enough to reach beyond tissue obstruction.

Oropharyngeal airways may be difficult to place in some patients with large or unusual tooth configurations, and placed improperly may force the tongue posteriorly and aggravate soft tissue obstruction. They also stimulate the gag reflex in conscious patients or may be impossible to place at all in those with masseter spasm. However, proper placement of an oropharyngeal airway usually yields a patent conduit for air flow and renders the mouth and teeth open to allow for further manipulation such as suctioning of secretions and laryngoscopy if necessary.

Positive pressure ventilation using an Ambu (or similar) self-inflating bag and face-mask is another method of providing airway patency. The soft tissues of the mouth and pharynx that are the most common cause of airway obstruction are often forced out of their obstructing position by a relatively small amount of continuous positive airway pressure (CPAP) or positive end-expiratory pressure (PEEP). This requires a tight-fitting face-mask that sits flush against the mouth, nose, and cheeks as well as a gas delivery system capable of sustaining a positive pressure flow. Careful placement of the mask upon the face and an even distribution of force to hold it in position can be achieved either manually or with the use of behind-the-head mask straps.

Of course, the success of achieving airway patency is made most probable by combining these various modalities described above as in the use of positive pressure with a mask along with an oro- or nasopharyngeal airway and, of course, proper head and mandibular alignment. Neither pharyngeal airways nor positive pressure face-mask systems provide any protection against aspiration of stomach contents.[3]

Laryngoscopy and intubation of the trachea

Intubation of the trachea can be accomplished in a variety of ways: blindly, or under direct or indirect vision of the larynx. It can be done blindly using tactile methods to identify the epiglottis and laryngeal opening, or by using auditory cues of listening for breath sounds from the connector end of the endotracheal tube.[4] Under direct vision, there are a number of laryngoscope blades which offer different views of the epiglottis and larynx – each having a particular line of sight and quality of anatomical perspective.[5] There are flexible fibreoptic laryngoscopes which allow direct visualization of the larnygeal structures through a powerful lighted tube.[6] Indirect methods of laryngoscopy involve the use of special mirrored laryngoscope blades that require practice and coordination to take advantage of the inverse images that appear.

Patients may either be awake or unconscious for endotracheal intubation. Awake patients usually require significant amounts of pharmacological sedation as well as generous application of local anaesthesia to the mucous membrane of the upper airway in order to co-operate in the procedure. If patients are in true respiratory distress, they may already be in a sedated condition from the effects of hypoxia and/or hypercapnia. Such a patient would need very little, if any, pharmacological intervention to co-operate in the procedure.

A tube into the trachea may be placed either via the oropharynx, the nasopharynx or directly into the trachea (tracheostomy). The advantages of nasally placed tracheal tubes are that they bypass the teeth and tongue and therefore cannot be occluded by the clenching of the patient's teeth. Also, the nasopharynx provides a rather snug anchor around which the tube is less likely to be moved, especially because the muscular tongue is also bypassed by this route. Disadvantages are that the tube size is often limited by the diameter of the nasal turbinates, and proper placement is somewhat harder to achieve. Bacteraemia may be produced. Contra-indications to nasal intubation include basilar skull fracture (*see* p. 130) and severe bleeding diathesis (*see* p. 46). Oral endotracheal tubes are more commonly placed using direct laryngoscopy techniques and nasal tubes are often placed using fibreoptic laryngoscopy or special (Magill) forceps if direct laryngoscopy is used.

If a patient is to be rendered unconscious for endotracheal intubation, there will probably be a need for some degree of muscle relaxation to allow easy visualization of the laryngeal structures. This can either be accomplished with the use of pure inhalation anaesthetics such as enflurane which offer a degree of muscle relaxation directly proportional to the depth of anaesthesia, or by the use of individual agents to cause unconsciousness, such as barbiturates plus other agents such as suxamethonium (succinylcholine) to produce muscle relaxation.

To produce muscle relaxation to facilitate endotracheal intubation, a powerful short acting agent with short onset is preferred. This is especially true in emergency circumstances, as failure to achieve speedy intubation might be complicated by continued muscle paralysis and continued ventilatory cessation by the patient. Therefore, suxamethonium (succinylcholine), a depolarizing neuromuscular junction blocking agent has been traditionally popular, while atracurium, a newer nondepolarizing neuromuscular junction blocking agent – also with quick onset, short duration, and elimination pathway independent of enzyme action – has great promise for use in emergency intubation without some of the untoward effects of suxamethonium (succinylcholine).

Management of acute (upper) airway obstruction

1. Establish/improve the airway:
- clear obstruction!
- head positioning
- jaw thrust – open mouth
- nasal or oropharyngeal airway
- O_2 to 100 per cent (spontaneous ventilation).

2. Ventilate with 100 per cent O_2 mask:
- control ventilation.

3. Intubate the trachea:

- failure of protective mechanisms of larynx
- failure of ventilation
- failure of oxygenation
- need for improved pulmonary toilet.

4. If intubation attempt fails:

- go back to step 2, then re-attempt intubation, modifying original technique.

5. If ventilation by mask and intubation fails, supply 100 per cent O_2 via transtracheal conduit (14G IV needle through cricothyroid membrane) DO NOT attempt to ventilate via transtracheal needle (transtracheal oxygenation *only!*).

6. Attempt to re-intubate the trachea, if this fails, proceed to emergency tracheostomy (*see* p. 203).

7. Once ventilation/oxygenation is established, treat any associated cardiovascular instability.

8. Diagnose and treat the underlying cause of airway obstruction.

Causes of difficult intubation

- Enlarged tonsils and adenoids (inflammation or tumour).
- Retropharyngeal abscess, tumour, or cystic hygroma.
- Nasopharyngeal tumours.
- Myxoedematous thickening or retropharyngeal soft tumours.
- Pharyngeal tumour.
- Laryngeal and upper tracheal tumours.
- Enlarged thyroid.
- Middle and lower tracheal compression.
- Patients unable to extend the head or flex the neck.
- Unable to open mouth widely – temporo-mandibular joint dysfunction.
- Short muscular neck with full set of teeth.
- Receding lower jaw with obtuse mandibular angles.
- Increase in posterior and anterior depth of the mandible (if ratio of effective mandibular length to the posterior depth of the mandible > 3.6 difficult intubation is unlikely).[7]

Other therapeutic measures

By definition, patients with respiratory insufficiency have lost their normal pulmonary reserve and there are a number of therapeutic modalities that can help improve their oxygenation potential and ventilatory efficiency.

Pulmonary toilet refers to the mobilization and removal of

respiratory secretions. Failure to deal properly with the normal or often increased secretions of the bronchial tree in respiratory insufficiency can lead to serious complications with retained secretory material, mucous plugs, atelectasis, and ultimately pneumonia. Inspired oxygen needs to be humidified to prevent drying of thick secretions and gases should be warmed if the normal heat exchanging mechanisms of the upper airway are bypassed by artificial airways or an endotracheal tube.

Oro/nasotracheal suction helps patients with poor cough to expel their secretions more completely, and occasionally fibreoptic bronchoscopy at the bedside using suction and saline lavage is indicated to dislodge or remove mucous plugs that have defied other forms of therapy. In particularly refractory situations, tracheal intubation becomes necessary solely to expedite removal of particularly copious secretions that have not responded to the above measures.

Positioning of the patient to enhance diaphragmatic function, and allow even expansion of all areas of the lung will minimize atelectasis and aid removal of secretions. Coughing and deep breathing by the patient will similarly oppose atelectasis and discourage pooling of secretions. Decompression of any thoracic or abdominal cavity fluid, or gas collections such as pleural effusion or gastric distension can immediately improve ventilatory function and diaphragmatic efficiency. In cases of splinting from thoracic and/or upper abdominal wounds causing pain, titration of narcotic analgesia to provide relief without significant CNS-induced respiratory depression is quite helpful. Bronchodilators can be used to improve ventilatory mechanics in patients with bronchospastic disorders, and positive airway pressure can oppose atelectasis and small airway collapse. Ultimately, mechanical ventilation may be necessary if the patient's ventilatory capacity fails to improve with the less invasive measures outlined above.

Care of patients during surgery

Patients with hypoxaemia who require therapy with continuous positive airway pressures (CPAP) or positive end-expiratory pressure (PEEP) to maintain oxygenation on a given FIO_2 need to have that positive pressure continued throughout the peri-operative period, even though they may be in transit or in the operating room. Special bag systems (e.g. Ambu) are available that allow PEEP to be maintained during the breathing cycle, and in the operating room special valve adaptors placed in the anaesthetic breathing circuit provide PEEP or CPAP at a specified level.

Patients who require mechanical ventilation pre-operatively will need to be similarly supported during transport to the operating room, either with a portable mechanical ventilator or manually by use of a self-inflating bag system. All patients with any degree of respiratory insufficiency should be transported with supplementary oxygen at the same concentration provided on the ward or in the emergency department and should be accompanied during transport by personnel experienced in diagnosis and management of respiratory problems.

Patients with chronic respiratory insufficiency will occasionally require operative surgical intervention and it is clear that any such procedure is undertaken at a higher risk of morbidity or mortality in a patient with respiratory insufficiency than a similar operation in a patient with normal respiratory function. This is because any operative intervention usually involves a number of factors which interfere with respiratory function, such as immobility, lack of ambulation, supine position (bedrest), and, especially in the case of abdominal and thoracic procedures, restriction of chest wall and diaphragmatic motion from pain or dressings. Additionally, there may be pharmacological CNS depression of respiratory function from narcotics, muscle relaxants, and/or general anaesthetics.

For an elective operation, a patient's postoperative pulmonary function may be predicted by the anaesthetist's pre-operative work-up including history, physical examination and laboratory tests – a predictive value. Therefore, a patient with chronic respiratory insufficiency is a relatively *known* risk, and preparations for appropriate care can be planned and undertaken. By contrast, a patient with chronic respiratory insufficiency who needs an *emergency* operation can be very difficult – unless, of course, he or she is well known to the anaesthetist and is in optimum condition; lacking this information, it is best to anticipate that the patient will require more rather than less measures of postoperative support.

Of course, pre-operative preparation of a patient with chronic pulmonary insufficiency, which can be so important and worthwhile in an elective setting for ensuring successful outcomes from operative intervention, will be quite limited in the emergency setting since there is usually not enough time for formal evaluation of pulmonary function. There certainly will not be time for initiation of therapeutic modalities designed to optimize pulmonary mechanics such as pharmacological trials or incentive spirometry. Nevertheless, if the patient is conscious and able to co-operate, a quick assessment of gross pulmonary function may be obtained by the use of a spirometer and a pre-operative arterial blood-gas analysis, preferably before the administration of any respiratory depressant drugs or supplemental oxygen.

Premedication

Premedication should not be given to patients with respiratory insufficiency before they have been seen by the anaesthetist and fully assessed. Antisialogogues are needed prior to bronchoscopy or difficult intratracheal manipulations, but are otherwise avoided in bronchitic patients to avoid the development of sticky secretions. Sedative, narcotic and hypnotic drugs are hazardous and should be avoided.

General or regional anaesthesia

It may be possible to employ local or regional anaesthesia for emergency surgery in patients with respiratory insufficiency e.g. in relatively limited operations on extremities such as debridement or abscess drainage, but the relative ease and simplicity that makes regional anaesthesia attractive in this setting must be weighed against the risk of pulmonary decompensation and loss of control over physiological function during and after operation. The main advantage in avoiding general anaesthesia in these patients is the added monitor of having an awake and responsive patient with whom to communicate in order to continually assess neurological, cardiac, and pulmonary function. The disadvantages of regional or local anaesthesia in this group of patients is that they require co-operation both to achieve the proper degree of anaesthesia and to provide the necessary operating conditions for the surgery to progress. Patients with respiratory insufficiency are likely to be uncomfortable in an emergency situation and therefore not able to co-operate fully for the successful completion of a regional or local anesthetic. If sedation is required to make a patient with respiratory distress comfortable, the effect of narcotics and/or anti-anxiety agents may be to depress ventilation.

General anaesthesia needs to be carefully planned not only for the intra-operative needs but also for postoperative considerations. Certainly, maintenance of adequate pulmonary function during operation is of the highest importance, and the fraction of inspired oxygen and possible use of CPAP or PEEP will depend upon individual patient needs. An important consideration will be postoperative goals in respiratory function that will affect the choice of anaesthetic agents and techniques employed. If a patient begins an anaesthetic with compromised respiratory function, there is little likelihood that function will be significantly improved by the end of the anaesthetic unless the operation deals directly with the cause of the pulmonary compromise; e.g. treatment of pneumothorax or repair of diaphragmatic rupture. In fact, most surgical interventions lead to a worsening of pulmonary function.[8] Any narcotics used should be administered carefully so that continued respiratory depression does not impede the patient's recovery. The same considerations apply to the use of muscle relaxants and potent inhalational agents. All these medications may be useful in providing a safe and reliable state of general anaesthesia intra-operatively, but their careful use dictates that their continued effects postoperatively be taken into consideration when planning a general anaesthetic technique. The level of post-operative support necessary should be dictated by the patient's underlying disease or the effects of operative intervention and not from sloppy anaesthetic techniques and residual drug effects.

Patients with acute respiratory insufficiency pre-operatively are not candidates for elective operations. When it becomes necessary for someone in this category to undergo an emergency procedure, the use of regional or local anaesthetic techniques should be avoided since these patients are almost always unstable, require a secure airway, and require close attention to ventilatory control. Postoperatively, the need for ventilatory support will depend on the patient's underlying pathophysiology and the nature of the surgical intervention.

References

1. Hlastala M. Physiological significance of the interaction of oxygen and carbon dioxide in blood. *Crit. Care Med.* 1979; 7: 374–9.
2. Donlon, JV. Anesthetic management of patients with compromised airways. *Anesth. Rev.* **VII**, 1980; 2.
3. Roberts JT. *Fundamentals of Tracheal Intubation.* New York: Grune & Stratton, 1983.
4. Waters DJ. Guided blind endotracheal intubation. *Anaesthesia*, 1963; **18**: 158.
5. Kaplan JA (ed). *Thoracic Anesthesia.* London: Churchill-Livingstone, 1983.
6. Taylor P, Towey, R. The broncho-fibrescope as an aid to endotracheal intubation. *Br. J. Anaesth.* 1972; **44**: 611–12.
7. Murrin KR. Intubation procedure and causes of difficult

intubation. In: Latto IP, Rosen M (eds). *Difficulties in Tracheal Intubation*. London: Baillière Tindall, 1985.
8. Zikria BA, Spencer JL, Kinney JM, et al. Alterations in ventilatory function and breathing patterns following surgical trauma. *Ann. Surg.* 1974; **179**: 1.

28

Postoperative Complications

Wendy Scott

Factors predisposing to postoperative complications
Types of complication
What to do should a complication arise
    General procedure
Casualty departments
Complications following local anaesthesia
    Poor positioning and/or long procedures
    Tourniquet
    Hypothermia
Complications following general anaesthesia
    Hypoxia from respiratory problems
    Hypoxia and cardiovascular problems
    Awareness
    Specific anaesthetic techniques and certain anaesthetic agents
    Specific surgical procedures
    Certain physiological conditions
    Certain pre-existing disease states
Pain
Psychological problems

Many potential postoperative complications can be anticipated (and hopefully prevented) by the anaesthetist making a pre-operative visit.

Factors predisposing to postoperative complications

- Very sick patients requiring immediate surgery.
- Inadequate pre-operative work-up.
- Insufficient information about a patient (because a patient is too sick to give adequate details of previous or current

medical history, medication and allergies or because notes may be unavailable or lost).
- Certain physiological states and pre-existing diseases.
- Poor operating conditions when certain facilities and equipment may be lacking.

Types of complication

Complications may be:

Minor – contributing to patient discomfort and distress.
Major – which may be potentially life threatening if not immediately dealt with.

They can happen:

Early – on the table at the end of a procedure,
    – *en route* to or in the recovery room,
    – back in the ward.
Late – hours after the procedure,
    – some days later.
    Patients may recover completely, partially or not at all.

The contribution anaesthesia makes towards surgical post-operative complications may depend upon the relative skills of the anaesthetist and surgeon concerned. It must be remembered that the complications of anaesthesia cannot necessarily be equated with the disease state or with the seriousness of the surgery performed. Patients can die from anaesthesia following emergency dental extraction yet there may be no adverse anaesthetic sequelae after emergency coronary artery by-pass surgery. However, the anaesthetic management of the severely ill patient requires greater skill to avoid potential postoperative problems.

What to do should a complication arise

Minor complications may:
- be immediately obvious, e.g. vomiting, restlessness, confusion,
- be reported by the recovery room staff, e.g. pain, extravasated infusion, complaint of a sore throat;
- not be elicited until the anaesthetist's postoperative visit to the ward, e.g backache, thrombosed vein.

Major complications are usually reported immediately they happen or are diagnosed. It is unlikely that an anaesthetist will *not* know, or be informed about, a major complication in a patient that he has anaesthetized.

General procedure

(a) Examine the patient thoroughly and assess the nature and severity of the complication.
(b) Treat as appropriate. Consult a colleague if necessary.
(c) Write full and comprehensive notes. Remember to date your entry.
(d) Make an entry in the incident book – if there is one.

Minor complications

(i)   Go and see the patient again a few hours after the operation when recovery from anaesthesia is complete and the patient is fully orientated.
(ii) Listen to any complaints from the patient, nursing staff and possibly relatives.
(iii) Explain truthfully the situation and any further treatment that will be necessary.
(iv) Reassure the patient.
(v)   Date and record this and any subsequent visit to the patient in the patient's case notes.
(vi) Either write to the patient's general practitioner or ensure mention is made in the discharge summary of any relevant information.

Major complications

There should be a prescribed hospital or departmental policy for dealing with cases of major complications. It is advisable to follow it!
The policy should be along the following lines:

(i)   The anaesthetist concerned should, having carefully examined the patient, discuss the matter as soon as possible with his superior and with the surgeon.
(ii) The treatment and further management of the patient should be the concern of the anaesthetic team and not of the individual anaesthetist.
(iii) The anaesthetist's Defence Society should be informed of 'unexplained' complications or where mismanagement or negligence could possibly be alleged. A telephone call may be all that is required. The Defence Society will advise should further information be necessary.
(iv) The patient's next of kin should be informed as soon as is practicable.

(v) The patient and/or the patient's relatives should be told the truth. It is better that this be done jointly by two qualified members of staff – one of whom should be senior. Ideally information should not, at least in the first instance, be given over the telephone, but if unavoidable then only to the next of kin or a named person with a witness present to verify any statement given out. Record the telephone call in the patient's case notes.

(vi) As before, any assessments, examinations and treatment must be adequately documented and appropriate follow-up after the patient is discharged should be arranged.

Casualty departments

Many people requiring anaesthesia for minor emergency procedures go home after a few hours whether they have had *local* or *general* anaesthesia. In these cases it is imperative that morbidity be minimum (and mortality negligible!).

It is the anaesthetist's duty to ensure that the patient has been warned about any anaesthetic postoperative complications that may still be present or might occur when the patient goes home, e.g. nausea, vomiting, tiredness, lethargy, stiffness, pain. Sore throat is a complication which may follow tracheal intubation. It is not usually recommended that small children who have been intubated go home soon after having had an endotracheal tube passed – especially if the procedure was long as laryngeal oedema may be a late complication. This effectively means that such children are admitted overnight.[1]

Any patient discharged the same day following an anaesthetic, is given verbal and, ideally, written instructions to minimize postoperative problems and to prevent more serious sequelae. After *local anaesthesia* these are that the patient:

- Should be escorted home by a responsible adult.
- Is given advice as to which analgesic may be taken. Remember to prescribe adequate analgesia while the patient is still in hospital if it is required.
- Is given a letter, if appropriate, for his general practitioner.
- Is advised about the specific complications of the surgery. e.g. toes 'going blue' with a plaster cast.
- Is given the name, address and telephone number of the hospital and told he can contact the casualty department if there is a problem, or that he may return in person.

After *general anaesthesia* the above provisions apply, but *in addition*:

- The patient must not drive a car or be in charge of any type of machinery for up to 24 hr after the anaesthetic; times vary according to the anaesthetic agents given.[2]
- The patient is advised not to drink any alcohol for the rest of that day as potentiation may be a problem, especially when the agent used is one where recovery depends on redistribution.

Complications following local anaesthesia

Poor positioning and/or long procedures

Minor problems

Backache, stiffness, painful pressure areas, pins and needles. (NB The operating table feels uncomfortable after lying on it for longer than 10 min.)

Major problems

Peripheral nerve injuries which may take some time to recover, and indeed may never recover.
Pressure sores, especially if they subsequently become infected.
Deep venous thrombosis (DVT).

- Pre-operatively assess the duration of the procedure and the skill of the surgeon. Would *general* anaesthesia be more appropriate? Put sponges and gamgee under heels and pressure areas. Ensure calves are not flat on the operating table – especially in obese patients (*see* p. 352).

Tourniquet

Minor problems

Those which occur after the cuff is deflated; i.e. redness or grazing of skin (especially 'fragile' skin as in the elderly), pins and needles or even temporary hyperaesthesia.

Major problems

Those which occur after sudden release into the general circulation of:

- *Large volumes of local anaesthetic* as after Bier's block or intra-operatively if the cuff is faulty. This causes feelings of apprehension, pallor, nausea, dry mouth, metallic taste, palpitations, fits, respiratory failure followed by circulatory failure.
- *Toxic acidic metabolic products* related to the duration of time for which the tourniquet was inflated. This could give rise to cardiac dysrhythmias, especially in already compromised patients.
- Ensure that the cuff(s) of the tourniquet, the aneroid gauge, and connecting tubing are in good working order. It is preferable to use a tourniquet with a double cuff for Bier's blocks (*see* p. 120) and ensure that it is not released until the local anaesthetic used is adequately tissue bound (*see* p. 254).

Hypothermia

Body temperature can fall rapidly during both local and general anaesthesia when shivering, the body's response to cold, is prevented. The return to normal temperature postoperatively may be accompanied by marked shivering – it is vital that oxygen be administered. Shivering greatly increases oxygen demand (p. 355). Patients who have undergone regional anaesthesia may be hypothermic for longer and so have to remain a greater length of time in the recovery room compared to those who have had general anaesthesia.[3]

Complications following general anaesthesia

Many minor complications can be prevented or modified by attention to detail.

Nausea and vomiting: if there is a history of nausea and vomiting after previous anaesthesia then prophylactic antiemetics may be prescribed with the premedication, or given either during the operation or immediately postoperatively.

Restlessness may be due to pain, in which case adequate analgesia is required. (May also be due to hypoxia, *see* Major complications.)

Dizziness may be due to the surgery performed (e.g. middle ear), blood loss or the residual effects of the anaesthetic agent used.

Shivering. Give oxygen (*see* p. 330).

Confusion especially in children and the elderly (*see* p. 297). Remember also hypoxia can cause confusion!

Thrombosis of superficial veins: avoid using small veins for the injection of agents known to cause thrombosis (e.g. IV diazepam), or pain (e.g. methohexitone, [methohexital], etomidate).

Tissue hypoxia is the primary threat to the patient in the immediate postoperative period.

- It is advisable that all patients are given oxygen-enriched air in the recovery room to aid in the prevention of postoperative hypoxia.

Hypoxia from respiratory problems[4]

Upper airway problems

Obstruction from tongue, blood, vomit or broken tooth.

- Ensure a clear airway.

Inhalation of vomit, blood or debris (distal atelectasis and subsequent infection).

- To avoid, turn patient on to side prior to extubation.
- Management: arrange chest radiograph, send sputum cultures, treat actively with O_2, appropriate antibiotics, physiotherapy; consider IPPV and/or corticosteroid therapy.

Obtunded cough reflex and secretions
Anaesthetic gases contribute to making secretions viscous and they depress ciliary action. Plugs of mucous may block airways causing distal atelectasis. Infection and bronchopneumonia may follow.[5]

- Consider using humidified gases or a condenser–humidifer for long operations. Give adequate analgesia to encourage coughing. Arrange physiotherapy as necessary. Bronchoscopy may be required to remove a mucus plug if it is in a large airway and physiotherapy has failed to move it.[6]

Hypoventilation

Chest wall injuries (see p. 193)

Residual neuromuscular blockade

Muscle weakness leads to feelings of panic at inability to breathe.

- Assess with nerve stimulator (*see* p. 86). Repeat atropine and neostigmine if indicated and ventilate lungs if blockade persists.

Central respiratory depression
Narcotic overdose with slow respirations and small pupils.

• Try naloxone, (titrate as required) (*see* p. 351.).

Hypocapnia: during intra-operative ventilation Paco$_2$ may be below that required to stimulate ventilation.

If patient has been hyperventilated intra-operatively consider adding 4 per cent CO_2 to the inspired gases at the end of the operation. (Ideally measure end-tidal CO_2 to prevent post-operative hypocapnia) (*see* p. 84). Great care must be exercised. Carbon dioxide administration can cause cardiac arrhythmias and acid–base disturbances, particularly in a debilitated, elderly or ill patient, and in the presence of serum electrolyte disturbances. Prevention of inadvertent hypocapnia: use Bain co-axial breathing system with appropriate fresh gas flow rates.[7]

Damage to the respiratory centre from trauma, surgery or emboli; seen clinically as delayed return to consciousness and inadequate ventilation.

• Consider postoperative ventilation – but only if there is hope of recovery.

Diffusion hypoxia

Nitrous oxide leaves the blood 30 times faster than oxygen enters causing a 'dilution' effect of the inspired air.

• Ensure oxygen in the inspired air is higher than room air for at least 5 min at the end of the operation to allow for this dilution effect.

Ventilation-perfusion abnormalities

Lungs with ventilation-perfusion ($\dot{V}/\dot{Q}$) inequalities are not able to transfer as much oxygen and carbon dioxide as those uniformly ventilated and perfused. Regional differences from top to bottom of the lung mean that the $\dot{V}/\dot{Q}$ ratio is greater at the apex. Low ratios occur when there is underventilation in relation to per-fusion as in atelectasis, chronic obstructive airways disease, pneumothorax and neuromuscular defects. High ratios occur when there is overventilation in relation to perfusion as seen in pulmonary embolus, shock and positive pressure ventilation.

• Consider whether sitting the patient upright in the recovery room (if fully awake) would improve the $\dot{V}/\dot{Q}$ ratio, by the effect of gravity. Check that cardiovascular function is adequate first.

Hypoxia from cardiovascular problems.

A decrease in cardiac output reduces oxygen transport and may result in tissue hypoxia. Causes include hypotension and myocardial depression.

Hypotension

This may be due to:
Hypovolaemia due to dehydration or blood loss

- Check fluid balance and look for other signs of blood loss. e.g. pallor, tachycardia, sweating.
- Insertion of a central venous line, if not already *in situ*, is advisable for management of the patient's IV fluid therapy.

Vasodilatation: many anaesthetic agents are also vasodilators. Hypovolaemic patients may remain normotensive until induction of anaesthesia.

Anaphylactic shock: a sudden collapse and unresponsiveness in a conscious patient following parenteral administration of a drug may be the only signs of anaphylactic shock in the postoperative period.

- Do not assume all cases of sudden collapse are due to myocardial infarction.

Myocardial depression

Anaesthetic drugs decrease the contractility of the heart and may reduce the body's ability to compensate for blood loss. Arrhythmias may occur.

- Postoperative ECG monitoring is useful in all patients, but essential in patients who developed serious intra-operative cardiac arrhythmias.

Myocardial decompensation
Congestive cardiac failure may be produced or exacerbated by fluid overload.

- Identification of at risk patients and ECG monitoring is required. Ideally the pulmonary capillary wedge pressure (PCWP) should be measured using a balloon flotation catheter; but when this is not possible a central venous line should be inserted for the measurement of CVP.

Arrhythmias

Bradycardias result from excessive β-blockade, residual effect of neostigmine and halothane, hypothermia, myxoedema and raised CSF pressure. Tachycardias are seen after certain anaesthetic drugs, e.g. gallamine and trimetaphan, and also occur due to blood loss, pyrexia, anxiety and thyrotoxicosis.

The need to treat arrhythmias depends on their systemic effect. If blood pressure and cardiac output are maintained it may be enough to treat the cause. For example a bradycardia which causes hypotension requires atropine, whereas a bradycardia due to hypothermia in a normotensive patient requires only correction of body temperature. Restoration of blood volume will reduce tachycardia in hypovolaemic patients.

- Hypoxia can produce arrhythmias.
- Arrhythmias can produce hypoxia!

Hypocalcaemia

Citrate prevents the ionization of calcium. Large volumes of citrated blood rapidly transfused can cause citrate intoxication; i.e. a metabolic acidosis producing cardiac dysrhythmias and tremors. Plasma K^+ increases as pH is reduced.

- Consider whether the addition of calcium would improve muscle contractility (including respiratory muscles) (*see* p. 21).

One gram of calcium gluconate can be given per litre of transfused blood, but some anaesthetists feel that calcium may be harmful.[8]

Awareness

The extent to which awareness (i.e. the patient being awake whilst supposed to be unconscious during anaesthesia) is a problem, from the patient's point of view, is determined by how much is remembered, at what stage of the operation it occurred, and whether there was subsequently distress. It is standard practice to have some patients awake in the operating theatre at the end of an operation. A few patients remember this and think they were awake during the operation. The vast majority remember nothing. The risk of awareness is potentially greater in emergency anaesthesia where there is often no premedication and where light anaesthesia is required as in emergency Caesarean section. Benzodiazepines reduce the incidence of awareness but must be used with caution.

Specific anaesthetic techniques and certain anaesthetic agents

Spontaneous respiration

Inappropriate patient selection for this technique can contribute to postoperative complications. The increased resistance and work of breathing through an endotracheal tube, especially for a long time, may compromise respiration and cause exhaustion, especially in obese patients (*see* p. 352). If, pre-operatively, a patient cannot inspire 80 per cent of his predicted vital capacity then spontaneous breathing during anaesthesia is inappropriate, as expansion of the lung will be inadequate.[6]

Intermittent positive pressure ventilation (IPPV)

When IPPV is employed there may be problems following the use of muscle relaxant drugs, i.e., residual neuromuscular paralysis, dual block, apnoea due to cholinesterase deficiency when suxamethonium (succinylcholine) has been given; use a nerve stimulator to differentiate the type of block. Long periods of IPPV can cause microatelectasis.

Certain specific agents with recognized postoperative complications

Ketamine
Complications include:
Amnesia for immediate post-recovery period. Emergence delirium phenomenon, bad dreams, confusion and irrational behaviour.

The incidence of emergence phenomena may be reduced by giving droperidol (with diazepam) as a premedication. Recovery should be in a quiet room and the patient left undisturbed until awake. Droperidol may be given as treatment in the recovery room if required – again with diazepam. Atropine may also be required. Transient blindness following ketamine is rare and lasts about half an hour after recovery of consciousness.

Halothane
Shivering; this is often referred to as the 'halothane shakes' but may be seen also with other anaesthetics, e.g. enflurane. Keep the patient warm and oxygenated.

Postoperative jaundice is described following halothane anaesthesia. Patients with unexplained pyrexia following halothane should never be given halothane again. Repeated halothane anaesthesia increases the risk of jaundice. Avoid repeating a halothane anaesthetic within three to six months.

Fentanyl

Itching – patients complain of an 'itchy nose' and will rub it immediately on waking.

Respiratory depression[9] – this results from overdose often achieved by administration of serial doses during anaesthesia. The patient will not breathe, or breathes very infrequently (although often quite deeply) at the end of the operation.

- Naloxone reverses the analgesic effects of fentanyl as well as the respiratory depression. Only use it if necessary and titrate the dose. The action of naloxone is short and it may be that the original fentanyl is still active after the naloxone has been metabolized. Therefore careful observation of the patient must be maintained for some time after naloxone administration; a repeat dose of naloxone may then be necessary. Late respiratory ('biphasic') depression may occur after an apparently normal initial recovery. The phenomenon may be due to redistribution of fentanyl between body compartments during recovery.

Rigidity is a rare complication thought to be related to the secondary peak in plasma levels. It is exacerbated by hypothermia and could interfere with postoperative ventilation should this be necessary. Treatment includes:

- neuromuscular blockade for ventilated patients,
- naloxone in non-ventilated patients.

Specific surgical procedures

Emergency anaesthesia is often required for surgery to trauma victims. The severity of the trauma, however, does not necessarily determine the eventual outcome. Although some trauma such as thoracic trauma increases the likelihood of certain complications, survival and recovery rates depend on the aggressive management of postoperative complications.

Hypovolaemia and blood loss, myocardial depression, aspiration pneumonitis, arterial hypoxaemia, fat embolism and renal failure may be contributing factors in the development of the very serious complication of post-traumatic pulmonary insufficiency (also known as shock lung or adult respiratory distress syndrome). The site of the incision and the nature of the surgery influences the incidence of postoperative complications. After upper abdominal surgery patients normally have a reduction in Po_2 levels for up to three days after surgery (longer after thoraco-abdominal operations). Patients with respiratory diseases are more likely to develop complications after upper abdominal surgery.

Head injury patients may require postoperative ventilation because of damage to the respiratory centre.

Certain physiological conditions

Obesity[10]

Minor

- Increased risk to pressure areas and peripheral nerves e.g. brachial plexus
- Backache

Major

- Hypoventilation:
  Stiff thoracic cage and fatty infiltrates in respiratory muscles causing increased work in compromised muscles.
  Reduced vital capacity with functional residual capacity approximating the closing volume (the level at which airway closure occurs).
  Pre-existing cardiorespiratory problems, e.g. obstructive lung disease.
  Pickwickian syndrome (8 per cent of extremely obese)[10]
  Diminished respiratory centre drive.
- Pressure sores with risk of subsequent infection.
- Deep venous thrombosis (DVT).

Prevention/management

Great care is necessary when positioning obese patients on the operating table or transferring them to the recovery room. There is a greater risk of an obese patient being dropped. Check the integrity of the canvas. If using two canvases ensure that the poles are both through the lower canvas. In the extremely obese when two operating tables are required side by side, ensure the brakes are on! Pressure areas should be meticulously protected. Arm retaining boards pushed too far through one side of the table can damage the brachial plexus on the opposite side.

Consideration should be given to mechanical or pharmacological methods of preventing DVT, i.e. inflation–deflation boots or 'mini heparin' regimens. Chest physiotherapy and early mobilization are required to prevent chest infections and DVT.

Hypoventilation is aggravated by central respiratory depression from narcotic analgesics. Therefore care is necessary to titrate analgesia against respiratory depression. Pharmacological stimulation may be required, e.g. naloxone for specific antagonism of narcotic agents or doxapram infusions for patients in whom postoperative ventilation is inadequate in the immediate postoperative period to avoid short term IPPV. (Many obese patients are hypertensive and doxapram is contra-indicated in severe hypertension – also in status asthmaticus, coronary artery disease and thyrotoxicosis.)

Neonates and very young children

There is so little margin for error when dealing with the very young that all problems are potentially major (*see* p. 287).

Hypothermia
Neonates are poikilothermic creatures when premature, sick or under anaesthesia – it is in these situations that stores of brown fat are depleted or not metabolized. Therefore it is necessary to maintain such neonates in an environmental temperature of 33°C, 'the neutral thermal environment', at which oxygen consumption and heat production are at a minimum. Maintenance of temperature in the recovery room is as important as during surgery. Hypothermia can lead to a metabolic acidosis and hypoventilation. Heated incubators are essential for the transport of babies along cold hospital corridors.

Apnoea
Failure of a neonate to breathe postoperatively can be due to:

Hypothermia – take baby's temperature.
Metabolic acidosis ⎫
Hypoxia ⎬ measure arterial pH and blood-gases
Hypercapnia ⎭
Hypoglycaemia – measure blood glucose
Overhydration ⎫
Infection (bronchopneumonia) ⎪ measure arterial pH and
Respiratory distress syndrome ⎬ blood-gases; take chest radio-
Pneumothorax ⎭ graph.

Relaxant overdose: the relative immaturity of the neuromuscular junction means that neonates are highly susceptible to neuromuscular blocking drugs. Potentiation of drugs and interaction with other drugs may also be a problem. Remember the possibility of intracranial haemorrhage in premature babies as a possible cause for apnoea.

- Babies born prematurely and who have a history of idiopathic apnoeic attacks will almost certainly require postoperative ventilation. Once the conceptual age of 46 weeks has been reached postoperative ventilation should not be necessary unless for another indication.

Laryngeal spasm; in neonates wait until the baby is 'crying' on the tube, i.e. fully awake, before extubation. Keep an open vein at least until the baby is ready to go back to the ward.

Fluid balance
Postoperative fluid balance must be carefully calculated. There are various methods of calculation, e.g. for neonates aged 1–7 days

$$\frac{\text{Age in days}}{7} \times 70 \text{ ml/kg/24 hr of (4.5\% dextrose/0.18 per cent saline)}$$

- replace vomit and gastric aspirate with isotonic saline
- include the volume of injectate of drugs in any fluid balance calculations.

Infection
Premature sick babies are very susceptible to infection.

- It is essential to be meticulous about technique.

The elderly (Chapter 24)

Difficulty in communication. Put in hearing aid and give patients their spectacles if required.

Ecchymosis; frail easily bruised skin with tortuous superficial veins susceptible to thrombosis. Avoid giving painful injections into small veins.

Mental confusion. Delayed recovery of mental faculties leads to confusion. Try to keep the number of personnel dealing with the patient to a minimum. A known face is reassuring.

Overdose problems due to delayed excretion from poor renal function and impaired liver metabolism. Normal adult doses of drugs may constitute an overdose. Hypoventilation as a result of drugs used in the anaesthetic further compromises respiration as, with increasing age, the closing volume approaches functional residual capacity (FRC). Any further reduction in FRC from surgery will result in closure of small airways in the dependent part of the lungs during tidal breathing.

- It is not the appreciation of pain that is diminished in the elderly, it is the amount of analgesic that is required to treat it that may have to be reduced.

Deep venous thrombosis is more common in the elderly. Give mini heparin and/or use mechanical inflation boots. Ambulate early if possible.

Chest infection and pneumonia. These problems occur more often in elderly patients when early ambulation is not possible. Sputum culture should be carried out early and antibiotics prescribed if appropriate. The physiotherapist has to work hard to prevent loss of mobility during hospitalization.

Hypothermia[3]. Patients over 60 years-of-age are more likely to reduce their body temperature during operations and they appear to have a decreased ability to regain thermoregulatory controls. Prolonged hypothermia in the recovery room and ward could further exacerbate the effects of parenterally administered drugs as their plasma half-lives may be prolonged. The elderly often suffer from multiple pathology. Shivering as a result of hypothermia is harmful in the presence of respiratory embarrassment or fixed low output states. Oxygen demand during shivering is increased by 400–500 per cent. Oxygen uptake is greater because of the increase in minute ventilation. Cardiac output also increases to ensure delivery of oxygen to the tissues. In the elderly in whom there is respiratory or cardiac disease, failure of the appropriate cardiopulmonary compensation results in anaerobic metabolism producing a metabolic acidosis. This further compromises cardiopulmonary function. There may be myocardial or cerebral ischaemia.

- A high level of inspired oxygen is necessary to meet the oxygen demand of shivering in the elderly – and in those with reduced cardiopulmonary function.
- Care is necessary when oxygen is administered for patients with chronic bronchitis as they need their 'hypoxic drive'.

Drug interaction. The elderly often require many different drugs. Drug interactions should be anticipated and avoided.

Pregnancy and lactation

Many emergency anaesthetics are given to women who are, or who have recently been, pregnant.

Epidural analgesia/epidural anaesthesia
Hyperalgesia: as the local anaesthetic wears off occasionally a woman experiences the feeling of not being able to bear anything to touch the areas previously numb. The legs feel hot, itchy and have painful 'pins and needles'. It can be very distressing and lasts 1–2 hr. It may be related to the number of 'top-ups', total dose of

local anaesthetic and duration of analgesia. Recognize the entity and reassure the patient.

Backache: if there has been some technical difficulty during insertion of the needle the patient may complain of pain at the insertion site for about 2–3 days.

Great care is necessary when patients who have had epidural blocks are manoeuvred into the lithotomy position. It is often difficult for the obstetrician and anaesthetist concerned to agree the exact cause of any subsequent backache (or neurological damage).

Hypotension: intra-operative hypotension may extend into the postoperative period. Check blood pressure chart kept during the anaesthetic.

- Ensure no other cause for low blood pressure e.g. bleeding.
- Give adequate IV fluids (*see* p. 269).
- Give ephedrine 5 mg IV and 5 mg IM if blood pressure continues to fall.

Neurological damage: obtain expert neurological advice immediately on recognition of this rare occurrence.

Direct injury: from needle or catheter – rare but may happen where an anatomical variation causes the spinal cord to terminate below the accepted L1 level. It may cause lower limb symptoms, e.g. jerking.

Epidural haematoma: rare but occurs in patients with coagulopathies or on anticoagulant drugs. The management is immediate myelography and surgical decompression.

Dural puncture: inadvertent dural puncture results in a high incidence of headache which can be severe and incapacitating. More dangerous is the accidental injection of local anaesthetic solution through the dura directly into the cerebrospinal fluid (CSF): this can produce a 'total spinal block' with cardiovascular collapse, respiratory arrest and loss of consciousness necessitating full emergency resuscitation. (This is extremely rare when the injection is made through an indwelling epidural catheter: it is more likely to occur during initial siting of the epidural needle and catheter.)

Management of accidental dural puncture:

- Lie patient flat for 24 hr in darkened room.
- Prescribe adequate analgesia.
- Keep well hydrated; oral fluids or reinstate IV fluids.
- Precribe laxatives to avoid straining.
- Infuse 500 ml isotonic saline through epidural catheter over 12 hr. For persistent headache a blood patch may be required (consult senior colleague before doing this).

- If accidental dural puncture occurs during an epidural block for routine analgesia in labour, the patient should have an elective forceps to prevent pushing which will increase the CSF leak and cause a worse headache.

Epidural abscess, this may lead to paraparesis or paraplegia. It may be iatrogenic from:
1. faulty technique
2. blood patch
3. blood-borne organisms.

Management:
1. recognition
2. laminectomy
3. antibiotics.

General anaesthesia
Inhalation of gastric contents (*see* p. 11).

Lactating women: emergency general anaesthesia may be necessary in post-partum women for such procedures as evacuation of retained products of conception. It is vital for the anaesthetist to know pre-operatively if the woman is breast-feeding in order to avoid the postoperative complications of:
1. sleepy babies
2. unwanted supression of lactation.

Prevention: explain pre-operatively to the patient what is to be done for the good of herself and her baby.

1. Avoid premedication (the anaesthetist's reassurance should work well in place of drugs).

2. Ask the patient to breast feed immediately prior to coming to the operating theatre. If possible ask her to express any excess milk which can be stored in a suitable refrigerator for use post-operatively. (Express by hand or pump and put into sterile bottles.)

3. The patient, with help if necessary, should express breast milk 4–6 hr *after* the operation; this milk should be *discarded*. Meanwhile the baby is fed on the previously expressed breast milk or soya milk. It is advisable not to give breast fed babies any form of cow's milk due to the increased risk of atopy.

4. The baby may be breast fed at next feed, i.e. 8–12 hr after the operation, but may be slightly sleepy. Mother and nurses should be warned.

Large doses of induction agents and narcotics should be avoided as should any postoperative drugs that are not essential. If large doses of, e.g. thiopentone (thiopental), have been required then breast milk should be expressed and discarded for 16–24 hr. Thiopentone is excreted in breast milk for up to 24 hr.

Certain pre-existing disease states.

Cardiac disease

Patients with a history of myocardial infarction have a 36 per cent reinfarction rate if anaesthetized within three months of a previous infarct. This rate has been reduced to 6 per cent by very aggressive management and by identification of those at risk, i.e. those who develop hypertension, hypotension or tachycardia intraoperatively.[11] Concurrent congestive cardiac failure increases the danger of reinfarction. The risk of reinfarction decreases with time after a previous infarct. Patients with any cardiac disease must be anaesthetized with great care (Chapter 1).

ECG monitoring must be continued in the recovery room and any change in ECG pattern can be identified and treated appropriately.

Respiratory disease

Chronic respiratory disease is often exacerbated by anaesthesia. There is increased sputum production, and incidence of postoperative infection and atelectasis – probably due to closure of small airways within the tidal volume, from reduced FRC. Postoperative radiography demonstrates pulmonary congestion and interstitial oedema.

Postoperative complications following anaesthesia can be reduced in patients with chronic obstructive airways disease by pre-operative work-up. The patient most likely to develop postoperative respiratory complications is male, over 50 years, a smoker, obese, with a history of chronic obstructive airways disease, having a long emergency anaesthetic for upper abdominal or thoracoabdominal surgery.

Asthma: drugs known to release histamine should be avoided in asthmatics. If bronchospasm occurs during anaesthesia adequate ventilation of the patient may be difficult. Postoperatively it is a problem to know when to extubate. Certainly an endotracheal tube should not be removed in a patient with marked bronchospasm. Postoperative ventilation should be avoided if possible.

Metabolic disease

Diabetes
Good pre-operative management and frequent intra-operative and postoperative blood glucose estimations are essential particularly

because hypoglycaemia is difficult to diagnose and may be the reason for a delay in regaining consciousness. Measure serum electrolyte and blood glucose concentrations. A 50 per cent dextrose solution should always be available to be given in the event of hypoglycaemia.

Avoid Hartmann's solution because it includes lactate. Blood sugar levels may be difficult to control in the first few post-operative days depending on how soon a patient can eat, whether there is any infection, or whether the patient is ambulant. Diabetes is a 'many systems' disease. Therefore a careful watch is necessary on all other measurements especially blood pressure, temperature, urea and electrolyte balance, urine output and specific gravity. Diabetics may have coronary artery disease, chronic respiratory disease, incipient renal failure, neuropathy.

Adrenocortical insufficiency

Adequate corticosteroid cover must be continued into the post-operative period.

Pain

Pain may be the aggravating factor, if not the cause, of many post-operative complications; e.g. nausea, vomiting, restlessness, sweating, anxiety, hypertension, tachycardia, failure to cough. The vasovagal effects may even mask signs of internal bleeding.

- Treat pain adequately and appropriately. There is a balance between the amount of analgesia necessary to relieve pain and allow coughing, and that which will cause respiratory depression.

Consider also the *intra-operative* use of local anaesthetics for post-operative pain relief, e.g. caudal, spinal and regional blocks used in conjunction with general anaesthesia, the effects of which extend into the immediate postoperative period. Epidural analgesia via a catheter allows postoperative 'top-ups' and the patient will require less parenteral analgesia. Intercostal blocks can be repeated as necessary after thoracotomy or trauma with fractured ribs. Adequate analgesia must be continued to allow the earliest possible mobilization of patients – as appropriate to the surgery performed. Early mobilization reduces the risk of respiratory problems, such as chest infections and pneumonia, and also the risk of DVT. It is important to give adequate analgesia to children, as short or long term psychological distress may ensue following a 'bad experience' in hospital.

Psychological problems

The pre-operative visit reduces anxiety. It is important to tell patients if they are going to wake up with a plaster cast on, catheter *in situ*, any numbness from local procedures, an IV infusion in an arm, a pin through a leg or their eyes covered.

Do not say 'it doesn't hurt' but assure patients that when they require it, adequate analgesia will be given. Anaesthesia may cause tearfulness and feelings of depression. Reassurance and understanding are required. Patients who have had an anaesthetic during which they were aware can be disturbed long after they are physically recovered from the original illness. They need extremely careful management for any subsequent anaesthetic.

Conclusion

Many postoperative complications can perhaps be anticipated if not prevented by an appreciation of a patient's medical history, his current illness, the surgery, the anaesthetic agent and the anaesthetic technique employed. However, even the most competent anaesthetists have patients who suffer postoperative complications. Knowledge of what can go wrong – and how to manage it if it does – is essential for the practice of safe emergency anaesthesia.

References

1. Berkebile PE. Postoperative care. *Int. Ophth. Clin.* 1973; **13**: 189–214.
2. Kortilla K. Minor operations, anaesthesia and driving. In: Matila M (ed). *Modern Problems in Pharmacopsychiatry.* 1976; **10**: 91–8.
3. Vaughan MS, Vaughan RW, Cork RC. Postoperative hypothermia in adults: relationship of age, anaesthesia and shivering to rewarming. *Anesth. Analg.* 1981; **60**: 746–51.
4. Adams AP. Respiratory problems in the postoperative period. In: Zorab JSM (ed). *Lectures in anaesthesiology* (World Federation of Societies of Anaesthesiology Lecture Series). Oxford: Blackwell, 1985; **1**: 51–62.
5. Stoddart JC. Postoperative respiratory failure: an anaesthetic hazard? *Br. J. Anaesth.* 1978; **50**: 695–9.
6. Taylor JP. Postoperative respiratory insufficiency. In: *Manual of Respiratory Therapy, 2nd ed.* St. Louis: C. V. Mosby, 1978, 46–51.
7. Henville JD, Adams AP. The Bain anaesthetic system: an

assessment during controlled ventilation. *Anaesthesia* 1976; **31**: 247–56.

8. James DCO. Blood transfusion and notes on related aspects of blood clotting and haemoglobinopathies. In: Scurr C, Feldman S (eds). *Scientific Foundations of Anaesthesia, 3rd ed.* London: Heinemann, 1982.

9. Bennett MRD, Adams AP. Postoperative respiratory complications of opiates. In: Bullingham RES (ed). *Opiate analgesia*. Clinics in Anaesthesiology. London: Saunders, 1983; **1** (1): 41–56.

10. Adams AP. Nutritional disorders. In: Vickers MDA, (ed). *Medicine for Anaesthetists, 2nd ed.* Oxford: Blackwell, 1982.

11. Rao TLK, Jacobs KH, El-Etr AA. Reinfarction following anesthesia in patients with myocardial infarction. *Anesthesiology* 1983; **59**: 499–505.

Further reading

Eltringham R, Durkin M, Andrewes S. *Postanaesthetic Recovery. A practical approach.* Berlin: Springer-Verlag, 1983.

Index

Abdominal
  distension in spinal cord damage, 148
  surgery, general anaesthesia and analgesia *see* Surgery
ABO blood group system, and grouping, 28, 30
  incompatibility, 40
Abscesses, dental, 165–6
Accident and Emergency department
  in civil disasters, 232–4
  complications following anaesthetics, 343–4
Acid-aspiration syndrome, 12
  in pregnancy, prophylaxis, 271, 272
  see also Gastric contents
  treatment, 12
Acute tubular necrosis, management, 308
Adrenaline (epinephrine) in cardiac arrest, 20, 24
Advanced paediatric life support, 21, 23
Adrenocortical insufficiency and anaesthesia, 359
Ageing, physiological changes, 290–93
  see also Elderly
Air embolism and orthopaedic surgery, 119–20
Airway
  complications, 346
  establishment in CPR, 15
  in head injury patient, 129–30
  management, cardiac arrest, theatre, 15
  paediatric, cardiopulmonary arrest, 23
  in neck trauma, 140–41, 146
  obstruction, 328, 331–6
    care and support of patients, 335–7
    in ENT emergencies, 160
    in facio-maxillary emergencies, 156
    treatment, controlling the airway, 331–3
      management of acute (upper) obstruction, 333–4
      supplemental oxygen, 330–31
    see also Intubation
Alcohol intoxication in emergency situation, 5

and orthopaedic surgery, 118
Alloantibodies, 29, 30, (*table*)
Alveolar disease, 329
Ambu suction booster, 3
Amniotic fluid embolism, management, 276
Anaemias, anaesthetic considerations, 49–52
  blood transfusion and surgery, 37–8
  developing countries, 237–8
Anaesthesia, Analgesia *see* General anaesthesia: Local anaesthesia: Local infiltration: Regional anaesthesia: and specific organs, regions and conditions
Anaphylaxis and transfusion, 40
Anesthesia *see* Anaesthesia
Aneurysm
  acute dissecting, 199–200
  leaking or ruptured, management, 180–91
  anaesthesia, and precautions, 184–6
  cross-clamps, and release, 186–8
  monitoring, 182–4
  postoperative care, 189–90
    instability, causes, 190
  preoperative preparation, 181–2
Angiography, 93–5
  cerebral, 93–4
  major and limb vessel, 94–5
Anti-Lewis antibodies, 29
Anti-Rh(D) immunoglobulin characteristics, 34
Antibody screening tests, 31
Anticholinergic drugs, general abdominal surgery, 104–5
Anticoagulants, oral, and surgery, 32, 48
Aorta, trauma, 199–200, *see also* Aneurysm
Aortic cross-clamp, 186
  release, 187–8
Apnoea, postoperative failure, 353–4
Arrhythmias, 349
Arterial
  blood gases, 204
  pressure, monitoring, 82
Assistance for anaesthetist, 2
Asthma history, and anaesthesia, 358
Atropine in cardiac arrest, 19
  children, 24

intravenous, during anaesthesia, 107
Auscultation, monitoring, 84
Autotransfusion, 42
Awareness, 349

Belladonna derivatives, danger in high environmental temperatures, 238
Benzodiazepines, for dental treatment, 166
  as premedicants, 105
Binding of drugs to protein, altered in liver disease, 319
Bleeding
  disorders, 44–9
    anaesthetic considerations, 45–6
    emergency tests, 44–5
    replacement therapy, 45
  following massive transfusion, 39
  in vascular surgery, 184–5
Block(s)
  brachial plexus sequelae, 262
  central neural, 254
    sequelae, 263
  emergency use, 258
  epidural, 106, 259, 268
  failed, 262
  field, 253
  intraoperative, 261–2
  lower limb, 259
  perineum, 259–60
  peripheral nerve, 253
  postoperative, 262
  during pregnancy, paracervical, pudendal, 268–70
  preoperative, 260–61
  regional, intravenous, in orthopaedics, 120–21, 254
  trunk, 259–60
  upper limb, 258
Blood
  disorders, 44–54
  donors, emergency collection, 31
  gases, monitoring, 85, 193
  groups, and grouping, 28–30
  loss, acute, 38
    massive, procedures, 7
    military casualties, 225
      replacement, 225–7, (table) 226
    and orthopaedic surgery, 118
  products, 31–6
    adverse reactions, 40–41
    important characteristics, 33–5 (table)
  tests, 44–5
  transfusion, adverse, reactions, 40–41
    autotransfusion, 42
    in burns, 211–14

metabolic water requirement, 213–14
  plasma, and whole blood, 213
  clinical aspects, 36–8
  degree of urgency, 37
  infusion flow rates, 37
  massive, conditions resulting, 38–40
  paediatric problems, 42
  plasma expanders and substitutes, 59–62
  preparation for surgery, 37–8
  procedures, 6–7
  in resuscitation, 193
  serology, 28–30
    laboratory aspects, 30–31
  sickle cell disease, 42
  see also Dextrans: Haemaccel: Hartmann's solution
Bradycardia and cardiac arrest, management, 18
Breathing, establishment in CPR, 15–16
Breathing in head injury patient, 130
Bertylium tosylate in cardiac arrest, 20
Bronchopleural fistula, 202–3
  dangers, 202–3
Bronchoscopy
  /laryngoscopy for inhaled foreign body, 161
  paediatric patients, 287
Burns, severe, 209–21
  anaesthesia, 214–18
  assessment, 215
  blood loss replacement, 218
  induction and intubation, 216
  Lund and Browder charts, 211, 212
  metabolic factors, 209–10
  monitoring, 217
  muscle relaxants, 216
  pathophysiology, 209–10
  pulmonary complications, 218–20
  resuscitation, 210
  size of burn, estimation, 211, 212
  transfusion, 211–14
  treatment of wound, 214
Burst abdomen, management, 114

Caesarean section under local infiltration, 271
Calcium salts in cardiac arrest, 20–21
Cannula, choice
  for central venous cannulation, 65
  large bore IV, in resuscitation, 17
  for percutaneous arterial cannulation, 70

Cannulation, central venous, 65–9
Cannulation, percutaneous arterial, 69–71
Capnography, 84
Carbon dioxide and hypercapnia, 327–8
Carbon dioxide and transcutaneous monitoring, 84
Carbon monoxide poisoning, 220
Cardiac
  arrest, in the theatre, 17–21
    adults, asystole, CPR, adrenaline (epinephrine) and sodium bicarbonate, 17–18
    defibrillators, 18–19
    drugs, 19–21
    internal cardiac compression, 19
    children, 21–5
    airway, 23
    complications, 25
    defibrillators, 24
    drugs, 24
    management, 23
  catheterization, anaesthetic considerations, 95–6
    infants and young children, 96
    neonates, older children and adults, 95–7
  emergencies, 192–207
  resuscitation, 192–3 see also Resuscitation
Cardiopulmonary resuscitation, 14–26
  see also Cardiac arrest: Resuscitation
Cardiovascular
  changes in ageing, 290
  disease in emergency situations, 5–6
  preoperative, general abdominal surgery, 102
  monitoring, 82–84
  system diagnosis, and anaesthetic procedures, 92
Cardioversion in ventricular tachycardia, 18
Casualty departments see Accident and Emergency department
Central venous cannulation, 65–9
  catheter over guidewire devices, 65–6
  difficulties, 68
  indications, 7
  multiple, 69
  techniques, 66–8
Central venous pressure monitoring, 82
Cerebral see also Head injuries
  angiography, anaesthesia, 93–4
  Function Analysing Monitor, 986

Function Monitor, 86
  physiology, 128–9
Cervical
  spine injury, and ventilation, 16
  cord drainage in facio-maxillary injuries, 157
Chest drains, insertion, 71–2
Chest trauma, 193
  blunt, and penetrating, 194–7
  resuscitation, 196
Child's assessment of risk in liver disease, 313
Chloroform, general and abdominal surgery, 108
Christmas disease, 47
Circulation establishment in CPR, 16
Circulation and head injury, 132–4
Citrate toxicity following massive transfusion, 38–9
  Citrated whole blood, characteristics, 33
Civil disasters see Disasters, civil
Coagulation factors in infants, 281
Colloidal osmotic pressure monitoring, 88
Colloids as intravenous fluids, 59–63
Communications, 2
Complement binding anti-IgA antibodies, transfusion reaction, 40
Compressed Spectral Array, 85–6
Computerization of monitoring, 88
Computerized tomography, scanning, emergency, anaesthetic scanning, 92–3
  general anaesthesia, 93
  Concentrated (packed) red cells, characteristics, 33
  Contrast medium, effects and reactions, 97–8
Cricoid pressure, 7, 9
Cricothyroidotomy, 72–3
  and cardiac arrest, 17
  technique, 73
Cross-match blood grouping tests, 30–31
Cryoprecipitate, in replacement therapy, 45
  characteristics, 34
Crystalloids, intravenous fluids, 55–9
  electrolyte content, 56 (table)
Cyanide poisoning, 220
Cyanosis, definition, 327
Cytochrome P450, 318

Deceiver syndromes, 103
Defibrillation in cardiac arrest, children, 24–5
Defibrillators in ventricular fibril-

lation and tachycardia, 18–19
Dehydration, developing countries, management, 237
Demerol see pethidine
Dental problems, 164–72
  anaesthesia, general, 167–71
  analgesia, 166–71
  bleeding, 165
  dento-alveolar trauma, 165
  fever, 168
  foreign bodies, 171–2
  general, 167–71
  infections, 171
  intubation, 170
  local anaesthesia, 166–7
  monitoring, 170–71
  packing, 170–71
  premedication, 169–70
  soft tissue abscesses, 165–6
  swelling, 168–71
  technique, 169–71
  toothache, 165
  trauma, 171
  trismus, 168–9
Developing countries, anaesthesia in, 236–45
  anaemia, 237–8
  anaesthesia, 231–4
  dehydration, 237
  environment, 236–7
  temperatures, 237
  training, 245
Dextrans, 59–61
  in blood replacement, 226 (table), 227
  complications, 61
  indications, 59–60
Diabetes history, and anaesthesia, 358–9
  and general and abdominal surgery, 112–14
Diagnostic procedures, 90–98
  angiography, 93–5
  cardiac catheterization, 95–7
  cardiovacular system, 92
  contrast medium effects, 97–8
  CT, 92–3
  dye studies, 95–7
  general considerations, 90–91
  magnetic resonance, 97
  nervous system, 91–2
Diaphragmatic hernia, congenital, 286
Direct compatibility blood grouping tests, 30–31
Direct current countershock in ventricular fibrillation, 18
Disasters, civil, 231–4
  anaesthetist's role, 232, 234
  developing countries, 238–45
  equipment, 238–40

cost, 238
  draw-over techniques, 238–40
  specific problems, 243–4
  techniques, 240–43
  sequence of events and arrangements, 231–4
Disseminated intravascular coagulation, treatment, 49
Drain, pleural, insertion, 71–2
Drugs used in regional anaesthesia, 247–50
Dural puncture, accidental, management, 356
Dye studies, anaesthetic considerations, 95–7
  infants and young children, 96
  neonates, older children, and adults, 95–7

Ear, nose and throat emergencies, 159–63
  airway obstruction, 160
  general problems, 159–60
  operations, 160–63
Electrolyte content of crystalloid solutions, 56
Elderly, anaesthesia, 288–99
  intra-operative management, 296–7
  pharmacokinetics, 293–4
  physiological changes, 290–93
  postoperative care, 297
  postoperative complications, 354–5
  preoperative assessment, 294–6
Electrocardiography, in patient monitoring, 83–4
Electroencephalography in patient monitoring, 85–6
Electrolyte balance, preoperative, general and abdominal surgery, 100–101
Electrolyte monitoring, 87
Embolism and orthopaedic surgery, 119–20
Emesis, vigorous and repeated, causing oesophageal rupture, 198, 199
EMO vaporizer, 238
Empyema, association with bronchopleural fistula, 202
Endotracheal intubation see Intubation, tracheal
Enflurane hepatitis, 321
Epidural
  abscess, 357–8
  analgesia, in pregnancy, 268–70
    caudal, 269
    lumbar, 268–9
      complications, 269
    spinal, 269–70
Epinephrine in cardiac arrest, 20, 24
Equipment, 2–3

Etomidate, military use, 229
Exogenous oxygen in head injury
    patient, 130
Eyelids, cuts, 173
Eyes, emergencies, 173-9
    foreign bodies, 174
    general anaesthesia, 174-5
        babies and young children, 174
        for perforating injury, 176-8
    intraocular pressure, 173, 176
    local anaesthesia, problems, 175
    major, 174-8
    minor, 173-4
    oculocardiac reflex, 178
    postoperative pain, 178
    pretreatment, 176

Facio-maxillary emergencies,
    155-9
    airway obstruction, 156-7
    anaesthetic technique, 158
    cervical cord damage, 157
    haemorrhage into airway, 155
    head injury, 157
    intubation, 156-7
    operations, 157-9
    recovery, 159
    shock, 156
Factors, coagulation, concentrates
    in replacement therapy,
    45
    in infants, 281
Factor VIII inhibitors, 47
Failed block, 262
Failed intubation drill, 272-4
Fat embolism and orthopaedic
    surgery, 120
Favism, 53
Femoral neck surgery, 121-2
    anaesthetic techniques, 122
    hypoxia, 122
Fentanyl, postoperative complica-
    tions, 351
Field, local anaesthesia, 256
    see also Military
Fluid balance
    during anaesthesia, general and
        abdominal surgery,
        109-10
    postoperative, 111
    preoperative, 100-101
    and head injury, 136
    in infants and children, 283
Fluorocarbons, 63
Folate deficiency, 53
Foreign bodies
    dental, 171-2
    eyes, 174
    inhaled, laryngoscopy/broncho-
        scopy, 161
Fresh-frozen plasma
    characteristics, 34
    in massive transfusion, 38

in replacement therapy, 45

Gas gangrene, developing coun-
    tries, 244
Gastric contents
    emptying in facio-maxillary
        emergencies, 155, 156
    before surgery, 101
    full, assumed, in trauma, 6
    inhalation, 11-12
        acid aspiration syndrome, 12,
        271, 272
        prevention, 11-12
    retained, pregnant patients, 271,
        272
Gastroschisis, management, 286
Gelatin derivatives, 61
    modified, 62
Gelofusine, 60, 61
General anaesthesia, complications
    following, 345-59
    see also specific headings
Glasgow Coma Scale, 124, 134, 135
Glucose, monitoring, 87
Glucose-6-phosphate deficiency,
    52

H$_1$ receptor antagonists, in contrast
    medium reaction, 98
H$_2$ receptor antagonists
    in contrast medium reaction, 98
    pregnancy, acid aspiration
        syndrome, 271, 272
    as premedicants, 105-106
Haemaccel, in blood replacement,
    60, 61, 226 (table)
Haematology in head injury, 137-8
Haemodynamic function subsets,
    205
Haemoglobins
    abnormal, 50-52
        anaesthetic considerations,
        51-2
    high affinity, 40
    level, lowest acceptable for
        anaesthesia, 49-50
Haemophilia A, 46-7
    factor VIII inhibitors, 47
    only life-saving surgery, 47
Haemophilia B, 47
Haemorrhage in neck trauma, 141
Haemostatic disorders, emergency
    tests, 44-5
    replacement therapy 45
Halothane
    in general and abdominal surg-
        ery, 109
    hepatitis, 320
    military use, 229
    postoperative complications, 350
Hartmann's solution
    in blood replacement, 226
    and diabetes, 359

HbS disease, 51
HbS/thalassaemia, 51
Head injury, 128–39
  anaesthesia, and anaesthetic agents, 137, 138
  evaluation of patient, 129–34
  support and resuscitation during, 134–6
  fluid management, 136
  haematology, 137–8
  neurological monitoring, 238
Heart disease during pregnancy, management, 276
Heart, effects, in spinal cord damage, 148
Heart, emergency surgery, 200–202
  myocardial infarction, 201
  re-exploration for bleeding, 200–201
  valve lesions, 201
Heparin and sugery, 48–9
Hepatic encephalopathy, risk, 312–13
Hepatitis
  halothane, 320
  virus, protection of anaesthetic team, 323
Human albumin solution, 35
  salt-poor, 35
Hydatid disease in developing countries, 243
Hydrocortisone, use before contrast medium procedures, 98
Hydroxyethyl starch, 61
Hypercapnia, definition, 328
Hyperkalaemia following massive transfusion, 39
Hypocalcaemia, 349
Hypocapnia maintenance, 109
Hypokalaemia, preoperative, 100–101
Hypotension, 348
  hypovolaemic, 317
Hypothermia
  as complication, 345
  effects on liver disease, 317
  and massive blood transfusion, 38
  and vascular surgery, 183
  in the very young, 353
Hypoventilation complications, 346
Hypovolaemia, 348
  correction, 225–27
  hypotension, 317
  prevention, liver disease, 322
Hypoxaemia, definition, 327
  prevention, liver disease, 322
Hypoxia
  from cardiovascular problems, 348–50
  diffuse, 347

  from respiratory complications, 346–8
Immunoglobulin(s), 29
  A deficiency, total, transfusion reaction, 40
  Anti-Rh(D), 34, 35
Induction, left lateral head-down position, 8–10
Infants, anaesthesia see Paediatric
Inhalation
  developing countries, 242–3
  of gastric contents see Gastric contents
  injury, 218–21
    management, 219–20
Inotropic agents, effects, 205
Intensive care unit, civil disasters, 234
Intermittent positive pressure ventilation, 350
Internal jugular vein, cannulation, 66–7
Intracranial pressure
  agents increasing, 91–2
  monitoring, 85
Intraocular pressure, 173, 176–8
  ketamine, and suxamethonium (succinylcholine), 176
  reduction, 176
Intravenous fluids, 55–63
  colloids, 59–63
  cystalloids, 55–9
  maintenance volumes, 56–7
Intubation
  burns, 216
  difficult, 73–9
    blind nasal, 74–8
    in ENT emergencies, 160
    in facio-maxillary emergencies, 156–7
    retrograde, 78–9
    under direct vision, 73–4
  nasal, in resuscitation, 17
    blind, under general anaesthesia, 74–6
    under local anaesthesia, 76–8
  in neck trauma, 147–8
  orotracheal in resuscitation, 16–17
  in spinal cord injuries, 126
  tracheal, in acute airway obstruction, 332–4
    difficult, causes, 334
    for dental anaesthesia, 170
    packing, 170–71
    in head injury, 131–2
    pregnant patient, 272–4
    rapid sequence, 7–8
      establishment and maintenance of anaesthesia, 10–11

Ion-selective electrodes, in monitoring, 88
Iron deficiency, 53
Isoflurane in general and abdominal surgery, 109
Isoprenaline (isoproterenol) in cardiac arrest, 19
Isoproterenol see isoprenaline

Jaundice and general and abdominal surgery, 114–15

Ketamine
 contraindications in ophthalmic surgery, 176
 developing countries, 242
 infants and young children, 96
 intravenous, during anaesthesia, 107
 military use, 229
 in neck trauma, 151
 postoperative complications, 350

Lactation, anaesthesia during, 357–8
Large bore IV cannula in resuscitation, 17
Laryngeal injuries, 162
Laryngoscopy, 332
 /bronchoscopy for inhaled foreign body, 161
Left lateral head-down position for induction, 8–10
Left ventricular function in emergency cardiac surgery, 202
Lidocaine see lignocaine
Life support, advanced paediatric, 21, 23
Life threatening situation, procedures, 6–7
Lignocaine (lidocaine) in cardiac arrest, 19–20 children, 24
Liver disease, 48, 310–24
 approaches to minor/major surgery, 321–2
 clinical assessment, 312–15
 drug-associated disease, 312
 dysfunction, acute, and chronic, 310–11
 hepatic blood flow problems, 317
 interaction with anaesthetic agents, 318–21
 intra-operative monitoring, 322
 liver failure, 313
 liver function after operation, 316–18
 possible complications, 314–15
 preoperative interventions, 311–15

protection, anaesthetic team, from liver disease, 322–3
 risk, classification, 313
 stabilization, 315–16
 surgery, timing, 315–16
Local anaesthesia (analgesia), 246–64
 agents, 247–50
 casualty department, 257
 complications following, 344–5
 equipment, 255
 in the field, 256
 methods, 252–5
 operating department, 257–8
 during pregnancy, 268–71
  see also Pregnancy, local analgesia during
 technique for blind nasal intubation, 76–7
 ward, 257–8
 see also Blocks: Epidural analgesia: Regional anaesthesia
Local infiltration in pregnancy, 271
Lund and Browder charts for burn areas, 211, 212
Lung abscess, 203

Magnesium trisilicate mixture, pregnant patients, 271
Magnetic resonance, anaesthetic considerations, 97
Mallory–Weiss lesion, 198
Mandibular fractures, 158
Mannitol, use, 59
Maxillary fracture, 158
Mendelson's syndrome, and treatment, 12
Methohexitone (methohexital), intravenous during anaesthesia, 107
Methoxyflurane hepatitis, 321
Metoclopramide as premedicant, 105
Metrizamide, risks, 98
Microaggregate infusion and massive transfusion, 40
Microsurgical techniques, 123
Middle-ear emergency, 162
Military conflicts, 222–31
 anaesthesia, 227–31
  induction, 229
  inhalation, and maintenance, 227–31
  regional, 228
  total intravenous, 228
 analgesia, 227
 blood loss and replacement, 225–7
 environment, 223
 evacuation to surgical unit, 223–4
 hypovolaemia, correction, 225–7

preoperative considerations, 224
receiving casualties, 224
recovery, 231
resuscitation, 225–7
triage, 224
ventilators, 230–31
Mobile Medical Team, 232–3
Monitoring, patient, 81–9
burns, 217
cardiovascular, 82–4
liver disease, 322
in neck trauma, 150–51
neurophysiological, 85–7
in head injury, 138
temperature, 87
vascular surgery, 182–4
Morphine, in premedication, 104
Munchausen syndrome, 103
Muscle relaxants
burns, 216–17
during general anaesthesia, 108
military casualties, 230
in neck trauma anaesthesia, 152
see also Suxamethonium
(succinylcholine)
Myocardial
depression, 348
infarction, emergency surgery,
201
history, and anaesthesia, 358

Nasal bones, fractured, 160–61
Neck trauma, 140–54
anaesthesia, 151–3
induction agents, 151–2
inhalation, 152
muscle relaxants, 152
cervical spine injury, 140–42
recognition, 142–9
repair, 149–53
resuscitation, 140
spinal cord damage, 147–8
tracheolaryngeal damage, 142–4
vascular damage, 144–6
airway control, 146
blunt trauma, 144
zone classification, 145–6
Neonates see Paediatric
anaesthesia
Nephrotic syndrome, management, 308–309
Nervous system, considerations for
anaesthesia, 91–2
Neuroanaesthesia, 128–39
Neurological changes in the elderly,
292
Neuromuscular function, monitoring, 86–7
Neurophysiological monitoring,
85–7
Normocapnia maintenance, 109
Nose see Ear, nose and throat
emergencies

Nuclear magnetic resonance see
magnetic resonance,
anaesthetic considera-
tions, 97
Nutritional status in the elderly,
293

Obesity, causing complications,
352–3
in the elderly, 293
Obstetric emergencies, 265–77
physiological changes, 265
Oculocardiac reflex, 178
Oesophagus, trauma, 197–9
varices, 198
Oncotic pressure, monitoring, 88
Ophthalmic emergencies, 173–9
minor, 173–4
general anaesthesia, babies
and young children, 174
major, 174–78
see also Eyes, emergencies
Omphalocele, management, 286
Orotracheal intubation in resuscitation, 16–17
Orthopaedics, emergency, 116–27
acrylic cement and blood pressure fall, 118
alcohol intoxication, 118–19
blood loss, 119
embolism, 119–20
IV regional block, 120
specific conditions, 121–7
tourniquets, 121
Oxford Miniature Vaporizer, 227,
238
Oximetry, pulse, 85
Oxygen
therapy, supplemental, 330–31
transcutaneous monitoring, 84

Paediatric anaesthesia, 278–88
cardiopulmonary resuscitation,
21–25
cardiovascular system, 279–81
for catheterization and dye
studies, 95–7
central nervous system, 281
fluid balance, 283
general anaesthesia, 283–5
ophthalmic emergencies, 174
P_{50} value, 280
postoperative care, 287
postoperative compliance, 353–4
preoperative assessment, neonates, 278–81
preparation, 282
preterm, normal heart, 280
respiratory distress, 279
specific surgical conditions,
285–7
ventilators, 284
Pain, postoperative, 359–60

Pancreatitis, acute and general abdominal surgery, 114
Pancytopenia, 53–4
Paracervical block during pregnancy, 270
Patient assessment, 4 *see also* Triage
  classification (ASA), 4–5
Percutaneous arterial cannulation, 69–71
  difficulties, and technique, 70–71
Peritonsillar abscess, 161
Pethidine (demerol), infants and young children, 96
Pethidine (demerol), premedication, 104
Phenothiazines as premedicants, 105
Physiotherapy following surgery, 112
Plasma
  abnormalities, acquired, 48–9
  expanders and substitutes, 59–62
  -reduced blood, characteristics, 33
Platelet
  abnormalities, 46
  concentrates, characteristics, 33
  in replacement therapy, 45
Pleural drain, insertion, 71–2
Polycythaemia, 54
Positioning, causing complications, 344
Postoperative complications, 340–61
  casualty departments, 343–4
  factors predisposing, 340
  general procedures, 342–3
  types, 341
Post-tonsillectomy haemorrhage, 161
Potassium
  content of IV fluids, 57
  depletion, replacement, 57
  excess, treatment, 58
Precordial thump, 18, 24
Pre-eclampsia, management, 275–6
Pregnancy
  general anaesthesia, 271–5
    equipment needed, 267–8
    failed intubation drill, 272–4
    induction, 271–2
    maintenance, 274–5
  post partum procedures, 275
  related pathology, 275–6
    retained gastric contents, management, 270
  local analgesia during, 268–71
    caudal epidural, 269
    local infiltration, 271
    lumbar epidural, 268–9

complications, 269
    paracervical and pudendal blocks, 270
    spinal, 269–70
  postoperative complications, 355
Premedication
  burns, 215–16
  for dental anaesthesia, 169
  in developing countries, 238
  general and abdominal surgery, 104–106
  ophthalmic emergencies, 176–7
Preoperative
  assessment, general and abdominal surgery, 100–103
  laboratory investigations, 103–104
  management for regional block, 260
Psychological problems and anaesthesia, 360
Pudendal block during pregnancy, 270
Pulmonary
  balloon flotation catheters, 205
  complications, burns, 218–20
  function in the elderly, 291
  lavage, 12
Pulse oximetry, 85
Pyloric stenosis, management, 285

Ranitidine and sodium citrate, protocol, pregnancy, 271, 272
Regional anaesthesia, 246–64
  blocks, 253–4 *see also* Blocks
    best emergency use, 258
    failed, 262
  chronic renal failure, 307
  drugs, 247–250
  equipment, 255
  in general and abdominal surgery, 106
    postoperative, 112
  intravenous, 254–5
  local infiltration, 253
  methods, 252–5
  peroperative, 261–2
  postoperative, 262–3
  preoperative, 260–61
  surface analgesia, 252
  toxicity, 251
Renal
  disease, 300–309
    acute renal failure, 307–8
    anaesthesia, general, 304–7
    chronic renal failure, 300–307
    complications, 300–304
    nephrotic syndrome, 308–9
    preoperative, general and abdominal surgery, 103
    regional analgesia, 307
  function, in the elderly, 297

and vascular surgery, 185–6
Replacement therapy for haemostatic disorders, 45
Respiration, spontaneous, 350
Respiratory
disease, history and anaesthesia, 358
preoperative, general and abdominal surgery, 101–2
insufficiency, 326–38
anaesthesia, general or regional, 337–8
causes, 328–30
obstruction, 328, 331–6
see also Airway obstruction
premedication, 337
treatment, 330–33
monitoring, 84–5
Resuscitation
in burns, 210–14
assessment of adequacy, 214
transfusion, 211–14
cardiac and thoracic, 192–3
cardiopulmonary, 14–26
adults, 15–17
airway, 15
breathing, 15–16
circulation, 16
other considerations, 16–17
cardiac arrest, 17–21
paediatric, 21–5
advanced life support, 21, 22
associated situations, 22
differences from adult, 21–2
management, 23
of military casualties, 225–7
Retrograde intubation, 78–9
Rhesus (Rh) blood group system, 29, 30
Right atrial pressure, balloon flotation, 205
subclavian vein, cannulation, 68
Road traffic accidents see Head injury: Neck trauma: Orthopaedics: Trauma

Salt depletion, replacement, 57
Sedation for emergency CT scans, 92–3
Seldinger method, 65–6
Sellick's manoeuvre, 7, 9
Sensory evoked potentials, monitoring, 86
Shock, in facio-maxillary emergencies, 156
Shock, in spinal cord damage, neck trauma, 148
Sickle cell disease, anaesthetic considerations, 50, 51
and blood transfuction, 42
Snake bites, 244
Sodium

bicarbonate, in cardiac arrest, children, 24
content of IV fluids, 56
Spinal
anaesthesia in femoral neck surgery, 122
cord damage in neck trauma, indications for early surgery, 147–8
heart effects, 148
shock, 148
temperature regulation loss, 148
injuries, management, 125–6
intubation, 126
spinal shock syndrome, 126
Stomach see Gastric contents
Succinylcholine see suxamethonium
Suction, 3
foot operated, 3
Supra-renal cross-clamp, 187
Surface analgesia, 252
Surgery, general and abdominal, 99–116
general anaesthesia, endotracheal, 107
induction, 106–7
intravenous agents, 107–8
maintenance, 108
muscle relaxants, 108
postoperative, 111–12
termination, 110
premedication, 104
intrathecal/epidural, advantages/disadvantages, 106
postoperative, 111–12
preparation and transfusion, 37
special, and postoperative complications, 351–2
see also Post- and Pre-operative: Premedication: and special conditions
Suxamethonium (succinylcholine)
contraindicated in burns, 216
during general anaesthesia, 108
and intraocular pressure, 176–8
and pregnant patients, 272

Temperature, environmental, in developing countries, 237
Temperature, monitoring, 87
Tetanus, developing countries, 243–4
Thalassaemias, anaesthetic considerations, 51, 52 3
Thiopental see thiopentone
Thiopentone (thiopental)
intravenous, during anaesthesia, 107
military use, 229
in neck trauma, 151–2

Thoracic emergencies, 192–207
  resuscitation, 192–3
Thrombocytopenia, 46
Thromboembolism and ortho-
      paedic surgery, 120
Tonsillectomy, haemorrhage fol-
      lowing, 161
Toothache, acute, 165
Tourniquet, complications, 344
  in orthopaedics, 121
Toxicity of local anaesthetic drugs,
      251
Tracheal injuries, 162
Tracheal intubation see Intubation,
      tracheal
Tracheolaryngeal damage in neck
      trauma, 142–4
Tracheo-oesophageal fistula,
      management, 285–6
Tracheostomy, 203–204
  emergency, 162
    and cardiac arrest, 17
  in neck trauma, 143–4
Transcutaneous O_2 and CO_2 moni-
      toring, 84
Transtracheal injection, 78
Trauma
  anaesthesia, establishment and
      maintenance after, 10–11
  chest, and intrathoracic arteries,
      193–202
  dental, 171
  multiple, 123–5
    score, 124–5
  neck, 140–54
    see also Neck trauma
  procedures, 6
  victims, full stomach assumed, 6
Triage, civil disasters, 232, 233
Trichloroethylene, general and
      abdominal surgery, 108
  for military use, 229

Urgent/emergency, considered
      synonymous, 1
Uterus, ruptured, developing coun-
      tries, 244

Vaporizer
  EMO, 238
  OMV, 227, 238
Vascular surgery, major, 180–91
Vasoactive drugs, 183–4
Vasodilators, administration after
      vascular surgery, 187,
      188–9
Vasopressors, administration in
      vascular surgery, 189
Vecuronium in ophthalmic surgery
      premedication, 177
Ventilation
  manual, of lungs, head injury
      patient, 130–31
  in neck trauma, 140–41
  in resuscitation, 15–16
    assessment of patient's com-
      plications, 16–17
    contraindications, 16–17
  -perfusion abnormalities, 347
Ventilator(s), 335–6
  alarms, 85
  for infants and children, 284
  military use, 230–31
Ventilatory failure, extrapul-
      monary, 329
Ventricular
  fibrillation, DC countershock,
      18
    drugs, 18
    precordial thump, 18
  tachycardia, precordial thump,
      18
Vitamin B_{12} deficiency, 53
Vomiting, preoperative, 100–101
Von Willebrand's disease, 47–8

Warfarin and surgery, 48
Water
  content of IV fluids, 56
  depletion, replacement, 57
  excess, treatment, 58–9

Yankauer suction, 3